WHAT PEOPLE ARE SAYING ABOUT

Great Expectations: Baby's First Year

"This book is a valuable resource and updated with details you will not find anywhere else. Well written and carefully researched, it complements the author's earlier books and adds to the important resources every new parent should have. Kudos to the authors."

—Stevanne Auerbach, "Dr. Toy," San Francisco

"The mother-daughter team who coauthored two other Great Expectations books open this outsized parenting manual with a chronology of what to expect—day-by-day, week-by-week, month-by-month—during baby's first year. . . . They're very modern in their trust-your-instincts advice, stressing that parents are wise enough to choose their own parenting style—comforting crying babies vs. ignoring them, etc. Likewise, they don't fret about boosting baby's I.Q. with fancy toys."

—*Publishers Weekly*

"In this follow-up to *Great Expectations: Your All-in-One Resource for Pregnancy & Childbirth,* mother and daughter Sandy Jones and Marcie Jones deliver a comprehensive overview of the first year of a baby's life with day-by-day, week-by-week, month-by-month details of what parents can expect. . . . The text is filled with useful tips throughout and contains a resource directory and a parent's dictionary."

—Dana Ladd, Community Health Education Ctr., Richmond, VA, in *Library Journal*

Great Expectations: Your All-in-One Resource for Pregnancy & Childbirth

"Emotions, physical changes, lifestyle changes, baby development, it's all there. Get ready: This book will get dog-eared from all your reading and then passed along to your best friends and sister."

—Peg Moline, Editor-in-Chief, *FitPregnancy*

"*Great Expectations* is terrific. The style of writing is clear, warm and very supportive. It's a great reference for any question that might arrive in pregnancy."

—Ann Stadtler, MSN, CPNP, Director of the Brazelton TouchpointCenter at Children's Hospital in Boston

"*Great Expectations* is the perfect resource for moms-to-be. Sandy and Marcie Jones speak to the expectant mother of today in a friendly, approachable tone, and present their thorough information in a way that's great for both quick look-ups and in-depth reading."

—Stacia Ragolia, VP, Community & Parenting, iVillage.com

G·R·E·A·T
EXPECTATIONS
BEST
BABY
GEAR

Sandy Jones and Marcie Jones

with a foreword by
Ann Brown

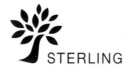

STERLING

New York / London
www.sterlingpublishing.com

STERLING and the distinctive Sterling logo
are registered trademarks of Sterling Publishing Co., Inc.

Library of Congress Cataloging-in-Publication Data Available

10 9 8 7 6 5 4 3 2 1

Published by Sterling Publishing Co., Inc.
387 Park Avenue South, New York, NY 10016
© 2008 by Sandy Jones and Marcie Jones
Distributed in Canada by Sterling Publishing
c/o Canadian Manda Group, 165 Dufferin Street
Toronto, Ontario, Canada M6K 3H6
Distributed in the United Kingdom by
GMC Distribution Services
Castle Place, 166 High Street, Lewes, East Sussex,
England BN7 1XU
Distributed in Australia by Capricorn Link (Australia) Pty. Ltd.
P.O. Box 704, Windsor, NSW 2756, Australia

Printed in China
All rights reserved

Sterling ISBN: 978-1-4027-3335-2

For information about custom editions, special sales, premium and
corporate purchases, please contact Sterling Special Sales Department
at 800-805-5489 or specialsales@sterlingpublishing.com.

Dedication

Sandy Jones and Marcie Jones would like to dedicate this book to the moms and moms-to-be who have posted thousands of questions to us on Happyhealthypregnancy.com. Thanks for giving us the opportunity to learn so much every day! And to Baby Jones Brennan, who we hope will be born as this book reaches the shelves. May your car seat be safe, your crib comfy, and your stroller easy to fold!

Acknowledgments

We would like to thank our amazing editor at Sterling Publishing, Jennifer Williams, for her warmth, support, and excellent judgment, and Jane Neighbors for her exquisite copy-editing input chapter by chapter.

We're also appreciative for the expert input of David Campbell and Joseph Colella for our car seat chapter, for Dr. Stevanne Auerbach for reviewing the toy chapter, for Fred Rivara, MD, of the Harborview Injury Prevention Center for feedback on the safety chapter, and Ann Brown, former chairman of the U.S. Consumer Product Safety Commission, for her expert review of the entire book with an eye toward baby-product safety.

In addition, we'd like to acknowledge Leonard Vigliarolo of Sterling's design department for giving the book an intuitive layout, accessible design, and beautiful pages; Emily Seese for her unswerving devotion to turning our book into a reality; and Gina Graham for her able assistance with photo research.

Finally, we would also like to acknowledge the valuable contributions of Michael Fragnito and Charles Nurnberg of Sterling Publishing and Alan Kahn and Steve Riggio of Barnes & Noble, who have offered us so much support and encouragement for the Great Expectations series over the years.

Table of Contents

A Word from the Authors

Babies don't come with instructions. They can't take care of themselves, nor do they have a choice about what car seat, high chair, play yard, or any other product their parents buy for them. They're entirely dependent upon you to make wise decisions.

That's where *Great Expectations: Best Baby Gear* comes in. It's a handy, easy-to-use reference to help you find the latest and best-quality products for your baby. Every chapter is loaded with all the information and tips you need to make wise choices.

Whether you're buying a car seat, a crib, diapers, a stroller—or even toys and clothes—*Great Expectations: Best Baby Gear* helps you make key decisions about what to choose. It also gives you the critical safety information you need to protect your baby from potential baby-product and household injuries.

Most parents assume that any product that is designed for babies, or has "baby" in the name, is inherently safe; but nothing could be further from the truth. Every year, baby-product-related accidents send nearly 60,000 babies and young children to hospital emergency rooms. That's why it's important to know what to look for and what to avoid when you shop.

Full-color photographs and charts throughout the book give you detailed examples of products in every important category to help you compare the features of real products in an easy-access format with product categories in alphabetical order. Not only that, but *Great Expectations: Best Baby Gear* gives you all the information you need to save hundreds of dollars when you shop for your baby.

You'll also find a detailed Internet directory in the back of the book that gives you instant access to product details online, and shows you how to locate important consumer information (including recalls) and contact manufacturers.

We've used our best, nonbiased judgment to select the products in *Great Expectations: Best Baby Gear.* We have not been influenced by manufacturers, advertisers, or information providers in making our selections, nor do we have any hidden agenda for promoting one product over another.

Instead, we have been guided by in-depth research into baby-product safety issues in every category, as well as our own—and other parents'—hands-on experience with products featured in our book.

However, product flaws or hazards that we were not aware of at the time of this book's publication could conceivably emerge. We caution you, our readers, to take full responsibility for choosing only the safest and best products for your babies (and yourselves), and to purchase these products only after careful, independent weighing of their quality, durability, and safety.

We always welcome comments and feedback from you. Please feel free to write to us in care of Sterling Publishing Co., Inc., 387 Park Avenue South, New York, NY 10016-8810. Although it may not be possible for us to respond to each of you individually, we are eager to hear your comments, and we will try to implement your baby-product suggestions in the next edition of our book.

—*Sandy Jones and Marcie Jones*

A Note from Ann Brown

Former Chairman, U.S. Consumer Product Safety Commission

If you are expecting a new baby or grandbaby, it's the most exciting time in the world! Having a baby can be a joy, and there's really no need to be fearful that you will do the wrong thing, or to convince yourself that danger lurks around every corner.

Shopping for your baby can become confusing, though, with so many baby products out there. And not all products are safe, right, or even necessary. At the same time, in our busy and demanding lives, it's challenging to do all of the research needed to make the best choices.

Baby safety is a critical issue. I see baby safety as a three-legged stool: Manufacturers need to make products that are continuously tested and proven safe. Government agencies charged with protecting families, and especially babies, need to be effective in ensuring that all products on the market are safe. And parents and others who buy baby products need to be well-informed consumers.

If any one leg of that baby-safety stool isn't working well, then the stool is broken. Baby products are not always made well. Government agencies, although they exist to ensure the safety of families, sometimes fail to do their protective jobs. And when those two legs of the stool are ineffective in guarding families and babies, an added burden is placed on parents to be aware of baby-product dangers and pitfalls.

Great Expectations: Best Baby Gear is a wonderful book. It's comprehensive and written in simple, straightforward language. It shows parents and gift givers what they really need and what they don't, and it offers great advice about where to cut corners and save money. More important: It includes the warnings parents need to heed to protect babies when manufacturers and government agencies fail to do so.

I recommend that you keep this valuable reference book close at hand and that you refer to it often during all the stages of your baby's development. Again, having a baby should be the most fun and exciting time in your life. Don't go overboard. Simply be normally thoughtful and concerned about the products that your baby uses, and make sure to keep up with baby-product recalls. Then relax and enjoy your baby!

—Ann Brown

G·R·E·A·T
EXPECTATIONS
BEST
BABY
GEAR

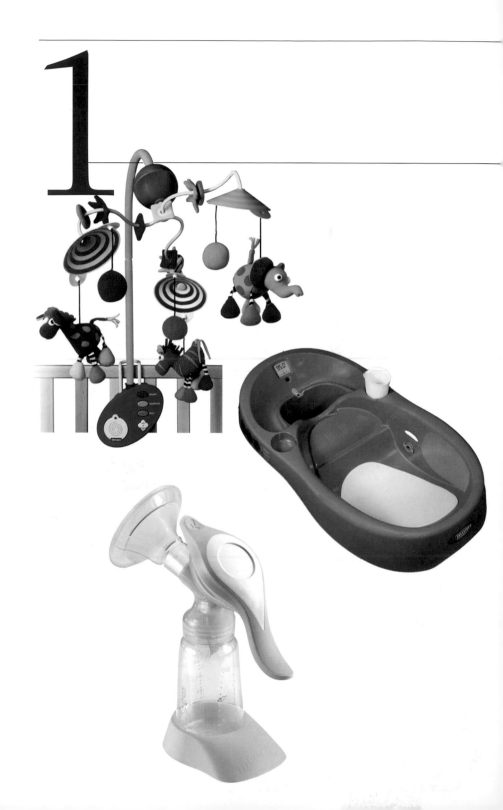

WELCOME TO BABY WORLD!

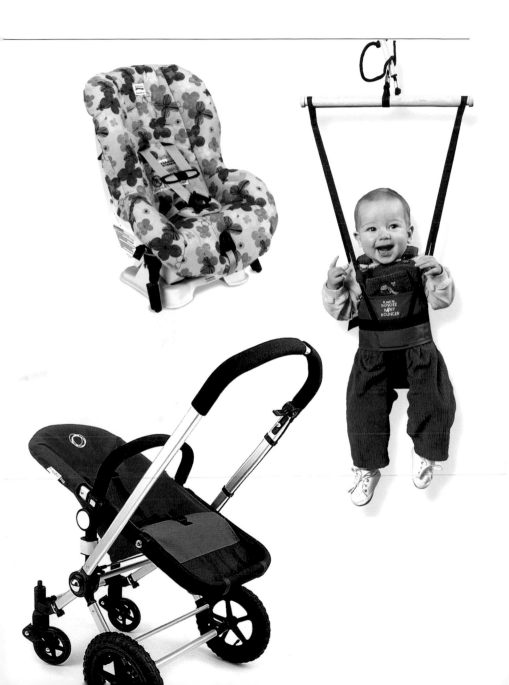

WELCOME TO THE BABY GEAR BUYING CLUB

Surprise! Equipping, feeding, and outfitting your small offspring is likely to cost you between $9,000 and $12,000 during pregnancy and the first year of your baby's life. Our handy gear guide is designed to help you figure out what to buy and what to avoid so you can save yourself hundreds or even thousands of dollars when you shop for your baby.

Expect to feel a bit overwhelmed by the thousands of baby items lined up on today's store shelves! Strolling down the aisles of giant big-box baby stores for the first time, like a Babies "Я" Us, or hitting the aisles of a big-ticket baby boutique can be dizzying. And surfing Target, Amazon, or any other huge site for baby items can make you shake your head and dream of being filthy rich.

Once you've caught a glimpse of your baby on a fuzzy sonogram, shopping becomes a more serious issue. Inevitably, there are those hormonal times when it's easy to load up your shopping cart while convincing yourself that "nothing's too good for our little Junior."

Layette, *schmayette*

Layette is the traditional word for all of the baby clothing and related paraphernalia that parents are expected to accumulate before their baby arrives. Baby magazines and stores love distributing long, detailed layette lists to unwitting parents for the sole purpose of driving them to buy more than they need (and probably more than they can afford).

When you start shopping for baby clothes, gear, and toys, it's important to keep in mind that your newborn couldn't care less how much you spend on him or feathering your nest. Your adorable little creature's primary needs will be first and foremost to be snuggled, kept warm, nursed, rocked, burped, and to have all damp and poopy diapers changed as quickly as possible. That's it—the bottom line.

Yes, baby products are helpful. Yes, they can be cute and clever. And no, you don't need to invest in an $800 stroller or a $1,500 sleigh-bed-style crib made of polished cherry, even if your heart breaks from yearning over it. At some point it dawns on you that the products you're buying don't need to last a lifetime. Two to three years from now your baby will have morphed into a child, and you may not need them for a while, if at all, especially if he turns out to be your one *magnum opus.*

Veteran parents have a leg up on first timers. They've got a different perspective on the whole business of having babies and childrearing. Plus, they have the added advantage of experience and the insight that stores will still be open after the baby arrives if they discover they really, *really* need something they don't already have. (They're also pretty cunning about waiting until after all of their baby showers have been thrown and all of the bounty from well-meaning gift givers has been counted up before seriously hitting the stores.)

Where to find the baby booty

Here's a big list of the places to shop for products. (Note: The Web addresses for many of these stores are listed in the *Web Resources* section that starts on page 338.)

■ **Discount chains.** Huge discount chains like Wal-Mart, Kmart, Sam's Club, and Costco are great places for saving money on *everything,* although their baby-product lines are usually limited to rather basic, no-frills models. The secret is to use "big box" discount chains for the stuff you have to replace often—disposable diapers, formula, and baby food, for example—and buy in bulk. You may be able to purchase items from the Web sites for these stores, but first have your product models in mind.

■ **Baby superstores.** The list of giant baby meccas includes Toys "Я" Us, Babies "Я" Us, Baby Superstore, Buy Buy Baby, and the Baby Depot sections found inside Burlington Coat Factory stores. Most carry a huge inventory of products, with advertised models you can purchase at substantial savings. But be sure to ask about their return policies before you buy, so you don't get stuck with a product that doesn't work for you.

■ **Retail chains.** National retail chains such as JCPenney, Sears, and Macy's carry limited stocks of mainstream baby products in their infant departments, such as cribs, strollers, potties, and clothing items. Prices are generally reasonable, and occasionally you may be able to grab a great bargain during special discount periods, such as advertised "baby weeks," or during end-of-season or change-of-model markdowns. (New baby-product models usually debut in late fall and the first of the year.)

■ **Internet stores and auction sites.** Baby-product "e-tailers" sometimes offer huge discounts, but these companies may come and go quickly. Make sure you're dealing with a reputable, enduring company or an auction seller with good feedback. Don't agree to back-order a product that's not in stock. Be aware that baby clothing and toys in good repair could be a good buy, but strollers, cribs, and car seats may be risky. They could be weakened from use, have hardware problems, or have been in recalls. When shopping online, don't forget to factor in shipping and handling costs when comparing prices, and look for written assurance that you can return the product if it isn't satisfactory.

■ **Baby boutiques.** Independently owned "stork shops," baby and children's stores found in malls, and luxury baby departments inside exclusive retail stores offer expensive baby goods, some with trim, colors, and accoutrements not found in standard retail outlets. If you're on a tight budget, don't shop here unless accompanied by a generous, rich relative, or plan to search out half-price sales and larger-size baby clothing on the off season by planning ahead for your baby's growth.

■ **Baby-product catalogs.** Direct-mail catalogs make for interesting browsing and can be a great way to get an overview of unique products without having to leave the house. If you're thinking of placing an order, again don't forget to calculate shipping and handling costs in the total price.

■ **Yard sales and consignment shops.** Clothing and baby toys are great finds at yard sales, but car seats, cribs, and strollers may not be. Ever-changing federal regulations make each new generation of car seat and crib safer than those manufactured even a year earlier, and strollers tend to deteriorate with wear. And a stroller may look okay until a baby sitting inside makes it veer to one side.

Bigger price tag, better product?

It's simply not the case that expensive top-of-the-line baby gear guarantees better quality and safety. Rigorous product testing appears to show that middle-of-the-line products often hold up equally well, and sometimes even better than pricey top-of-the-line models.

If you buy the highest-priced stroller, for example, you're most likely paying for a heavier frame, thicker padding, a removable U shaped infant head support, embedded earphones for playing CD or iPod music, or weather shields—all of which make the stroller bulkier and less portable.

Sometimes manufacturers pay to use well-known logos and brand names from other companies just to make their products sell better. Then they jack up the price of the product—10 percent or more—to cover their licensing expenses.

If you buy car seats or strollers with labels such as Eddie Bauer, Jeep, or Carter's, it doesn't mean the products are a higher quality or any less vulnerable to serious flaws and safety recalls than other models made by the same companies but without the well-known logo. To save money, stick to plainer, more generic models from the same respected manufacturers.

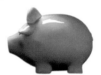

30 tips to save $3,000 (or more!)

1. Buy a "convertible" car seat. Infant car seats for babies weighing up to 20–30 pounds let you remove your baby without having to wake him up, but they're bulky and a huge strain to carry around. A convertible seat will be good from 5 to 40 pounds, or more. These seats can ride facing backward or forward, and will remain useful for two to three years, so take a look at them. (For more information on convertibles see page 102.)

2. Convert your baby's car seat into a stroller. If you decide to go with an infant-only car seat, don't buy it as half of a costly travel system that also includes a stroller. Instead, buy an inexpensive rack on wheels made just for supporting and rolling that type of car seat. (For more information on wheeled car seat carriers see page 296.)

3. Be stroller savvy. Simply because a stroller has a huge price tag doesn't mean it's a better baby hauler. Shop the lower end of a respected brand, such as Graco, Kolcraft or Cosco; then purchase extra accessories as needed. When choosing the stroller, go for something that's lightweight, with a reclining seat back, that can handle an uneven path, rather than a giant and very expensive baby bed on wheels.

4. Breastfeed your baby. You can save your family about $40 per week, or more than $2,000 a year, just in the cost of formula and bottles. Expect to spend a few thousand more if your baby turns out to be allergic to infant formula and requires hypoallergenic versions. Plus, your breastfed baby will be less likely to be an obese child or have digestive issues, get juvenile diabetes, cavities, or need braces later on.

5. Postpone buying a breast pump. Babies are the best breast pumps in the business! If you know you're going to be staying at home for a while, let your baby do all the work, instead of spending hundreds of dollars on a pump. But if you decide you need one, a good breast pump can be had for under $200. Buying (or renting) a breast pump is still a great deal compared with the monthly costs of formula feeding (not to mention the baby-wellness factor). An economical option in the early months is to temporarily rent a highly efficient, hospital-grade pump until you're sure you really need to own your own pump. (For more information on breast pumps see page 19.)

6. Use a front carrier. All your baby really longs for is to be close to you—to be nursed, rocked, carried around, and talked to. So forget about stoking up on costly baby toys or buying an $800 stroller, and plan to use a soft, hammock-like sling or a front carrier (a little fabric baby seat with straps) for the first few months after birth. Your baby will probably be soothed by the motion of your walking, and you have free use of your arms. Then, once you've gotten on your feet and know your baby better, start shopping around for strollers.

7. Cash in on (or exchange) unneeded baby items. Don't store baby gifts you don't need or want. Instead, return them for cash, sell them on eBay, put them up for sale at a consignment shop, or exchange them for goods you *really* need.

8. Dress your baby for comfort instead of fashion. Sure, it's cute to dress your son in miniature camouflage fatigues or your daughter as a little pink princess, but your baby will probably be grateful for old-fashioned cotton knit tee shirts, gowns, and footed sleepers that are considerably less costly and also a lot more comfortable.

9. Beg and borrow baby duds. Babies outgrow their clothes and move on to the next size in a matter of months (and sometimes in just weeks). Buy baby clothes one or two sizes larger than you currently need and let your baby grow into them. Better yet, negotiate for a carton or two of friends' leftover baby duds that you clean up with an oxygen-based detergent.

> **"We got a huge discount on a top-of-the-line imported stroller that was on sale as a floor model in a well-known store chain. It was none the worse for wear, but we had to make a trade-off: The store had a strict 14-day return policy, which meant we'd be up the creek if something went wrong with it. Fortunately, it held up well for as long as we needed it. "**

10. Convert your favorite over-the-shoulder pouch into a diaper bag.
There's no need to waste money on a designer diaper statement when your favorite roomy leather bag or backpack will work just fine. Folding diaper pads and clear plastic pouches are all you need to turn any satchel into a diaper container.

11. Let the crib just be a crib. You don't need to spend extra bucks to get a crib that converts into a love seat, a double bed, or a computer table, when a simple crib with a single lowering side works great for those first two years. Then purchase a toddler bed frame and use the crib's mattress for another year. Finally, once your child's old enough, you can buy a single twin bed to save space.

12. Nix baby armoires and other furniture that matches your baby's crib. Nursery furniture is usually overpriced and often of lower quality. Consider shopping in antique malls and thrift stores to find a quality chest that you adapt for your baby's room. (Protruding knobs on the drawers should be changed to flat handles. You'll need to install drawer stops, and the chest should be attached to the wall with L shaped brackets to keep it from falling over on your future toddler if he tries to use the drawers as steps to get to the top.)

13. Change diapers on top of a chest. Inexpensive cushioned diaper-changing pads with raised sides are available that let you convert any chest into a "changing station." Just be sure to firmly attach the pad to the chest using the provided screws and to always use the safety belt. A cushioned diaper pad on the floor works, too.

14. Skip the baby bathtub. Use the kitchen sink lined with a folded towel to do the job, or take the baby into the shower or tub with you. Placing the baby in a baby seat on the bathroom floor can help with getting in and out.

15. Don't fall for so-called "baby life insurance." Your baby doesn't need life insurance (though you might!). Instead, work with a financial advisor to set up the best savings plan for your baby's future.

16. Use your ears as baby monitors. You don't need to hear your baby's every snuffle. Just keep the doors open. Your baby will sound the alarm if he needs you.

17. Make your own baby food. There's nothing exotic about jarred baby food. How hard can it be to mash up a banana or a sweet potato, to stir up some instant oatmeal, to open a jar of unsweetened applesauce, or to run some cooked veggies through a blender or food processor? Go organic if you're concerned about pesticide residues.

18. Use a booster seat. If your kitchen is crowded, consider using a baby bouncer until your baby outgrows its weight limits, then sit him in a molded plastic booster seat that straps securely onto the seat of a regular chair. Some have front trays and operate just like a regular high chair but cost $50 (or more) less.

19. Be your baby's best toy. Babies have very limited attention spans and aren't all that crazy about activity centers or mobiles that play tunes and do tricks. So don't be seduced into spending hundreds of dollars on baby toys when the type of stimulation your baby *really* needs is the multisensory kind provided by grown-ups when they walk, talk, and respond to their offspring.

20. Use a family practice physician. If pediatricians' fees are exorbitant in your neck of the woods, explore using a physician in family practice. He or she will be trained to treat not only your baby but

Checklist

Basic shopping rules

It's possible to save literally thousands of dollars by following a few shopping rules.

✔ **Seek out advice from other parents.** Ask your friends what they liked and didn't like about their stroller, high chair, crib, etc. They may also offer to part with their leftover baby clothes, which can save you a bundle.

✔ **Do your homework.** Check out baby books with what-to-buy sections from the library, or buy your own. Copy and print out parents' baby-product reviews from www.ePinions, www.babybargains.com, and other Internet sites that offer candid product reviews.

✔ **Browse first.** Check out several stores for big-ticket items, and give strollers a test drive. If one folds, fold it. If there are removable items, remove them to troubleshoot potential problems. Keep a notebook, and when you find items you like, write down model names, numbers, and prices so you can comparison shop later.

✔ **Postpone buying until after your baby shower (or after your baby arrives!).** People love buying for babies. Spread the joy (and expense) by signing up for gift registries, and telling relatives and friends. Of course, save gift slips and tags so you can return or consign what you don't need. Postpone buying a high chair, splurging on baby clothes, or piling up baby toys until after your baby arrives. You may discover you don't need everything you thought you did.

✔ **Shop at consignment shops and thrift stores.** Consignment shops sell used clothes and goods on behalf of clients, and then split the profits with them. Not only can you find great clothing and gear deals, but you can also recycle your own kids' unwanted or gently used stuff later, saving hundreds of dollars in the process. (Note our cautions about car seats, strollers, and cribs, though).

✔ **Mistrust salespeople.** When you're ready to start accumulating baby gear, remember that even mild, grandmotherly shop clerks may be experts at subtly guiding you toward buying more than you need. Sometimes stores purposely mark down a limited quantity of low-end product models from well-known manufacturers as "loss leaders," just to get parents into the store to buy more. Don't let them "upsell" you into things like expensive mattresses, matching bedding sets, pricey imported strollers, car seats, or video baby monitors on impulse.

✔ **Look for bargains.** Big-box stores sometimes offer good deals on no-frills baby products. Also keep your eye out for newspaper ads announcing sales and special deals at the big megastores for babies. You may also be able to find supersoft, luxury baby clothing in upscale stores and trendy Internet boutiques at half price as the season changes, but keep in mind that your baby will outgrow anything you buy.

also you and everyone else in your family. You may be able to combine both appointments.

21. Plot your baby's growth. Stock up on disposable diapers—buy them by the case from giant warehouse chains. Use a copy of your doctor's growth chart to plot your baby's growth curve so you won't buy too many size 2 diapers when your baby is about to graduate to size 3. (The same goes for baby clothes.)

22. Use coupons. Get on lists to receive money-saving coupons for diapers and formula by signing up for baby clubs sponsored by drugstore and supermarket chains and on manufacturers' Web sites and Internet coupon sites. Use coupons at grocery stores that double them. (Quick trick: If you check "planning to breastfeed" on surveys sponsored by formula manufacturers, you're like to be mailed formula coupons worth more, receive them more often, and be given cartons of formula samples than if you check "planning to formula feed.")

23. Attend baby fairs. For an inexpensive admission ticket you may be able to strike a deal with manufacturers' sales reps to buy display products at a substantial savings, since they don't want to have to pay shipping to send the products back to the warehouse.

24. Take advantage of freebies. Search around and you may be able to skip the car seat purchase. Some community organizations, car dealerships, and muf-

fler companies offer free loaner car seats.

25. Skip the play yard. Millions of units of play yards have been recalled over the years. Not only that, they just don't work as well as baby beds. Use your baby's crib or a less expensive bassinet as a baby sleeper for the early months.

26. Use a pet gate. The same manufacturers that sell baby gates also manufacture pet gates. And usually pet gates add extra inches at the top, which could be an advantage if your child's a climber. Just make sure the gate's mesh can't be scaled by small feet and that the gate's frame fastens into the wall with screws if you're planning to use it at the top or bottom of a staircase.

27. Use reusable bottles. Although disposable bottles seem like a good idea on the surface, it's much less expensive to wash the same bottles over and over. The best bottles are made of non-polycarbonate material and have smooth sides that are easy to clean, without straws or nooks and crannies that could trap milk residue.

28 Treat disposables like garbage. Retailers make their money on selling the liners of diaper-disposal systems designed to seal off diapers so they won't smell. Besides, the disposal systems are a challenge to operate (especially with diapers in larger sizes). A simple kitchen-size trash receptacle with a plastic bag for a liner and some spray deodorizer (out of baby's reach) or inexpensive Ziploc resealable bags will work just fine.

29. Buy a firm, inexpensive foam mattress. Your baby doesn't need a 750-coil Baby Beauty mattress with a lifetime guarantee. A simple firm foam mattress will work well, is easier to make up, and could be hundreds of dollars cheaper.

> **"As painful as it might be to sit down and actually go over your financials, having a strong dose of reality will help quell your urge to buy on impulse."**

30. Use regular detergents and avoid fabric softeners. You don't need to buy special baby detergents for laundering your baby's clothes. They're more expensive, and those that are powdered can clog up fabrics, making them less absorbent. Use a liquid fragrance-free detergent to keep from irritating your baby's nose and skin, and don't use liquid or sheet-style fabric softeners for the same reason.

Debunking the junk

Almost as soon as you read the "pregnant" sign on the wand of your pregnancy test, your name, your due date, your address, and many other details about you will start motivating people wanting to sell you things, which translates into lots of junk mail and even dinnertime phone calls to sell you everything from condos to baby insurance. If you want to keep your news and personal information to yourself, think twice about divulging your real name, home address, e-mail address, or your due date, and don't sign up for contests, giveaways, or any free subscriptions to baby or pregnancy magazines. Get on your state's do-not-call list and dedicate a unique e-mail address to handling all of your newsletters and special deals, so you don't waste time with unwanted solicitations.

Handling unwanted gifts

It's inevitable that you're going to receive a few baby gifts that you honestly don't want or can't use. Worse yet, everyone may decide to give you nearly identical gifts, and there's really not a whole lot of use for three baby monitors or crib mobiles. But don't just store the unwanted items on the top shelf of the closet where they'll gather dust. Here are our suggestions for handling unwanted (or unneeded) baby gifts:

Be kind. If you're given a dud or a duplicate, focus your attention on the gift giver, rather than the gift. "How thoughtful of you!" "This is so sweet," or just a warm "Thank you!" will do.

Decide what to dump. Hold on to gifts that you know are going to be sought out by the donors later but get rid of items that are duplicates, that you don't think are safe, or that you know you won't use.

Regift with care. Don't attempt to recycle the gifts at other baby showers. It could backfire if another shower guest recognizes her present.

Don't break open the packaging. If the product comes in sealed packaging, don't break it open as a way of feigning excitement. The more seals you break, the harder it will be to convince a store to take the product back.

Speed the gift back to the store. If you know the store where the gift came from, return it quickly. Some stores have iron-clad return policies that are measured in days, not months. And if you postpone until next season, retailers may be more reluctant to accept your return. Some stores won't take the product back at all, even though it's a gift.

Negotiate for cash. Hopefully, gift-givers have been thoughtful enough to include a gift slip inside the package. Returning gifts for cash will give you more flexibility when it comes to choosing what you need and for shopping around for the best bargains. Without a receipt, you may have to settle for an exchange. (It helps to deal directly with the store's manager.)

eBay it. The baby gift you hate may be just what another mom or showergoer is looking for. But don't expect to recoup

WARNING

Baby products hurt babies!
The shocking truth is that baby products and baby toys send over 150,000 babies to emergency rooms with injuries every year! Leading this list are car seats (when they are not involved in car accidents), strollers and carriages, cribs, walkers, and jumpers. Babies routinely fall out of products, fall into them, have their hands and feet or bodies injured by them, or have other baby-product related accidents. Always stay close to your baby and don't ever rely on a baby product or toy to be a babysitter!

the full retail value of the product. Buyers want bargains and will stop bidding once the price gets anywhere near the gift's actual value.

Swap online. If you receive a gift certificate or gift card from a store that you don't want to shop in, you may be able to swap it for one you'd prefer using. Check out www.certificateswap.com, www.cardavenue.com, and www.swapagift.com.

Donate it. You may be able to donate your unwanted gifts to a charity thrift store, feel good about helping a less fortunate family, and get a tax break at the same time. Make sure to ask for a receipt.

7 ways to prevent baby-product accidents

1. Shop carefully. Make sure the product is right for your baby. Check out the manufacturer's age and weight recommendations and read all the product warnings in the brochure that comes with the product before you buy.

2. Follow the directions. Honestly, now, did you read the directions? There you'll find the information that's critical for your baby's safety, and who to contact when there's a problem. Put all your baby-product receipts and literature in a single file so you can find them when you need them.

3. Mail the registration card. Even though it may make you a target for junk mail, it's also the way that manufacturers locate customers who have bought faulty products to inform them there's been a recall, and there are many every year. Skip the questions that don't directly apply to the manufacturer's getting in touch with you—such as your family size, income, and hobbies.

4. Keep up with recalls. Periodically check the Web sites of the Consumer Product Safety Commission, the National Highway Safety Administration, and other federal agencies that regulate baby products to see if you own recalled items.

5. Use those straps. The seat straps in strollers, car seats, high chairs, booster seats, swings, and changing tables are there for an important reason: They protect babies from falling out or getting strangled. Use them every time you put your baby inside.

6. Stay nearby. Stay in the same room if your baby is in a stroller, high chair, play yard, car seat, or other contraption. Feed your baby in your arms; never use a bottle-propper.

7. Always hold your baby during bathing. Rather than using a dangerous suctioned bath seat that could topple over and cause your baby to drown, always stay right by your baby when he's near or in water.

Where to report baby-product problems

Baby products are the number one cause of product recalls by federal agencies. Manufacturers are obligated by law to report product flaws and parents' reports of injuries or potential injuries from products. And in some cases, manufacturers have been slapped with multimillion-dollar fines when they've attempted to hide potentially dangerous product flaws from the government agencies that regulate product safety.

If a baby product hurts your baby, or even if he has a near miss and barely escapes injury, report the problem to the appropriate federal agency that governs product safety. That will put the agencies on alert that something could be wrong with a product, and your reports along with those from other parents could eventually lead to a product recall or ban.

Consumer Product Safety Commission (CPSC)
The federal agency in charge of monitoring and regulating products, including those for babies and young children. It issues product recalls, and it accepts parents' reports of unsafe products. Hotline: 800-683-2772. Web address: www.cpsc.gov.

Food and Drug Administration (FDA)
The branch of the U.S. Department of Agriculture that regulates baby food and baby skin-care products. The Web site offers brochures on baby feeding and health. Hotline: 888-463-6332. Web address: www.fda.gov.

National Highway Traffic Safety Administration (NHTSA)
A branch of the U.S. Department of Transportation (DOT) that oversees the crashworthiness, testing, accident reporting, and recalls involving babies' and children's car seats. Maintains a database of car seat recalls and offers buying guides, installation tips, and other pertinent car seat safety information. Also offers a free product-registration form. Some offerings in Spanish. Hotline: 888-327-4236. Web address: www.nhtsa.dot.gov.

Steps to take when a baby product goes bad

If your baby is injured by a stroller, crib, high chair, bouncer, or other baby product, or he has a near miss, stop using it and report the hazard to the appropriate agency. (See previous section "Where to report baby-product problems".)

Before you report the problem, be sure to have available the product's brand name, the exact model name, and the serial or identification number found on the product.

If your baby has been injured and you feel that you should receive compensation for the injuries and medical care involved as a result of the product-related accident, hold on to the product. Don't seek to have it replaced or exchanged, since you may need to produce it as evidence in court. If you win your case, you'll probably get your money back, plus any legal fees you've paid.

However, if your baby's injury was not serious or costly, then you may decide simply to have your money refunded or the product replaced.

You should still report the problem to the correct governmental agency, so other children won't be exposed to the danger.

Also call the manufacturer's toll-free customer service line to notify them about the product problem.

In addition, file a formal written complaint, addressed to the president of the company. The address of the company may be on the product; or try its Web site, usually under "contact us" or "About (name of co.)." If you can't locate it, ask your local librarian for help. Most will respond to a telephone inquiry.

In your letter to the president, enclose a duplicate copy of your receipt for your purchase. If you have a camera with close-up capabilities, include photos of the product's problem. (But not with your baby using it.) Give your address and a telephone number or e-mail address where you can be reached.

State clearly that you're asking for a full refund of the purchase price of the product and not a replacement of the same model, which could have the same serious flaw.

Take your letter to the post office, register it, and request a return receipt (to prove it was received). Make several photocopies of your letter, your post office forms, and your sales receipt, should you need them later.

By law, companies are required to

report serious product failures to the CPSC. The reason for sending a "hard copy" to the company's head is that the consumer complaint departments of some less-than-forthright companies may attempt to minimize the seriousness of your complaint or to persuade you that a product's dangers are somehow due to your negligence, and ask you to return the flawed product to them, in order to defuse a potential lawsuit.

But typically, manufacturers will refer unhappy consumers back to the retailer where the product was purchased, for replacement or exchange of the product. If the manufacturer fails to respond to your complaint within a reasonable amount of time—say three weeks—return to the store where you bought the product.

Take a copy of the letter you wrote to the manufacturer, your original store receipt, and the product. Insist upon talking only with the manager about the product's problem. Show him or her your letter, your receipt from the post office, and your store receipt. Then demonstrate the product's problem.

It may be wise to initially ask for a full refund, and inform the store manager that you don't wish to replace that particular model with an identical one from the same company, since the replacement could potentially harm your baby, too. You will likely either be given a refund of your money so that you can purchase another (and safer) substitute, or you will be offered an exchange for a product of equal value from another manufacturer that is satisfactory to you.

Hopefully, everything will get satisfactorily resolved with the store's manager, particularly since retailers don't want to create ill will with customers.

If you're still denied a refund, you have several options. You can threaten to report the store to the local Better Business Bureau, to contact the consumer reporters for local news stations about what you feel is unfair treatment by the store, or you can threaten to hire a lawyer. Federal laws and the Federal Trade Commission place the responsibility for replacing a defective or failed product primarily on the shoulders of the retailer that sold you the product. The legal term is "breaching the implied warranties of merchantability and suitability for purpose." The attorney general's office in most states will also help consumers to resolve complaints, but expect delays in getting a response or action on your case.

2

BABY FEEDING

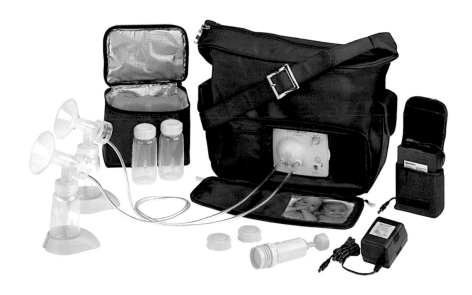

One of the first decisions you'll make is how to feed your baby—something you'll be doing night and day for your baby's early months. This chapter describes feeding-equipment options for both breastfeeding and bottle-feeding. Also included is useful information about baby food and feeding accessories.

FEED ME, I'M YOURS!

It's a joy to finally have your baby outside your body, but certainly a challenge to have to get up over and over to feed your little sucker. Your baby's stomach is about the size of a walnut, and she's born to be a high-octane nursing machine that needs frequent nourishment just to survive.

One of the earliest choices you'll make is whether to put her to your breast or go the baby-bottle-and-formula route. There are lots of solid health and nutrition reasons for at least starting breastfeeding, and the more weeks your baby gets human milk the better. Consider getting help and coaching from a La Leche League leader or certified lactation consultant. (To find one, refer to *Web Resources* starting on page 338.)

Now we're going to jump straight into breast pumps, nursing bras, and nursing accessories to help you find the best buys, then we'll discuss baby bottles and formula. That will be followed by baby food and baby feeding accessories for when your baby is getting ready to start solids, at about six months of age.

Breast pumps and breastfeeding aids

It's commonly believed that every mother who plans to nurse should prepare in advance by buying a breast pump. But that's simply not the case. Your newborn will be the best possible breast pump you could have. (But you'll probably need some baby bottles on hand in case you decide to express milk for your baby.)

For the uninitiated, a breast pump is a hand-operated or motor-driven device that creates a gentle tugging action to collect milk for storage and to feed the baby later. Pumps usually come with several basic components: a shield to cover the nipple and areola (the colored ring around the breast), a tube into which the milk flows, and a container for storing the milk.

Motor-driven pumps use batteries or they plug into an electrical outlet to run the small motor that creates suction, rather like a miniature vacuum cleaner. Instead of a steady suction, they have a rhythmic tug-and-release action that mimics the way babies pull in, tongue the breast, and swallow.

Most pediatricians and lactation consultants recommend that babies not be given bottles for the first few months, to prevent nipple confusion, so mastering breastfeeding and hand-expression techniques come first, with pumping later. And you may discover you don't need a pump, after all. Manual expression is similar to a massage technique, and you can find instructions for how to do it from a variety of breastfeeding books and also online at breastfeeding sites such as www.breastfeeding.com.

If you know in advance that you'll be returning to work, or you expect hours of separation from your baby most days, or

if your baby arrives early and is hospitalized and could benefit from the infection-fighting powers of human milk, then an effective breast pump may help to keep your milk supply up and going and allow you to collect it and store it in the freezer until it can be fed to your baby.

There are five basic kinds of breast pumps—some more efficient than others. Inexpensive and also very ineffective bulb models resemble bicycle horns with a suction bulb connected to a single-piece horn and collection area. Hand-operated pumps use a spring-action handle or a syringelike cylinder that allow mothers to control the strength and rhythms of suction.

Small battery-operated models, usually with wall-outlet adapters, are compact enough for carrying in a diaper bag or purse. Midsize all-electric pumps are the mainstream workhorses for pumping, and some models are able to collect milk from both breasts at the same time, which speeds up the process. Large, hospital-grade electric pumps, available for rental from hospitals, clinics, and some pediatricians' offices, are the most efficient of all pumps and allow dual pumping.

When to Buy

A baby is the most efficient breast pump! There's no need to purchase an electric or manual breast pump until after your baby has arrived and you're sure you really need one, either because your baby has sucking problems or you want to store your milk for feedings while you are away from home.

What you get for the money

If you discover you truly need a pump, it doesn't pay to scrimp on the price. Cheap bicycle-horn pumps with a bulb on one end (under $10) and flimsy battery-operated pumps that baby-product manufacturers use to extend their baby-product lines ($30–$40) simply don't do the job effectively, and in some cases they can be downright painful and even damage delicate breast tissue.

Manual pumps that are hand operated allow you to create and control the suction yourself by squeezing a handgrip or pulling on a syringelike cylinder attached to a bottle or container ($25–$50). Short of expressing your milk yourself, they are the most economical option.

Midsize electric pumps ($200–$300) are the most popular for in-home or at-work use when you're sure you'll be missing some (but not all) daily feedings. These models can run on batteries or use an adapter for electrical outlets. They're reasonably efficient and quiet, and lightweight enough to carry around. Most come with a discreet carrying case and an insulated compartment for keeping bottles of milk cold. Models that pump both sides simultaneously may cost more, as do adapters to tap into your car's electrical system, but both extras may be worth the added convenience they offer. Models generally require 6 to 10 batteries, and pumping quickly eats up batteries, so the adapter for the electrical outlet should be used as much as possible.

By far the most effective pumps are hospital-grade models that can cost thousands of dollars. Fortunately, many lactation consultants and hospitals offer these pumps for rent for around $30 to $50 per month. The sheer size and weight of these pumps (11 to 22 pounds) and sometimes their noise can be disadvantages if you're planning to use the pump away from home.

But if you have a hospitalized preemie or a special-needs baby, such as one with sucking problems or a cleft lip or palate, or you're facing illness or hospitalization yourself, then a big efficient pump can help keep up your milk supply until your baby is able to do the job herself.

Most manufacturers of midsize and hospital-grade pumps offer a one-year warranty on defects in workmanship for the pump itself, and a limited (90-day) warranty on the system's other components.

Shield comfort is important

The shield is the horn-shaped part of the pump that fits over the areola and nipple. Many women experience discomfort with the breast shields that come with pumps, and it's often caused by standard shields that are too small for ample breasts. Many breast-pump manufacturers offer adapters to help make the shields fit better. Signs that the shield is the wrong size are rubbing on the sides each time there's a pulse in suction, your nipple filling up the air space at the end of the shield nearest the pump, and soreness around your nipple and areola (but not on the tip).

The Federal Women, Infants and Children (WIC) Program

WIC is a federally funded program overseen by the U.S. Department of Agriculture. Currently, it serves over 8.2 million pregnant mothers and those with infants and children through over 10,000 clinics across the U.S. WIC programs provide education, supplemental foods,

Checklist

Breast pump shopping

The best person to advise you about breast pumps is a certified lactation consultant. Ask your baby's pediatrician for a referral, or use a lactation-consultant locator online, such as the one found on www.ilca.org. Here are our suggestions about what to look for when you shop for a pump:

✔ **Efficient.** The best pumps are those that are the most effective at getting the job done. A well-designed manual pump can do the job but is tiresome.

✔ **Quiet.** Especially if you plan to pump at work and there's no private place to do it, the more nearly silent the better.

✔ **Easy to clean.** You'll be cleaning everything but the pump motor itself each day, so it should be easy to assemble and disassemble and to sterilize.

✔ **Adjustable vacuum strength.** Make sure that you can adjust how strong the vacuum is on the pump for your own comfort. Being able to control the cycling speed (how fast the suction pulses) is also a plus.

✔ **Electric adapter.** Pumps eat up batteries, so don't just rely exclusively on them to run the unit. Instead, make sure the pump offers an adapter for electrical outlets, and also consider purchasing an optional adapter for the cigarette lighter outlet in your car.

✔ **Comfortable shield.** If you have large breasts, standard shields that fit on the breast may not fit comfortably. Try special adapter inserts.

✔ **Portability.** Unless you're pumping only at home, the pump should come with an easy-to-tote carry case and be lightweight enough so you can carry it to work each day.

✔ **History of reliability.** Trust a name-brand pump manufacturer of hospital equipment, such as Medela or Omron, rather than trusting manufacturers of other baby-product lines, such as strollers and high chairs, who manufacture pumps simply to enlarge their baby-product lines.

nutrition and breastfeeding counseling, and some programs offer breast pumps for working mothers who meet the program's low-income criteria. Income guidelines for WIC eligibility vary from state to state and by family size. Check with your local department of human services to see if you qualify.

HAND-OPERATED PUMPS

These pumps use your muscle power to run. You hold the pump to your breast and then you either use a pump that creates suction, using a fitted cylinder that is drawn in and out like a piston, or you squeeze a spring-action hand-grip attached to a collection bottle that produces the needed tugging action.

Most manual pumps are designed to screw onto a standard baby bottle for milk collection and storage. And some offer adjustable suction controls and soft shield adapters to fit most breast sizes.

A manual pump should come complete with everything you'll need: a breast shield with possibly a small insert to ensure proper fit, the pump assembly with valves or a membrane, a bottle, a one- or two-piece lid, and some have tubing that drains from the pump to the bottle. Useful extras include feeding nipples for the bottle and a stand for keeping the bottle upright.

It can be handy to have a manual pump around, especially if you become engorged or you have an overactive letdown that causes your baby to struggle or choke. The pump can help to "take the edge off" so your baby is more comfortable.

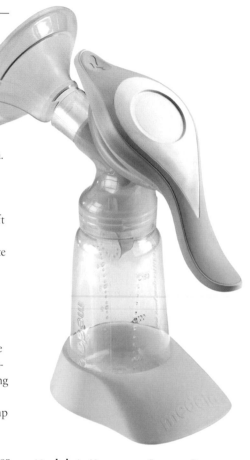

Medela's Harmony Breast Pump ($35)

This manual pump can be set to accurately mimic your baby's nursing. The letdown mode simulates the baby's initial rapid suckling to stimulate the "letdown." The expression mode simulates the baby's slower, deeper sucking, for maximum milk flow in less time. It's easier to clean with fewer parts than other, more complex manual pumps, and it fits most standard baby bottles. The kit comes with the pump, two breast shields, two 5-oz. containers, 2 lids, and 1 bottle stand.

Philips' Avent Deluxe Isis Breast Pump

(S50)

The Avent Isis Pump has a soft silicone cushion that features 5 petal-shaped cushions that flex in and out to massage your breast and stimulate the letdown reflex for gentle, reliable milk extraction. The drawback is that there are so many parts to assemble and dis-assemble for cleaning that some moms become discouraged and give up.

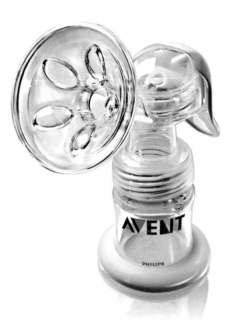

Highs & lows of hand-operated pumps

Highs. They're lightweight, silent, rela-tively inexpensive, and they're easier to tuck into a purse or briefcase than bat-tery-operated or electric models. Those with pistol-grip action and adjustable suction strength work well to collect milk once you have a milk letdown, and they can help to soften overactive letdowns by draining off the first heavy flow.

Lows. They work on your muscle power, and that can be tiring— especially since it takes 15 to 20 minutes to empty each breast, and they're able to empty only one breast at a time. They're not nearly as effi-cient at milk gathering as mid- and large-size electric pumps.

SMALL ELECTRIC PUMPS

These small pumps are usually sold as kits in baby stores and drugstores. Most come with a battery-operated motor unit and/or AC adapter, a manual pump, breast shield and insert, collection container, bottle stand, and lid for the bottle. Some include an insulated carrying case and cooling packs, or those may be offered as an optional purchase.

A good pump in this category should operate at a minimum of 30 cycles per minute (CPM), which is an effective level of sucking and releasing for occasional use. The strength of the suction varies with the unit, and some models, rather than having a knob to control vacuum strength require that you make the vacuum pulse by tapping your fingertip over a hole in the unit.

Small battery and electric pumps eat up batteries, so having an electrical adapter can be helpful. This type of pump might do a reasonably good job for short-term use or during occasional separation from baby such as a night out, relief of temporary engorgement, even a part-time job. But they're effective only if your milk supply is well established and your baby is still able to directly feed at the breast for most daily feedings to ensure that your breasts receive sufficient natural stimulation from the baby to sustain your milk supply.

Highs & lows of small electric pumps

Highs. They're small, fairly quiet, easy to carry around, and less expensive than larger, more "professional" versions.
Lows. They don't work as well as larger pumps, and their small motors have a history of breaking down. They usually have only one milk receptacle instead of two, which makes pumping slower than pumping both breasts at once. As batteries lose their charge, the pumps' cycling and vacuum levels are reduced, causing the pump to become increasingly less effective. (Get one with an electric outlet adapter and keep extra batteries on hand!)

Medela's Swing Breast Pump
($150)

Both a battery-operated and a plug-in pump, the unique 2-phase letdown action mimics a baby's natural nursing rhythm. In the stimulation mode, it simulates a hungry baby's rapid sucking motions to start milk flowing. The expression mode is similar to slower, deeper sucks after milk begins to flow. The unit has adjustable speed and vacuum settings. Components include a soft breast shield, 2 bottles and caps, a bottle stand, an AC adapter, tubing, a valve, and a membrane, in a drawstring bag. Requires 4 AA batteries (not included).

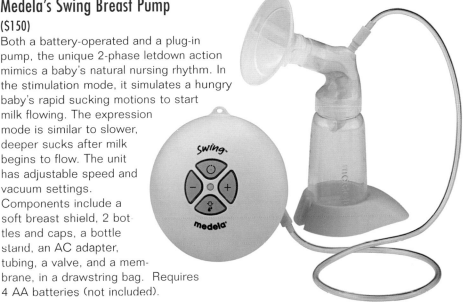

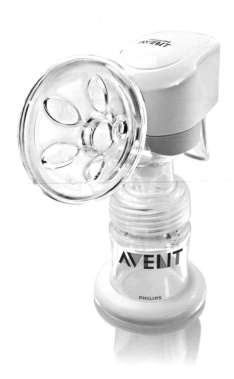

Philips' Avent Isis iQ Uno Breast Pump
($120)

This compact handheld pump is not inexpensive like "drugstore" models, but it is lightweight and runs on batteries or an AC adapter. It provides infinite pumping-speed and suction settings and allows manual setting of unique pumping rhythms, which the pump then mimics. The pump's shields have massage cushions to gently stimulate a letdown. Its closed system helps to prevent milk from backing up into the motor. A battery booster ensures uninterrupted power for effective pumping, and a light that changes from green to orange when battery power is limited to only one more pumping. The kit comes with the pump, 2 Avent feeding bottles, 2 sealing discs for milk storage, a battery pack, and a power cord.

MIDSIZE ELECTRIC PUMPS

These are the "workhorses" of the breast-pump world. Some are designed for pumping a single side, while others are able to pump both breasts simultaneously, which saves time. They are normally sold as a kit that includes a small motor encased in a zippered, insulated carry case. Also included are washable tubes that lead from the motor to the breast shields, and collection bottle(s). Units offer adjustable speed and vacuum levels and can run on either batteries or an electrical adapter. Some cases also have a special freezer-pack section for holding bottles of breast milk until they can be refrigerated or frozen. Breast shields ("horns") may have adapters for larger breast sizes. An optional cigarette lighter plug is usually available for pumping in the car and on trips.

Highs & lows of midsize electric pumps

Highs. Although not very lightweight or quiet, these units offer excellent efficiency when it comes to collecting milk, and they stimulate the breasts adequately to keep up a mother's milk supply. They're expensive, $100–$200, but if you're planning to express milk at work every day, the investment will be worth it over the long haul.

Lows. They eat up batteries in a hurry, so you will probably need an electrical outlet nearby. They're noisy, so people drifting in and out of the ladies' room or health suite at work will know something's going on. Occasionally mothers have problems with the fit of the breast shields, and cleaning the tubes and components can be time-consuming.

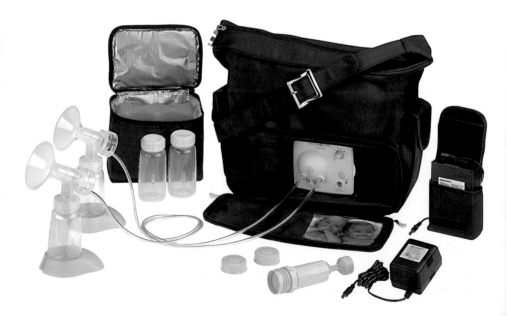

Hollister/Ameda's Purely Yours Electric Breast Pump
($215)
This pump offers flexibility and portability for moms, especially those planning to return to work. It offers 8 adjustable suction levels and 4 cycle speeds. Its milk collection kit has a patented silicone diaphragm that acts as a solid barrier between the pump tubes and the milk to prevent milk or moisture from entering the pump motor or tubes. Three power options are available: AC adapter, 6 AA batteries, or a car adapter (included with some models). Higher-priced models, including the new Ultra version, come with a carrying case or backpack. Optional flange adapters available for larger- or smaller-than-usual nipples. (Batteries not included.)

Medela's Pump In Style® Limited Edition (left)
($300)
All Medela electric pumps work well. This particular version is a relatively quiet dual-action pump suitable for working moms who need to pump both sides several times a day, with each pumping cycle lasting about 15 minutes. The pump has an internal chip that controls the speed and suction settings to more closely mimic the way a baby stimulates milk letdown, and then it nurses more slowly and deeply thereafter. It offers adjustable suction pressure and variable speed settings. The package comes with 4 collection containers and lids, cooling elements to chill expressed milk, an AC adapter, a small manual pump, a removable battery pack for cordless operation (uses 8 AA batteries, not included), and a manual conversion kit—all packed into a black microfiber bag with an insulated section. Similar products include the Metro, which comes in a designer backpack or shoulder bag, and the Pump In Style limited edition with a roomy messenger bag and extra milk-storage options.

LARGE HOSPITAL-GRADE ELECTRIC PUMPS

These are big, heavy units, about the size of a car battery, that are used in hospitals and cost $500 or more. They're considered the "Mercedes-Benz" of pumps and are designed for quiet, smooth operation with adjustable cycles per minute and vacuum pressure. They're most effective for mothers who are initiating breastfeeding and for those who want to sustain lactation during such special circumstances as when babies are unavailable to nurse because of hospitalization or sucking problems.

Some hospital pumps may have a smoother pumping cycle than others, but all are designed for both single and double pumping. Double pumping normally does not affect the vacuum levels on these strong pumps, which gives them a more consistent feel and operation than lighter-weight (and lower-grade) pumps.

The pumps can be used by multiple mothers because of special membranes that keep the milk from contacting the pump itself. Each mother using the pump purchases her own single or double kit for the particular model she is using. Components are easy to clean or sterilize.

Medela's Symphony Breast Pump
($1,200–$1,500)

This hospital-grade pump is comparatively quiet and efficient. The pump offers single or double pumping, and the user can switch between single and double pumping simply by applying or removing the second collection kit to the breast. It starts off with the option of several minutes of activated stimulation to help with letdown before settling down to a regular pumping rhythm and vacuum strength that can be adjusted by a knob. The pump's LCD display indicates the pumping mode, vacuum level, battery status, and other handling and service information. The pump comes with breast shields, connectors, bottles with lids, a valve and membrane, and collection connector tubing, as well as a vehicle lighter adapter.

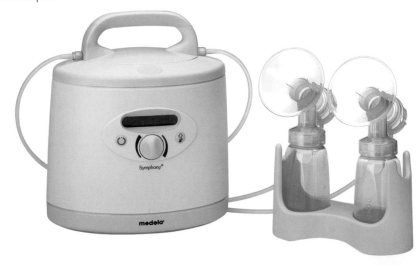

How to store breast milk for your baby

When you're gathering milk to be stored, make sure that your hands are clean and, if you use a breast pump, that the components and bottles have been washed in hot soapy water and allowed to air dry. It is best to store milk in a plastic or glass bottle with a sealable top, or in a sterile sealable bag, although those are more difficult to use than rigid self-standing bottles. You can add fresh milk to frozen milk as long as there is less fresh than frozen.

Human milk doesn't resemble formula. It appears thinner and more transparent, and it can have a bluish, yellowish, or brownish tint and still be normal and healthy for your baby. Cream from the milk can also gather at the top, so shake the bottle or bag before giving it to your baby.

The safest way to store breast milk is to:

✔ Keep at room temperature (less than 77° F) for 4 to 8 hours
✔ Keep at the back of a refrigerator for 3 to 8 days
✔ Keep at the back of a freezer for up to 3 months

The milk will expand when it freezes, so allow adequate space in the bottle. Date bottles or bags by writing on masking tape with a marker or ballpoint pen. Thaw the container with milk slowly by swirling it in warm water or by putting the container in the refrigerator the day before it is to be used, but don't use hot water or microwaving, which can destroy valuable milk proteins. Microwaved milk could also burn your baby. Thawed breast milk can be refrigerated for up to 24 hours, but it should not be refrozen.

Highs & lows of hospital-grade pumps

Highs. They're highly effective and rapid in gathering milk, and they're useful for emergency situations, such as providing milk for a hospitalized baby when nursing is interrupted temporarily. (Breasts require frequent strong stimulation and sucking to keep producing milk.)
Lows. They're heavy, not very portable, and prohibitively expensive for purchase, but short-term rentals are available. They require an electrical outlet, and some make a noticeable churning sound that may be embarrassing to you if you are pumping in a less-than-private setting.

NURSING BRAS

Choosing a nursing bra

A good nursing bra is important for supporting your breasts and holding your nursing pads in place to help absorb leakage. Any store with a good bra department will help you get the right fit.

Finding the right bra

Trying on bras (like bathing suits) is the only way to really know how well the bra will fit and how comfortable it will feel. There should be no overhang under your arms or spilling out over the top of the bra. Underwire bras are not recom-

mended, because they can constrict your milk ducts, which could cause them to get plugged up. If you can't live without the underwire, just make sure that the U shaped wires do not compress any breast tissue. Carefully fit yourself into an underwire bra by bending over every time you put one on.

Bras and support

A well-fitted bra can help your heavy breasts feel more comfortable, but it probably can't prevent sagging and stretching. Breast shape and firmness are mostly determined by heredity, and even women who don't choose to breastfeed

---

 # Checklist

Nursing-bra shopping

You'll need at least three bras: one to wear, one in the laundry, and one in the drawer. And your breast size may be larger at first and smaller after a few months. Try out more than one style to settle on the one that you like best. Here are tips on choosing a good nursing bra:

✔ **Comfortable fit.** Make sure that the cup is roomy enough to hold breast pads and won't put pressure on any part of your breast that could interfere with milk flow. (Note: Milk-making tissue goes all the way up to your armpit and even around your torso.)

✔ **Easy to open.** You should be able to fasten and unfasten the bra flap with one hand and without having to fiddle with it, especially when you're breastfeeding away from home.

✔ **Washability.** The bra's material should be able to withstand repeated washings without stretching, pilling, or shrinking.

✔ **Breathability.** The fabric should allow your skin to breathe without trapping moisture inside.

✔ **Special features for large breasts.** Look for extra support features, and avoid bras that open completely, which could make it a hassle to close up shop. Choose bras that continue to support the breasts from underneath when the bra flaps are open. Choose well-padded, adjustable shoulder straps that aren't stretchy, for more support.

find that their breasts change after pregnancy. After you wean your baby, your breasts may appear to shrink and seem droopier, but they firm up somewhat as months pass.

Avoid:

✗ Bras that are too tight or have underwires (unless you fit them carefully).

✗ Synthetic bras or those lined in plastic that don't "breathe."

✗ Bras with difficult-to-operate latches.

When to Buy

Purchase a nursing bra during the final weeks of pregnancy so you'll be sure to have a couple of bras on hand at the hospital and for those early sleepless days at home with your new baby. Your rib cage and cup size will remain substantially the same.

Bravado! Designs' Nursing Bras
($25–$50)

Bravado! makes a variety of extremely comfortable maternity and nursing bras in a series of patterns and sizes from B all the way up to double E. Most feature a secure band under the bra as well as stretchy soft cups with a plastic fastener on the strap. They're great for everyday comfortable wear, but not great for strong support, such as for jogging. You can visit their Internet site to view choices: www.bravadodesigns.com.

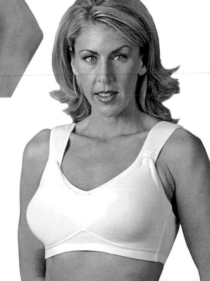

Fancee Free's Molded Nursing Bra
($30)

If you're fuller-figured and seeking good support without lots of bulkiness and seams that show through knitted shirts, then this may be the bra for you. The thick straps help to give your breasts support. Sizes range from 34 D to 48 H.

Other breastfeeding accessories

Here's a list of other breastfeeding accessories besides pumps and bras that you may want to check out:

■ **Baby bottles.** These will be useful for storing expressed milk in the refrigerator or freezer and feeding your baby while you're away. (But wait to do that until breastfeeding is well established.)

■ **Nursing pads.** Washable, reusable cotton nursing pads are usually sold in pairs, or you can buy disposable leak-resistant nursing pads by the box. Both designs tuck inside your bra to help absorb leaks between feedings. (A folded cotton handkerchief works, too.)

■ **Nipple creams.** Nipple creams, such as Lansinoh, may help to soothe sore or chafed nipples.

■ **Support pillows.** A C-shaped nursing pillow, such as a Boppy, is extra firm and wraps around your waist to take pressure off your shoulders and arms while you're nursing. Some pillows are inflatable to different heights. (Note: Pillows present a suffocation hazard, and a baby should never be left alone on one.)

■ **Stool or hassock.** To help to support your feet as you nurse.

■ **Nursing clothing and privacy items.** Many maternity and online breastfeeding sites carry specialized nursing clothing such as tee shirts, blouses, and dresses that have hidden side panels for discreet nursing and other specialty cover-ups to hide, or at least make it less obvious, that you are breastfeeding.

Baby formulas

Babies' bodies aren't able to absorb pure cow's milk, because it doesn't contain the right mix of nutrients and proteins. For the same reason, skim milk isn't recommended for babies, because it doesn't contain the fat that babies require to thrive and to maintain the insulation of nerve cells in their brains.

Modern-day formulas could be called artificial milk. They're created from homogenized vegetable and animal fats, oils, and skim milk to closely imitate the fatty-acid content of human milk. Liquid formulas may also contain thickening and stabilizing agents for uniform consistency, and they often contain additional ingredients, such as lecithin, carrageenan, and mono- and diglycerides, which are added to ensure that the formula doesn't separate with standing.

Most formulas come in three versions: powdered, premixed, and ready-to-feed bottles. Powdered is the least expensive, and ready-to-feed bottles are the most expensive. (**Note:** Powdered formulas are not sterile, and some have been recalled because they were suspected of being tainted with food-borne contaminants.)

Breast milk or formula should be your baby's primary source of nutrition and hydration for the first year. In rare instances, a baby may have an allergic reaction to the proteins or sugars in the cow's milk portion of a formula. And even more rarely, a baby's

When to Buy

Baby formulas
If you know you'll be bottle feeding, it's a good idea to have a supply on hand when you bring baby home. Your baby's pediatrician is the best source for advice about what brand to buy, in what form, and how much to have on hand before your baby arrives.

allergic reaction to formula can be serious and even life threatening, causing vomiting, hives, and breathing problems. But typically, allergic symptoms are much milder—a constantly runny nose with clear mucus, diarrhea, a tendency toward ear infections, or unexplained bouts of fussiness or colic.

Alternative formulas for allergic babies are made with soy protein (not the soy milk found in health food stores), or with more refined (and also more costly) predigested formulas called protein hydrolysates. Your baby's physician may prescribe one of these formulas if your baby shows symptoms of being allergic to regular formulas. Ask your healthcare provider about recent research that links soy formulas with an increase in vulnerability to peanut allergy and the way soy could affect your baby's processing of certain minerals.

Ask your baby's doctor about the particular brand of infant formula to use and whether you need to boil the water for formula, the bottle, and the nipple assembly.

DHA and ARA in formulas

DHA (docosahexaenoic acid) and ARA (arachidonic acid) are substances found in human breast milk. Both are long-chain, polyunsaturated fatty acids, which appear naturally in certain fish oils, eggs, and some algae and fungi. They're thought to play a part in babies' visual functioning and neural development. Some formula manufacturers are now adding DHA and ARA to their formulas, but the long-term benefits of these substances are not completely clear. Your baby's pediatrician is the best source for advice about choosing formula.

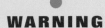

WARNING

Don't microwave formula
Never heat bottles of formula or breast milk in a microwave oven. The formula will heat unevenly and develop hot spots, which could burn your baby's mouth, Instead, use a bottle warmer or immerse the bottle in a bowl of warm water.

Don't prop your baby or the bottle
Some parents believe that the sooner their baby can hold her own bottle and feed herself, the smarter and more independent she is. And every year, another couple somewhere in America invents yet another contraption for holding a bottle in a baby's mouth so parents don't have to do it. Not only do these less-than-loving contraptions not work, they can be dangerous if your baby begins to spit up or choke on formula, and you're not there to help. Your bottle-fed baby deserves the same loving closeness and attention during feeding that breastfed babies get each time they nurse. So relax in a comfortable rocker or recliner, and hold your baby close.

How to prepare formula

Be careful to follow the formula manufacturer's instructions to the letter when you mix formula. Formula that's too concentrated can put a strain on baby's kidneys. Formula that's too diluted with water can deprive your baby's body of critical nutrients.

Prepare formula only in small batches, so that you're sure it's fresh. Keep it refrigerated, or use an ice pack in your diaper bag so it can't spoil. Discard leftover formula rather than serving it a second time. Baby's mouth and saliva contaminate the formula with bacteria.

There's no medical reason for heating formula, but babies appear to prefer it at body temperature. Most parents opt to rotate the baby's bottle under warm tap water for a few minutes until it becomes comfortably lukewarm. You can also buy bottle warmers for the same purpose. (Note: Adult fingers and hands aren't sensitive enough to distinguish minor heat differences. Always test a sprinkle of the milk on your wrist to make sure it's not too hot.)

If you use powdered formula and your tap water comes from a well, be sure to have your well tested periodically, especially during hot weather, for the presence of contaminants. You may want to consider investing in a water filtration system if you suspect that your water contains nitrates, lead, or other contaminants.

WARNING

Counterfeit formulas

The FDA recommends that parents always look for any changes in formula color, smell, or taste. And to always check "use by" dates on the containers, to never buy damaged cans, and to call the manufacturer's toll-free number with any concerns or questions. The FDA warns consumers about counterfeit infant formulas that may bear a false "use by" date to obscure the fact that the product may no longer contain the amounts of nutrients listed on the label or may otherwise not be of acceptable quality. Sometimes these formulas may be relabeled to disguise the true contents inside, and these misrepresentations may affect babies who are allergic to mislabeled ingredients. If you have any doubts, check that the date on the individual container and the case are the same.

Choosing a safe baby bottle

Most baby bottles are molded from clear, shiny plastic. That makes them less breakable than old-fashioned glass bottles and less heavy. Plus, the plastic allows them to be molded into helpful shapes such as angle-necked versions that make it easier for parents to hold the bottle and allow breast milk or formula to pool around the bottle's nipple as the baby drinks, to help her swallow less air.

Some studies show that rigid, shiny, clear baby bottles could contain low doses of certain plastics known as polycarbonates, and specifically a chemical called bisphenol-A (BPA) that has been shown to leach into milk or formula in minuscule amounts. Animal studies have shown that large amounts of the chemical could potentially have a hormone-disrupting effect, particularly when the container is heated, such as when sterilizing formula on top of the stove. The lowest safe amount of BPA that babies can ingest without being harmed is still unclear.

Plastic baby bottles may also contain polyvinyl chloride (PVC) as well as substances known as phthalates, also used as plastic softeners in nipples, pacifiers, and teethers. These substances are thought to be toxic and can leach out of the product when they are chewed and come in contact with babies' saliva. On the other hand, bottles made of polyethylene or of polypropylene don't contain hormone-disrupting chemicals or other known toxic additives.

If you're concerned about buying baby-safe bottles, here are our suggestions for what to do:

✔ **Use tempered glass.** Select glass bottles that have been tempered to make them less likely to shatter. Immediately discard

When to Buy

Purchase a newborn starter set of 4 (or more) standard bottles and nipples in the 4 to 6-ounce size before your baby arrives, and plan to change the system later if the bottle or nipple designs don't work well with your baby.

any bottles with chips or cracks. Evenflo glass bottles are available in some pharmacies and online from a number of sources, including Amazon.com.

✔ **Look for a different plastic.** Choose plastic bottles that the manufacturer says contain no polycarbonate, or select those made of polyethylene or polypropylene, which are generally less shiny and more opaque than clear plastic bottles.

✔ **Avoid scratches.** Don't use bottle brushes to clean clear plastic bottles, and replace bottles if scratches show up inside.

✔ **Don't use hard-to-clean bottles.** Bottles with built-in straws aren't very practical. They pose a sanitation problem, because it's next to impossible to scrub the entire milk residue from the inside of the straw. Also beware of bottles shaped like doughnuts, bears, animals, soda bottles, or sports equipment, which are also hard to keep clean.

✔ **Don't store milk in disposable bags.** Avoid disposable nursers. Not only are they more costly than reusable bottles, their plastic bags may contain fine plastic dust inside. And there's a risk the bags could leak or burst when someone mistakenly microwaves them, showering your baby with hot milk. Plus, babies have choked on the tabs of some bags.

Nipples

Nipples, like bottles, come in a variety of shapes and materials. Most nipples are molded from latex, a form of rubber, or from silicone, a clear material used widely in the medical world. Silicone is durable, is easy to clean, and isn't likely to cause allergic reactions. On the downside, it's more likely to rupture and tear if you try to enlarge the nipple hole with a needle or when your toddler chews on the nipple. The surface of silicone nipples can also be slippery when wet, making it harder for young babies to grasp.

Latex, on the other hand, can cause allergy problems in babies, and nipples made from it are more likely to rot over time from exposure to saliva and the acids in milk. Whichever material you choose, inspect each nipple closely every few days for tears or abnormalities, and replace old nipples with new ones every three months or so.

When bottle-feeding your baby, make sure the nipple hole is the right diameter. If your baby seems to be sucking too hard, then you may need to change to a fast- or medium-flow nipple. A nipple with too tiny a hole could collapse under your baby's strong sucking motion. On the other hand, if your baby seems to be sputtering and gulping a lot, she may need a slower nipple. One test is that the formula comes out in a spray for a second or two when the bottle is inverted, and then trickles down to drops. Buy new nipples rather than trying to change the hole yourself.

When it comes to nipple shape or feel, babies seem to have their own individual preferences. Some babies prefer firm, short nipples, while others like nipples that are softer or more elongated. Special nipples are available for premature babies with

Q I have a problem with the pump I'm using: it hurts! It's a small battery-operated model. It makes me not want to use it. What should I do?

The biggest problem with inexpensive "drugstore" battery and AC pumps is they can really hurt when you use them, and pumping shouldn't hurt at all. Other problems mothers face are that small, flimsy motors burn out quickly and eat up batteries. We suggest exploring pump-rental options from a local hospital or lactation consultant's practice or investing in a midsize pump. Then make sure that you're using the proper-size shield for your breast. (See our discussion of shield fit on page 20.)

Q I've gone back to work, and pumping just isn't working for me. I'm pretty confident that I need to wean my baby. Can you suggest the best way to do that?

The breastfeeding experts at La Leche League International have a large collection of articles on weaning on its Internet site: www.lalecheleague.org. The organization suggests that weaning be done gradually, and with love. If you wean cold turkey, your breasts will likely become painfully engorged, and you might develop a breast infection. Your baby will probably fight the switch from your warm, soft breast to the bottle, and she may mourn the loss of "her" breasts. Try substituting a bottle for her least favorite feeding. Let the baby have a few days (or weeks, if possible) between each time you substitute a breastfeeding session with a bottle. For your own comfort, keep expressing a little milk from your breasts at first, just to take the pressure off. For babies older than one year, try substituting a cup of water, juice, cow's milk, or solid food in place of your toddler's least important feeding. Nighttime feedings are usually the last to go.

Q My grandson always has to have his pacifier popped in his mouth. I think it looks awful. When it falls out of his mouth, he has a fit, and his mouth always has a red rash and ring around it. Plus, I never know what his expression might be behind his constant plastic "plug." Are pacifiers harmful? Have you any suggestions for how to handle this with my daughter-in-law?

Some babies become positively addicted to their "passys" and won't leave home (or go to sleep) without them. Weaning a baby from a pacifier can be a tricky business. But most babies outgrow them on their own at some point. You could try "losing" your grandson's pacifier while you're babysitting, but it could backfire by reinforcing how important his pacifier is to him. Ultimately, it's your son's and daughter-in-law's responsibility to deal with the pacifier issue, and any tampering on your part could be viewed by them as an unwelcome intrusion.

Q I am in a work situation that makes it especially inconvenient to use a pump, and I hate the thought of using some kind of gadget on myself. I've heard that some mothers know how to get milk using their hands. Can you explain how to do that?

Manual expression, as it's called, takes some practice. It's best to start standing over a sink to experiment with what works best for you. Once you get the hang of it, all you need is some milk storage bags, a place to wash your hands and a private space. The most popular way to do it is called the Marmet Technique, which uses pressure from the pads of two fingers and a thumb and a rolling action to rhythmically drain milk reservoirs. You can find it described online, or you can read about it in La Leche League's manual *The Womanly Art of Breastfeeding*.

weak sucks or those with mouth and jaw deformities, for pulpy juices, or for feeding toddlers formula thickened with cereal.

So-called orthodontic nipples are elongated, almost hourglass-shaped. Advertisers claim they're better for baby's jaw development, but the center of the nipple is also hard to get clean, and if the nipple is made from latex, it may rot over time, causing it to become sticky and interfere with milk flow. We suggest starting first with a standard newborn-size nipple, and then experimenting with other versions if your baby seems to have problems feeding.

Be sure to read the directions for the nipples after you get them home. For example, some nipples come with neck rings that can be adjusted to regulate the volume of milk flow according to how tightly you screw on the plastic bottle ring. All nipples should be boiled out of the package for about five minutes before using them the first time, to remove dust and chemical residues.

Pacifiers

All babies appear to have a need to suck, even when they've had enough nourishment. A pacifier (called a dummy in some countries) is a nipple mounted on a shield that lets babies suck contentedly even when they're not being fed.

Just as with bottle nipples, pacifiers come in a variety of materials and shapes,

WARNING

Avoid pacifier accidents

There have been numerous pacifier recalls due to unsafe designs. Pacifiers can break apart, allowing a baby to choke on the rubber section or to suffocate when a pacifier shield is too small and gets lodged in the baby's throat. Numerous babies have died in pacifier-related accidents, mostly from choking on pacifier parts that have come loose. Or they have accidentally hung themselves when strings or ribbons tying pacifiers around their necks have gotten caught on the ends of cribs or play yards. Pacifiers also harbor germs, and studies show that babies using pacifiers are more vulnerable to inner-ear infections. Frequently inspect pacifiers to be sure the shield hasn't cracked, and the nipple hasn't started to pull loose, and replace them every few months. Never tie a pacifier around your baby's neck using a ribbon or string. And wash pacifiers in warm, soapy water or boil them for 5 minutes after use to keep them clean and germ-free.

and babies have distinct preferences about the kind they like to use. You may want to buy several types to try with your baby. And again, boil them for five minutes before letting your baby suck on one.

Using a pacifier with your baby has both good and bad points. On the plus side, babies seem to enjoy mouthing them, and at least one recent study appears to show a connection between the regular use of a pacifier and the reduced chance of a baby dying from Sudden Infant Death Syndrome (SIDS). On the down side, prolonged and intense pacifier use, as prolonged finger sucking, can lead to dental-arch deformities and misalignment of the front teeth after the first few years.

When to Buy

Have a set of 2 newborn-size pacifiers on hand before your baby arrives, sterilize them, and pack them for the hospital.

When to start solids

Your baby's physician is the best source of information about when to start solids and what foods to introduce first to your baby. Typically, pediatricians recommend that babies start a mild iron-fortified instant baby cereal mixed with breast milk or formula at around five to six months of age. Foods such as dairy products, tomatoes, strawberries, and citrus fruits are thought to be more likely to cause allergic reactions in babies and are usually delayed until after the first year.

Allergy-symptoms include clear mucus or other coldlike symptoms that run from the nose; wheezing (chest rattling) and asthma like symptoms; frequent ear infections; red, itchy eyes; vomiting, constipation, or diarrhea; skin rashes, hives (swollen welts), or a sore bottom.

There's another danger in starting solids too early. Babies younger than 5 months of age have immature intestinal tracts, and their bodies may react to foreign proteins and other food substances by establishing allergies that can cause problems later. And the baby's kidneys may not be mature enough to adequately remove excess waste products from foods such as meats.

By six months of age, most babies' bodies will have begun to produce enough protective immune substances that the chances of having a serious allergic response to foods are lessened. But a bigger issue is that it's important not to trade off the valuable nutrients found in breast milk or formula for less adequate foods at the very time when your baby's body needs maximum nourishment.

Here are some signs that your baby may be ready for solids.

✔ **Sitting up.** Your baby is able to sit up on her own with some support and can hold her head steady.

✔ **Trying to grab your food.** When you eat, your baby is very interested in watching you eat and tries to grab your food and put it in her mouth. She may lean forward like a baby bird waiting to be fed.

✔ **No tongue thrusting.** Tongue thrusting—pushing food back out of her mouth—has diminished.

✔ **Lip skills.** Your baby shows signs of chewing food and can draw her lower lip in to keep food inside her mouth.

✔ **Accepting a spoon.** Your baby is open to having a spoon in her mouth and is able to swallow food without choking.

✔ **Ravenous appetite.** Your baby has reached the 5- or 6-month stage and can't seem to get enough to drink, but that doesn't seem to be related to a temporary growth spurt, teething woes, or coming down with an illness.

On the other hand, if your baby spits food out or clamps her jaws shut and turns her head to the side, she's signaling that she doesn't want to participate. Our suggestion is to ease off and wait a few weeks before trying a different flavor. The rejected food may be accepted by your baby later on when it's mixed with other food flavors.

Getting started with solid food

The best approach is to nurse your baby first or let her have her bottle, and then offer her a spoonful of smooth, easy-to-swallow food. That's because a really hungry baby isn't going to be very cooperative; plus, breast milk or formula should continue to be the mainstay of your baby's diet during that first critical year of growth and brain formation. Set your sights low: offer just a quarter of a teaspoon of the new food several times a day, then gradually increase amounts as time passes.

Start with a single pure food, not a mixed stew or other combination of ingredients, and stick with the new item for a few days so you can identify the culprit if your baby's body has an allergic reaction, such as stomach upset, diarrhea, or a runny nose and coldlike symptoms with clear mucus. (Note: What goes in one end will likely come out the other—so there may be a new color to bowel movements.)

Once your baby has mastered eating skills, it's very simple, economical, and healthier to puree your baby's food yourself from fresh ingredients, whenever you have the time, rather than relying solely on baby food in jars for feeding.

Exposure to light and heat in clear glass jars can kill valuable nutrients, including vitamin C. The money you save when you make your own baby food can help make up for the expense of selecting organic produce that is likely to contain fewer toxic pesticides and other unwanted chemicals. Certain foods, such as beets, broccoli, carrots, cauliflower, green beans, spinach, and turnips, aren't recommended for young babies because of their high levels of naturally occurring nitrates that may affect a baby's ability to use oxygen and result in a serious health condition called "blue-baby syndrome."

If you use jarred baby food, remove a portion from the jar for your baby and serve it in a separate container. Never feed your baby from a used jar that's had the chance to be contaminated by your baby's saliva and bacteria. If you want to prepare your own baby foods, our suggestion is to get baby-food cookbooks from the library or a bookstore and try out a few recipes.

WARNING

These foods can choke

Some types of food should be completely avoided because they have a history of choking babies: tough meat, whole peanuts or other nuts and seeds, hard candy, marshmallows, popcorn, hot dogs, canned Vienna sausage or toddler sticks, potato chips or corn chips, fish with small bones (such as trout), raisins and other dried fruits if they're uncooked, peanut butter, and raw fruits and vegetables if they're hard or crunchy, whole pieces of canned fruit, or fruit that has seeds.

Feeding your older baby

Once your baby has passed her first birthday and has acquired eating skills, you can make unseasoned family foods palatable for your baby by using a baby food grinder, blender, or food processor and adding a little liquid to make it smooth.

Be forewarned, though, that baby feeding can be a real mess! Initially, you might want to try covering your front with a towel and feeding your baby while she sits in your lap so you have better control of her and the feeding process. You may want to spread a towel or other "splash guard" under the high chair, too.

By the time your baby reaches 8 to 12 months of age, she may be able to handle finely chopped meat and other high-protein foods such as legumes and cheeses, as well as grain products, such as crackers and breads. Finger foods should be small enough for her small hands to manage, and soft enough so that she can chew on small pieces without choking on them.

Here are some suggestions: cooked macaroni or noodles, small pieces of ripe fruit such as bananas or cooked apple, white or sweet potatoes, or other easy-to-chew vegetables, small slices of mild cheese, crackers, teething biscuits, and Cheerios.

Baby-feeding accessories

Here's a list of baby feeding accessories you may want to have on hand as your baby starts solids.

■ **Spoons.** Soft-tipped spoons with padded bowls are great for feeding new eaters because they help to protect baby's gums.

■ **Baby dish.** Feeding-dish choices include plain unbreakable bowls and high-sided bowls with suction cups underneath so your baby can't toss them over the side of the high chair; hollow warmer bowls with an internal compartment to hold warm water are nice, but make sure the cap on the filling hole can't come loose and potentially choke your baby.

■ **Baby-food grinder.** Some parents find that a small handheld baby-food grinder with a turning handle that pushes food through the blades and into a feeding cup is an easy way to mash up vegetables and meats with juices.

■ **Bibs.** A soft, flexible plastic bib that buttons or fastens with Velcro on the back and with a trough in the front can

---

When to Buy

Baby-feeding accessories
Your baby doesn't need solids until she has good mouthing skills and expresses an interest—usually around 5 to 6 months. A soft spoon, a small dish with steep sides and some washable bibs are all that's needed.

---

be used over and over and is great for catching spills.

■ **"Splat" mat.** A large bathtub mat or a square of plastic sheeting serves as a good catchall under baby's high chair.

■ **Suctioned high-chair toys.** Toys with strong suction cups on their bases can be handy to fasten on the high chair's tray while you're fixing baby's meal; plus, they put an end to the "drop it over the side and watch Mom pick it up" game.

Overrated juices

The nutritional value of fruit juices is mostly overrated. According to the Food and Nutrition Service of the USDA, apple, pear, cherry, peach, and prune juice contain a lot of sorbitol, a type of carbo-hydrate sometimes called sugar alcohol, which is hard to digest and can cause babies to experience diarrhea, abdominal pain, and bloating.

Citrus fruits are high on the list of allergy-causing foods. Orange juice, or juices from citrus products containing ascorbic acid, may cause her to have allergic reactions, such as rashes.

Juices are acidic, and if you give them to your baby at naptime or bedtime, the acid from the juices may pool in your sleeping baby's mouth, causing baby-bottle mouth—a form of tooth decay that causes the front teeth to rot from the inside and then to crumble and break off.

In addition, fruit juices aren't nearly as nutritionally complete as breast milk and formula. If your baby has a lot of juices in her diet, she will naturally cut back on drinking the breast milk and formula that are so important to her nutrition. Offer juices very sparingly and only toward the later part of your baby's first year, when her body is mature enough to handle them.

SAFETY CONSIDERATIONS

Baby food and formula are regulated by the Food and Drug Administration under the U.S. Department of Agriculture (www.fda.gov), and it should be noted that the FDA does not test formulas for compliance with their regulations prior to their being marketed. Breast pumps are overseen by the Food and Drug Administration (www.fda.gov/cdrh/breastpumps/) as well as the U.S. Consumer Product Safety Commission (www.cpsc.gov). For accidents or near accidents related to feeding dishes, bottles, or other baby-feeding equipment, use the CPSC's product hotline, 800-638-2772, or report product problems at www.cpsc.gov.

3

BACKPACK CARRIERS

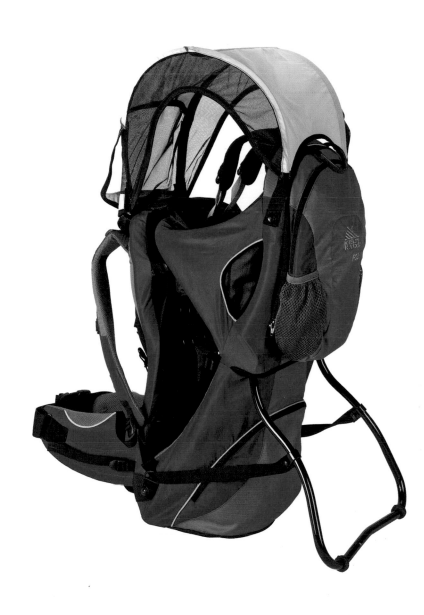

Backpacks are framed baby carriers that let you tote your larger tot hands-free, with the weight distributed across your back, shoulders, and hips. They're suitable only for babies five months of age or older who have gained strong sitting skills. This chapter gives you all the ins and outs of backpacks to help you pick the best model for your needs. It also has tips for how to use them and safety suggestions.

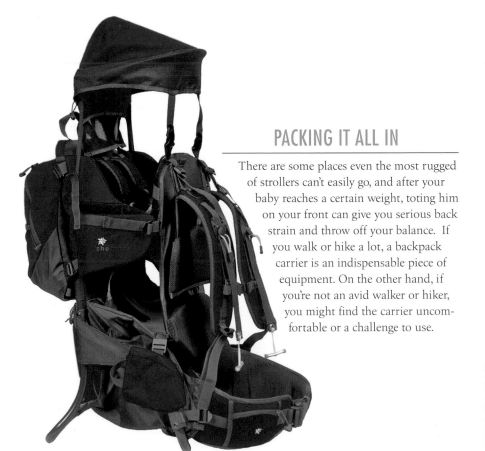

PACKING IT ALL IN

There are some places even the most rugged of strollers can't easily go, and after your baby reaches a certain weight, toting him on your front can give you serious back strain and throw off your balance. If you walk or hike a lot, a backpack carrier is an indispensable piece of equipment. On the other hand, if you're not an avid walker or hiker, you might find the carrier uncomfortable or a challenge to use.

What you get for the money

Frameless soft carriers (starting as low as $30) are generally less costly than framed versions, and some manufacturers have models that can be worn on the parents' backs. Granted, fabric models are lightweight and less bulky than carriers made with metal and molded plastic supports, but without the firm structural support from tubes or molded plastic, the all-fabric versions put more strain on parents' shoulders and backs. (See our chapter on soft carriers, page 250.)

Some popular baby-product manufacturers offer simple framed carriers with prices starting at about $90 to $100. They aren't made to distribute weight for long trips or to withstand heavy wear—but might work for you if you plan to go only on short jaunts about town or a brisk walk to an airport gate.

A basic baby-carrying backpack will have a frame made of lightweight aluminum, padded shoulder straps, a hip belt, and straps to hold baby in. Dense rip-stop, quality nylon fabric with mesh vents will be more comfortable for both you and your baby in warm weather than packs covered in heavyweight canvas or other heavyweight materials.

Extra features are added as the price of backpacks rises. More money translates into denser foam, higher-quality construction, more durable tubing, and extras such as a support stand, a detachable fanny pack, water-bottle holders, an arching sun/weather shield, more pouches, pockets, and blanket straps, and roll-down mosquito netting. (It helps if the backpack has roomy pockets that you can reach with the baby still on your back, or a generous detachable fanny pack to strap around your waist with the zippered pouch in front.) Also, in the top price ranges there are more ergonomic frames and frame adjustments.

The best-quality frame backpacks don't carry the brand names of traditional juvenile-product manufacturers. Look for manufacturers specializing in outdoor gear, with brand names such as Kelty, REI, and Sherpani Alpina. Parents praise these brands for durability and comfort. However, even their entry-price point (marketing-speak for cheapest) models retail for more than $100.

Comfort counts

If you plan to do serious trekking with your baby, comfort features for both of you are almost certainly worth the extra money. Look for thick, dense padding everywhere, and a wide, comfortable pelvic belt to help distribute weight. Safety features are important, too, such as shoulder and waist straps to hold baby down, so he can't stand up or possibly fall out.

The more adjustable the pack, the better—and those with adjustable frame lengths can make a huge difference in comfort. A model that you can adjust while you're actually wearing it is a huge boon, but you may have to pay more for that convenience. Any kind of customizable fit is worth the money, especially if

When to Buy

When your baby can sit up sturdily – around 5 to 6 months of age and after that until he's too heavy to be comfortably toted on your back, usually when his weight exceeds between ¼ and ⅓ of your weight.

more than one family member (or child) will be using the pack.

Baby comfort features include cushioned leg holes, and the bottoms of the holes flush with the seat so your baby's legs won't be squeezed. A cushioned back bar that keeps the pack from bumping your baby in the face as you walk is an important feature, too (and gives a teether something to gnaw on!).

Even the best-designed backpacks can be a real challenge when it comes to putting the pack on and off and getting the baby in and out. A freestanding pack can be unstable and tippy while you're trying to strap baby inside. And getting the pack swung around and the shoulder straps on is an art to be mastered.

Check your strength

Before you invest hundreds of dollars toward the dream of introducing your baby to Mother Nature, a reality check is in order. Honestly now, are you strong enough to tote on your back for hours at a time? Uphill? Or even upstairs? What about later, when he gets heavier?

By necessity, your baby's weight isn't carried close to your body but juts out from

> **"Make sure the place where you buy your baby's backpack has a liberal return policy. Thankfully, our baby didn't spit up on it, and we were able to take it back when we discovered our baby hated being inside it."**

the back where the baby is seated, and even the costliest frame with high-density foam padding on all body contact points can't make your baby weigh any less.

The more comfort features piled onto the carrier, the more pounds will be added to your body's burden. Then add in all the pounds of diaper-changing paraphernalia stuffed into every pocket, extra baby duds, bottles, formula (if you're not breastfeeding) and baby food, plus the sweaty heat of having your back covered all the time, and you may find yourself feeling enormous sympathy for donkeys, camels, llamas, and other beasts of burden!

The basic rule of thumb is that the pack must be useful and tolerable for you until your child gets big enough to walk on his own or his weight exceeds about a quarter to a third of your own weight. After that, your child will need to ride in a stroller or use his own two legs (unless he balks and buckles at the knees because he's tired, hungry, or distraught).

It's not that backpacking with a baby can't be done, and enjoyed, but some considerations are in order first. Wearing a backpack for any length of time takes practice and getting used to. So don't plan to buy a pack today and go on a three-day trek with your baby tomorrow. Start gradually. Make sure you're strong enough to do it. Build up your endurance with practice. While a hefty muscular dad may be able to tote a tot without a lot of discomfort for hours at a time, a short bantamweight mom may find wearing one comfortable for only brief periods.

Checklist

Backpack shopping

A backpack carrier for your baby needs to be comfortable for you and also comfortable and safe for your baby, too. Here are our suggestions for what to look for when you shop:

✔ **A comfortable frame.** One that doesn't press into your back or hips as you walk, or jar the baby.

✔ **Adequate spacing for straps.** Not so close together that they rub your neck or so far apart that they slip off your shoulders.

✔ **A padded pelvic belt.** To distribute some of the weight from your shoulders.

✔ **Thick padding.** For straps, leg holes, and the components surrounding your baby's face.

✔ **Sturdy baby seat belts, shoulder harnesses, and hardware.** To keep baby safely seated inside. Straps should be attached with multiple layers of stitching.

✔ **Roomy storage pockets.** For diapers and other baby gear.

✔ **Clear directions for use.** Weight and size limits, and how to put the carrier on correctly.

✔ **Comfortable leg holes.** Wide enough to not bind the baby's legs, but not so large that a baby might slip through (a common reason for backpack recalls).

✔ **Quality fabric.** Moisture resistant and easily wiped clean with a mild detergent. A detachable, washable bib is nice, too.

✔ **Storage pouches.** For extra diapers, wipes, pacifiers, and so on. A waterproof area for bottles, dirty diapers, and/or clothes can be handy.

✔ **Support stand (optional).** A flip-out stand in the back can help with mounting the baby on your back, but it will also add weight to the pack.

✔ **Open return policy.** So you can return the pack if it doesn't work well for you or the baby. (Be sure to save your receipt.)

✔ **Safe model.** Not on the recalls list—a good thing to check before you buy any baby product.

Avoid:

✗ **Used models.** Unless you can inspect them first to be sure all the hardware and seams are intact, and you do a search on CPSC.gov to make sure the model hasn't been the subject of a recall.

✗ **No safety belt.** Your child could be seriously injured if he stands on the seat and falls to the ground. (You can't see him behind you.)

✗ **Unsafe stand.** Hinges without spacing to protect babies' fingers and narrow stands that tip over easily are dangerous.

✗ **Packs with wheels.** Although being able to roll your baby in a backpack sounds good, the wheels add substantially to the pack's weight and bulkiness.

✗ **Flimsy shoulder and hip padding.** If they're too thin, your shoulders and hips won't be comfortable.

✗ **Poorly designed seats.** Raised leg holes may inhibit leg circulation. Your baby's bottom should be level with or higher than the seat's leg holes.

Note: Don't shop for a backpack for your baby on the Internet until you've had a chance to try out the exact model in person.

Quick tip

Don't shop for a backpack for your baby on the Internet until you've had a chance to try out the exact model in person.

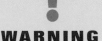

WARNING
Backpack safety issues
Never use a backpack carrier while in a car, on a bicycle, when jogging or skiing, while cooking, or in other situations where your baby might be injured. And don't prop his backpack on the outside of your car to load your baby inside. The surface is slippery! If the backpack slides off, your baby could sustain serious head injuries.

Highs & lows of Backpacks

Highs. Backpacks are great at distributing the weight of an older baby or toddler who's too big for a front carrier or sling, and they can go places strollers can't. Some babies really enjoy getting to sit up high and look out.

Lows. Backpacks can be complicated to use and awkward to take on and off. Not all babies like riding in them. With your back to baby, you won't be able to see what he's up to, and your baby could manage to stand up and fall overboard, especially if you haven't properly fastened the safety belt. If baby's a hair puller, the trip could be very annoying.

Q/A

Q We bought a backpack—is it worthwhile to spend more money on a sun/rain hood?

Most parents say yes. If you're going to be outside for more than about 20 minutes at a time, you'll want to protect baby's head from the elements. However, if you're not sure how much time you'll spend using the carrier, you can wait and order the accessory from the manufacturer later.

Q How am I supposed to get this thing on and off with a baby inside?

Very carefully! The easiest way is to have someone else help you while you practice putting it on and taking it off. If you're on your own, try putting the pack on the ground using the stand (if it has one) and kneeling or squatting with your back to the front of the pack. While it might not be the most graceful approach, it's the safest way to keep from dropping the baby!

Q Our son is 5 months old, and we're itching to get back on the trail again for a couple of nights. He's still breastfeeding. Do you have any suggestions about what to carry?

Your baby is the ideal age for camping—while he can sit up but doesn't insist on walking. It's also great if he's settled into a regular day–night sleeping pattern. Breastfeeding makes things so much easier! The baby's pack needs to be very, very comfortable for both you and baby, and like a new pair of shoes, you have to try it for a while to make sure it fits. Your baby will need protection from the elements, including rain, wind, and sun. (A strong sunscreen will be critical!) Mosquito netting and a rain canopy are good accessories, especially during insect season. If you're in cold weather, dress your baby in layers, but make sure that he's not so padded that he can't move his legs and arms freely and that his legs will fit through the pack's leg holes without hindering his circulation. If you have a soft carrier, take it along for those times when your baby gets uncomfortable and needs a postural change. Use a blanket on the ground when your baby's out of the pack. Don't forget to bring lots of diapers and a way to store and carry them out of the woods when you leave. As with all hiking expeditions, let others know your plans, carry some powdered formula (just in case), plenty of water, diaper rash cream, baby Tylenol, adhesive bandages, and the usual backup supplies (map, compass, signaling mirror, whistle, waterproof matches, a tarp). Plan short jaunts at first, in case your baby gets cranky in the wilderness. There's always the Comfort Inn down the highway.

"I bought the backpack for my baby and me, but it turns out that my husband is the one who really loves it. "

Sherpani's Rumba Unisex Backcountry Baby Carrier
($200–$250)

This 7.8 lbs backpack carrier is slightly higher priced than other models, but the big advantage is that the torso length of the carrier can be adjusted 6 inches up or down while it's being worn, a big plus if other family members use it. It also has a suspension system to soften jarring. The seat height for the baby is also adjustable, and smaller babies' feet can be tucked in. Then for older babies there are stirrups for the feet. Both options are more comfortable and better for baby's circulation than dangling. It comes with a removable daypack. The baby's 5-point harness system features a unique padded chest plate to provide support and prevent slouching. Included is a sunshade and rain cover. The low storage areas shift more weight onto your hips and off your back for extra comfort.

Kelty K.I.D.S.'s Pathfinder FC 3.0
($200)

This top-of-the-line aluminum-framed baby trekker weighs only 7 pounds 14 ounces and can carry up to a 50-pound load. It's made from high-density moisture-resistant poly fabric that cleans easily. It offers numerous excellent features, including a sliding back panel length-adjustment, curved, molded shoulder straps, carry and lift handles, a sternum strap, load-lifter straps, 2-layer curved waist belt with a zippered storage pocket, padded molded back panel, a cinching waist belt, reflective tape on all sides, a spring-action stand with no-pinch hinges, a sun/rain hood, and a 5-point safety harness and removable, washable seat pad for the baby. Dimensions: 30 inches high and 15 inches wide for torsos measuring from 12 to 20 inches. A zip-off diaper back with shoulder pads and changing pad are included. Available in cherry, black, or blueberry. Optional accessories include a diaper daypack and insect netting. (Kelty also makes scaled down, less expensive models.)

SAFETY CONSIDERATIONS

The most common baby injuries happen when a baby stands up and falls out, or when a parent trips or falls with the baby on his back, causing the baby to hit the hard components of the frame.

There have been a number of recalls for both soft and framed carriers, so be sure to check for recall information for backpack carriers before buying a used model. Recalls are typically for product hazards that allow a baby to fall out of the unit as safety belts fail, when leg holes are too large and allow the baby's body to fall through, or when hardware, such as buckles used to fasten the pack to the parent, gives way. You can locate backpack recalls by product category or by specific models at www.recalls.gov and access the Consumer Product Safety Commission's (CPSC) link.

At the time of this writing, the voluntary certification standard for backpack carriers administered by the Juvenile Products Manufacturers Association (JPMA) and the American Society of Testing and Materials (ASTM) was in the process of being implemented. Certified backpacks will carry the JPMA/ASTM sticker showing that they have passed rigorous safety and durability tests as well as carrying safe use warnings. Note, though, that certified products also undergo recalls when dangerous product flaws surface, and not all manufacturers elect to go through the certification process, although their products may be durable and safe.

4

BASSINETS & CRIB ALTERNATIVES

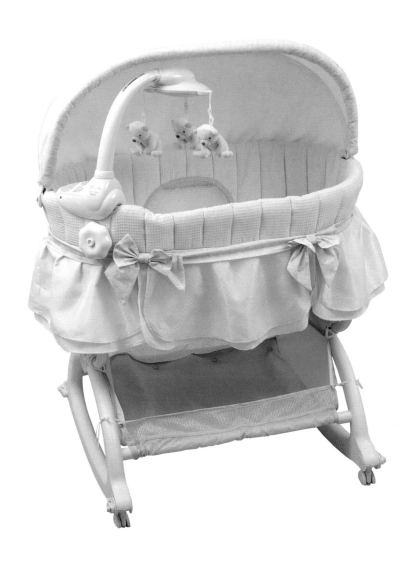

Most parents want to keep their newborns close at hand during the early months, instead of having them in a big crib in another room. Partly, it's the natural urge to keep close watch over their babies, and it's also to keep from having to rouse to full wakefulness when their babies cry and need to nurse over and over again in the night. This chapter presents all the options for keeping your baby at your bedside and gives you important safety and recall information.

GOOD NIGHT, BABY, SLEEP TIGHT . . . *PLEASE?*

Small-size baby beds can be a real convenience. They keep your baby nearby, and most are small enough to be moved through doorways, something that can't be done with standard-size cribs. Plus, a small bed for the first few months after your baby arrives won't eat up a lot of space in your bedroom, and new babies seem to feel safer being put down in small, confined spaces. After all, they've just come from living in pretty cramped quarters.

You have a variety of choices when it comes to shopping for a compact sleeping place for your new baby. A non-full-size crib resem-bles a standard crib complete with wooden (or metal) bars, but it's smaller. (And it may not have all of the extra features that the big models do.) Portable cribs are priced between $90 and $200.

A bassinet is a small baby bed supported by a frame with legs and usually with wheels. Bassinets come in a wide variety of price ranges from about $30 to over $200. You can expect to pay around $50 for a bare-bones model, $60 to $150

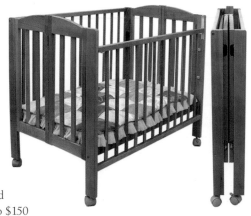

for models with fabric skirts, a hood, and a storage compartment underneath. Models priced at $150 and above come with advanced electronic features, such as lights, sounds, vibration, and a moving mobile, as well as novel designer shapes and plush fabrics.

Bedside sleepers attach onto the side of an adult bed and keep an open side toward the bed so a baby can easily be lifted from sleeper to bed and back. Some allow the open side to be closed for use as a portable bed or changing station. Prices range from $100 to $300. The lowest-priced models are made of tubular metal and mesh; the highest-priced versions are made of wood and are convertible to children's desks and other kinds of furniture.

Cradles are rocking baby beds, and bassinet/cradles are the newest product combination. They combine the comfort features of a bassinet's basketlike bed area with the rocking capability of old-fashioned cradles. These bassinets can be made of wood or molded plastic, and they offer just rockers or combine rockers with wheels that fold into the rocker frame.

Hand-carried baby beds, sometimes called carrycots or Moses baskets, are small rectangular boxes with carry handles used for transporting a sleeping baby. Some safety warnings are in order for these beds. Not all are made with the same quality and durability as full-size cribs. Often the mattresses supplied with them are flimsy, thin, and overly soft, and could be covered in inexpensive vinyl that isn't breathable and traps moisture. They're also difficult to balance, since the heaviest part of the baby is her head, putting the most weight at one end of the carrier.

Pets and baby beds

If you have large dogs in your home, keep in mind they could tip over the bassinet or cradle. Cats can also climb inside and lie over the baby's face, which could lead to suffocation. With pets in the house, keep the door to the room where your baby sleeps closed, put bells on collars, and use a baby monitor to help you keep tabs on where the animals are. Use a pet gate to discourage animals from entering your bedroom, and consider transferring your baby to a regular crib and purchasing a mesh tent that fastens over the crib if you need to shield your baby from cats. (It's available in baby specialty stores.)

When to Buy

Purchase a non-full-size crib, bassinet, or other crib alternative during the latter months of your pregnancy to allow your newborn to sleep in your bedroom with you; then use it only as long as recommended by the manufacturer.

✔ Checklist

Baby bed shopping

There are definitely lots of choices for where to put baby down for sleep, but no matter what type of sleep arrangement you use—whether a bassinet, a small crib, a standard crib, or a cradle—it's important to follow some basic safety and convenience rules, including these:

✔ **Sturdy construction.** Firmly put together with no wobbling when jiggled.

✔ **Stability.** Childproof leg and frame locks if there are other children in the house. Check that it can't be pulled over sideways.

Quick tip

Plan to invest 30 minutes or more to assemble the many components of most units.

✔ **A quality mattress.** An extra-firm quality mattress won't create a suffocation pocket around your baby's face if she accidentally turns over—try punching your fist into it. And if you can fit 2 fingers between the bed's edges or corners and the mattress, it could pose an entrapment or suffocation hazard.

✔ **Solid rather than fabric sides.** For safety, solid, unbending sides in a bassinet's sleep area, rather than fabric over a tubular frame. Loose fabric sides could allow the baby's neck, head, or limbs to get trapped in fabric pockets.

✔ **Washable fabrics.** Bedding and liner fabrics that are completely washable. (Read manufacturer's instructions.)

✔ **Safe rockers.** Rockers with rounded tips help keep it from tipping over. They should not stick out so far that they pose a tripping hazard. Beds that swing by hanging from a frame should have a locking mechanism to make them stationary.

✔ **Locking casters.** To make the bed more stable and to keep children from pushing the unit around. Keep casters locked except when you're moving the bed.

✔ **Fitted sheets.** Less likely to pull loose and entangle your baby. Buy 3 to 4 extra sheets in exactly the same size.

✔ **Storage and travel option.** Consider a compactly folding non-full-size crib if you have limited storage space or plan to use the bed for sleepovers away from home. (Plus it can be used a lot longer than smaller baby beds.)

✔ **Assembly.** Plan to invest 30 minutes or more to assemble the many components of most units.

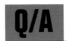

Q/A

Q **I know that everyone says that we should plan to have our baby sleep in our bedroom, but the room is tiny, and I think we'll both prefer to have privacy and put our baby down in her new crib in another room. Is it okay to do that?**

Sure. Where your baby sleeps is your decision. (And the stores will still be open after your baby arrives if you decide to change your sleeping arrangements.) Some parents find they sleep better when the baby isn't so close. In most cases, they get a baby monitor so they can hear their baby's sounds from another room. If there's space in your baby's room, create a comfy nursing station, preferably with a rocker/recliner or a comfortable footstool so you can rest. Put night-lights along your path so you can see where you're going in the night without having to turn on overhead lights. (Baby monitors are discussed on page 208.)

Q **We've bought a non-full-size wooden crib for our bedroom, but we can't find a bedding set (quilt, sheets, and bumpers) to fit it. Do you know of a place we can go online to buy special-sized bedding?**

Try www.sheetworld.com, which offers a wide variety of fitted sheets for both standard and nonstandard baby-bed mattresses in a large variety of colors and textures. Be sure to get the identical size to fit the mattress, and don't "cheat" by putting the mattress in a pillowcase, or using anything but a fitted sheet. (Also, don't be tempted to wrap the mattress in a plastic garbage bag or the clear bags that come from the dry cleaner. They pose a deadly suffocation hazard.)

NON-FULL-SIZE CRIBS

Non-full-size or "portable" cribs are small-scale, three-quarter-size rectangular beds with bars, and closely resemble standard cribs. Most have legs that adjust to more than one height, and some offer several mattress heights, too, including a playpen position for later use with toddlers. A few models have a side that can be lowered to help put the baby in and take her out.

Manufacturers' recommendations for the maximum weight and age of the baby vary, but general guidelines are that they can be used from birth until around 24 months of age or about 50 pounds (depending upon the model). Use whichever limit your baby reaches first. Those upper limits make them usable for much longer than bassinets, cradles, and other small baby beds.

Stringent federal safety regulations apply to portable cribs, just as they do for full-size cribs. The space between the bars can't exceed 2⅜ inches, to prevent the baby's body from sliding out and leaving her head caught, which can strangle the baby. The crib's mattress is required to fit tightly on all sides to keep parts of the baby's body from getting trapped. The hardware must not present harm to the baby, wood surfaces should be smooth and without splinters, and there should be no crossbar halfway up the railing that could allow a toehold for climbing out. In addition, to prevent babies from falling out, regulations state that there should never be less than 22 inches between the mattress support at it's lowest position and the crib's top rail. Also addressed are the assembly instructions for parents and a label on the crib with model information and how to reach the manufacturer.

Dream On Me's 3-in-1 Folding Portable Crib
($150)

The biggest advantage of a portable crib such as this one is that it takes up 35 percent less space than a full-size crib, so it can roll through doorways and be folded compactly for easy travel or storage. Unlike most portables, this model offers a single lowering side and also has locking casters. Depending upon the position of the mattress support, it can be used as a crib, a changing table, or a playpen (mattress included). Hinges allow the end boards to fold inward, and the mattress support folds up inside the crib's frame to store in the standing position. Available in natural, white, or cherry.

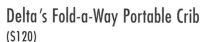

Delta's Fold-a-Way Portable Crib
($120)

A small crib that also offers one side that can be lowered by sliding down, just as a full-size crib's side works, using a lift-and-release mechanism. There are two floor heights, and the legs can be lowered to make a playpen configuration. The thin mattress (1 inch) is somewhat flimsy and covered with nonbreathable vinyl. We suggest replacing it with a firmer mattress no thicker than 2 inches.

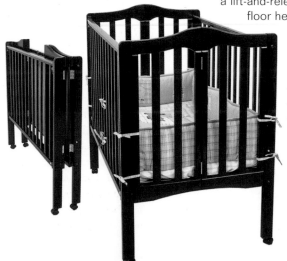

Highs & lows of portable cribs

Highs. These are simply miniature cribs, and they come under both strict federal regulations for safety and a voluntary certification program overseen by the Juvenile Products Manufacturers Association. (See "Safety Considerations on page 67.) They're slender enough to roll through most doorways, and unlike bassinets and most cradles, they offer a clear, unrestricted view of the baby from all sides. Typically, they can be used with a baby of up to about 2 years of age and weighing between 40 and 50 pounds, for much longer use than a bassinet. Most have a lowering floorboard to allow the crib to be used as a small playpen later.

Lows. They're heavier than bassinets and some other small baby beds, and they also cost more. Only a few models have sides that lower, so you will have to reach over them to put your baby in or lift her out. Some models come with soft mattresses rather than rock-hard versions that fit firmly against all sides. They require non-standard-size sheets. Some models offer only a single mattress height. Hardware may have sharp edges, and there is a risk that the floorboard could fall through if it warps or is not well secured.

BASSINETS

Bassinets are little beds on a stand. They're much smaller and more compact than portable cribs. The rectangular bed part of the bassinet, called the basket, sits on a wooden or plastic frame with four legs underneath. The basket may be permanently affixed to the stand or, in some models, may be removed so the frame can be folded for storage. Baskets can be constructed from rattan, flat wood reeds, or heavy-duty plastic material. And at least one new model has a circular shape.

Bassinets usually come in standard (12 –14 inches by 27–29 inches) and jumbo (15–30 inches) sizes. Basket depths can vary from 8 to 12 inches. Most manufacturers recommend that bassinets not be used once a baby reaches 15 pounds, or be discontinued when the baby is able to roll over or push up on her hands and knees on her own—whichever comes first. (Compare that to the 40- to 50-pound limit of some portable cribs.)

Least-expensive bassinets ($25–$35) are simple oval-shaped wicker baskets with no frills, fabric, or hood, and possibly no wheels. More expensive versions use the same basic basket design but have a rigid hood that's usually removable and covers a little less than half of the bassinet. Bassinets come with various fabric options: a fabric liner, a short skirt that covers the basket but not the stand, or a long skirt that cascades to the floor.

More-expensive models ($45–$50) may use molded-plastic or metal frames. At the top of the line ($65–$100+) are ones with a variety of extra add-ons that include not only the rounded hood but a long flowing skirt in a quality, all-baby-looking fabric that envelops not just the basket but also the hood. The bassinet may have not only wheels but also rockers on the base that work when the wheels are retracted. There may be a sizeable storage bin underneath the basket for supplies, and battery-powered extras such as vibration, a night-light, and musical sounds, and even moving mobiles that swing out of the way to make it easier to lower the baby inside.

It's worth noting that extra electronic perks eat up a lot of batteries, and you (and your baby) may not find them all that pleasing. On the other hand, having a bed that rocks itself or vibrates could help temporarily to soothe your baby when you're at your wit's end. Just don't expect it to convince your baby she's not hungry!

Bassinets come under a voluntary JPMA certification program. Special tests address suffocation, tip over, collapse, and hood detachment for both bassinets and cradles. If a bassinet meets the qualifications for certification, it will display "JPMA Certified" somewhere on the unit.

WARNING

Bassinets can fall over or collapse

Bassinets with folding legs that have flimsy hardware or don't lock in the upright position, and those with wheels that can't be locked, are unstable. They can fall over if a child leans in or tries to climb inside to see the baby. Keep the wheels locked, and don't allow children to play around the bassinet. Check frequently to make sure the legs are completely locked in the rigid, upright position.

Highs & lows of bassinets

Highs. When they're dressed in ruffles, they personify "baby." Wheels and the bassinet's narrow dimensions allow it to be rolled through doorways, something full-size cribs can't do. Some newborns appear to prefer being in small, enclosed spaces.

Lows. Bassinets are generally limited to babies weighing only about 15 pounds. Mattress pads tend to be soft and cushy, which could affect a baby's air supply if she accidentally rolls facedown. Closed sides shut out airflow, potentially making the bed stuffier. Fitted sheets may be hard to find in off sizes, and loose sheets pose an entanglement or even a strangulation danger. The long, narrow design of bassinets makes them vulnerable to being pulled over by siblings, and sometimes leg locks fail, causing legs to collapse. You may strike your baby's head on the rigid hood, especially if you're using the bassinet in low-light conditions. Bassinets with tubular frames that rely on fabric liners to keep the baby in place have had recalls when the liners have allowed babies' bodies, limbs, or heads to become trapped between component parts.

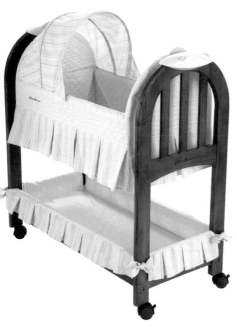

Eddie Bauer's Musical Rocking Bassinet

($130)

This combination bassinet and cradle comes with a quilted liner, a machine-washable pad and sheet, a storage area, and locking casters underneath. It has a rocking mechanism and timer so it can gently rock itself, or it can be manually rocked. The bed portion can be locked into a nonrocking stationary position. The hood is retractable. A sound unit plays 5 lullabies and has a volume control. Note: To improve stability, lock the casters unless the unit is being moved. From birth to 6 months. Requires 3 AA batteries (not included).

Kolcraft's Easy Reach Rocking Bassinet with Light Vibes Mobile

($100)

A molded plastic bassinet with an innovative back hood to allow for easy side entry. The wheels can be locked or can be folded into the rockers, so it can be either rolled or rocked. It comes with a removable, electronic mobile that can be rotated out of the way for easy entry and removal of baby or attached to the side of a crib. The basket can be vibrated using a variable speed control, and the music device plays a choice of 8 classical tunes and 4 ambient sounds. Comes with a night-light so you can look in on the baby. The walls of the basket are padded and quilted. The firm mattress is vinyl covered and comes with a single washable fitted sheet. Storage basket underneath. From birth to 3–4 months and/or 15 pounds. Stop using when baby can roll from side to side or starts to pull herself up. Requires 4 AA batteries (not included).

> **❝I didn't like the 'half bed' we got that strapped onto the side of our bed. It made it hard to get in and out of the bed, and, besides, the baby woke up every time I tried to lower her into it. ❞**

BEDSIDE SLEEPERS

These small, low, three-sided cribs constructed of metal or wood let newborns sleep within arm's length of their parents. Long straps secure the sleeper flush with the side of the adult bed by looping between the bed and the mattress springs. The concept is to give parents easy access to their babies without the dangers of SIDS and suffocation when babies actually sleep in their parents' beds.

Highs & lows of bedside sleepers

Highs. They're handy, especially if you're nursing and want to be able to move the baby in and out of your bed without having to get up.

Lows. Fasten bed firmly to the side of your bed. They take up a lot of space on its edge, which can make it tricky for you to get in and out of bed. Babies tend to fall asleep at the breast. Arousing them by removing them from the warmth of the parent's body to put them onto the cold sleeper surface is likely to awaken them (but placing them in a crib or other bed can do the same thing).

Arm's Reach's Mini Co-Sleeper
($160)

The Mini Co-Sleeper is a compact bassinet (24 x 34 x 31 inches) that attaches securely against the adult bed by passing straps under the top of the adult mattress. The straps are designed to fit all beds from twin to Cal king with bed heights up to 24 inches. Fabric and mesh sides allow for air ventilation. The unit adapts for use as a portable play yard, a sleeper, a diaper changer, or a freestanding bassinet and comes with a mattress and fitted cotton sheet. It has 2 locking wheels on one end. Storage or travel case included. Fabric liners are available in a variety of colors as are optional leg extensions that allow the unit to be raised 26 inches to 30 inches in 2-inch increments. From birth to 28 pounds in the sleeper position, or until the baby can pull up on hands and knees.

CRADLES

Cradles are a traditional rocking bed for newborns. They're typically constructed of wood and come in two basic styles: those with rockers on the base, and those that suspend the baby's bed from a hook or fastener at each end so the bed rocks pendulum-style or can be locked into a nonswinging position. (Just make sure the hooks that support the cradle's bed don't stick out over the bed part. They could hit your baby when you're lifting or lowering her.)

Cradles, like bassinets, come under a voluntary certification program overseen by the JPMA and manufacturers that outlines performance requirements and test methods to address suffocation, tip over, collapse, and hood attachment. Cradles that meet the certification standard will have a "JPMA Certified" sticker somewhere on the unit.

> **"We decided to use only a small crib for the first half year. It worked out great. Later, we invested in a convertible crib that also could be made into a toddler bed and full-size bed for later, so we're covered for quite a while."**

Antique cradles may be unsafe, particularly if bars or mattress support are loose, the mattress doesn't fit flush on all sides of the interior of the bed, or the bars are more than $2^{3}/_{8}$ inches apart. (If the top of a can of soda will pass through the bars, they're too far apart.)

These defects can cause suffocation if the baby gets wedged between the sides and the mattress or her body slides

through the bars with her head still caught inside. Being able to stabilize the cradle to prevent rocking helps to keep the baby in the center of the cradle.

Highs & lows of cradles

Highs. They have a romantic, all-baby feel to them. They offer a rocking motion that can be soothing to a baby.

Lows. The rocking motion is only side-to-side (rather than head-to-toe), and as the baby rolls back and forth, she could get trapped against one corner of the bed when her weight shifts to one side.

Parents often stub their toes when tips of the rockers stick out beyond the edge of the frame.

C&T International's Sorelle Dondola Cradle
($150)

This all-wood cradle (18-by-36-inch interior) gently glides back and forth from underneath. It has a lock at the base of the bed portion. It comes with locking casters that we recommend stay locked except when moving the bed, to ensure adequate stability. The cradle comes with a mattress and is available in cherry, white, natural, and caramel wood finishes. Somewhat complicated assembly is required. From birth to 25 pounds.

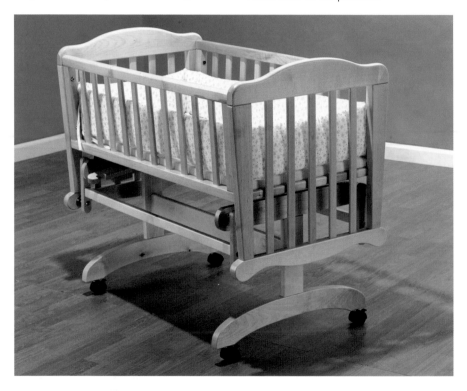

Angel Line's Gliding Cradle and Loveseat

($140)

This 37-by-24-inch hardwood cradle is available with either round spindles or flat slats. It has a smooth glider mechanism in the base, and the mattress height is adjustable. Once your baby moves to her regular crib, it can be converted into a loveseat with one side removed, and it can support up to 100 pounds in that configuration. Available in 4 finishes.

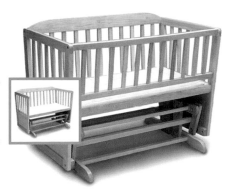

HAND-CARRIED BEDS

Hand-carried baby beds, also called carrycots or Moses baskets, are small rectangular baby carriers designed to sit directly on the floor. Typically, they're sewn of thick fabric, or from woven natural materials such as rattan or palm. They usually come with a soft inside pad and a washable sheet and liner. Parents use them as an alternative sleeping space for babies. Some large baby carriages come with both a stroller seat for the baby and the carrycot that can stand on its own for baby napping.

The designs of these carriers that have fabric or woven handles present some serious safety problems. Mattresses are often unacceptably soft and mushy—a suffocation threat. Handles can loosen, fray, and break while the baby is being carried, causing injuries. Since babies' heads are much heavier than the rest of their bodies, the carry bed can become unbalanced if the baby isn't positioned exactly in the center of the inside. With no safety harness to secure her inside, the baby could be dumped out.

For these reasons, we cannot recommend these hand-carried baby beds as a safe option for carrying or as a sleeping place for babies.

Safety checklist

Your baby will be spending more time in bed than awake during her first years. Whatever baby bed you choose for your baby, make sure that it's completely safe. Here are the most important things to remember when it comes to baby-bed safety.

✔ **The right size bed for your baby.** Follow the manufacturer's weight and age instructions for the best time to graduate your baby to a full-size crib (usually

WARNING

Antique beds and cradles can be unsafe!
Old-time baby beds, with carved headboards and spindles, and wooden baby cradles often are passed down from one generation to another. It may feel like an important family rite of passage to allow your daughter (or son) to sleep in the same baby bed as her grandparents did. Unfortunately, these beds are usually better suited to hold baby toys and stuffed animals. They may have missing or broken parts or loose screws, and the mattress may not fit flush against all sides, leaving gaps that could compress your baby's airway. Plus, the bed could harbor irritating dust mites. Bars spaced more than 2 3/8 inches apart (wide enough to allow a soda can to pass through) could strangle your baby if her body slides out, leaving her head caught in the bed.

than that could allow your baby's windpipe to be compressed by the edge of the mattress and suffocate her.

✔ **Suffocation.** For safety's sake, always place baby on her back for sleep, and keep soft pillows, quilts, and stuffed toys out of the bed. Don't add towels or other padding to the bed, and never line the mattress pad with plastic dry-cleaning or garbage bags. Your baby could suffocate.

✔ **Properly fitted bedding.** Use the right size sheets for the bed and make sure they're always tucked in, so the surface is smooth and sheets and blankets can't bunch around your baby's face.

✔ **Carrying.** Don't carry or roll the baby bed with the baby inside, since motion with weight inside could stress the mattress support and frame.

✔ **Protection from children and pets.** Don't let children play with or around the bed, and use barriers to keep pets away.

✔ **Correct assembly.** Carefully follow the manufacturer's directions for assembling the unit and never use a baby bed that has missing parts or hardware. Contact the manufacturer's customer service department if you run into problems.

✔ **Registration card.** Mail in the registration card or register the product online so that the manufacturer can contact you should there be a recall. (But note that not all manufacturers go to the trouble of notifying individual owners. When in doubt, go to www.recall.gov and search the Consumer Product Safety Commission's link.)

when she is able to roll over and get up on all fours), and never use the bed with more than one baby.

✔ **Firm, well-fitting mattress.** Avoid a smaller-than-standard baby bed if it has a mushy, poorly fitting mattress. The mattress should be at least 1- inch thick and nearly as firm as a brick, to protect your baby's face from being buried in a suffocating pocket should she accidentally turn facedown. It should fit snugly against all sides of the bed, and you shouldn't be able to insert more than 2 fingers between the mattress edge and the inside of the bed frame. A gap any wider

SAFETY CONSIDERATIONS

Full-size and non-full-size cribs come under stringent federal guidelines from the Consumer Product Safety Commission (CPSC.gov), and since cribs figure in more baby deaths than any other baby-product category, federally-based recalls are usually fast and rigorous when crib models are found to pose hazards to babies.

Full-size (standard) and non-full-size cribs, plus bassinets, cradles, and handheld infant carriers, are all covered by voluntary safety standards overseen by the American Society of Testing and Materials (ASTM) and the Juvenile Products Manufacturers Association (JPMA). "Voluntary" means that companies can elect to participate or not in the extra testing required.

Simply because a product is JPMA certified does not make it immune to being recalled, and many certified products have been recalled over the years. On the other hand, the manufacturers of perfectly safe products sometimes elect to not undergo the costly testing process that requires products to be tested by an independent testing facility for compliance with specific standards. If a product passes the tests, JPMA allows the manufacturer to label it with the "JPMA Certified" seal, which usually appears somewhere on the frame.

5

BATHING SUPPLIES

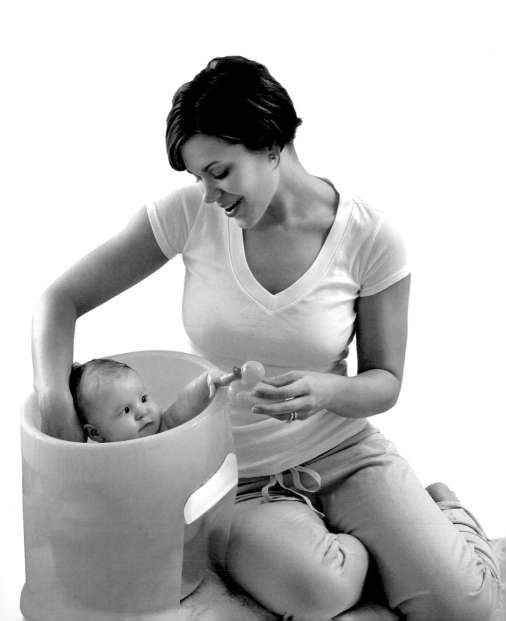

After you bring your baby home, and his belly button and circumcision sites have healed, the time will come when baby's first bath can no longer be postponed. Parents dread it and babies often cry! This chapter is about choosing a tub and other practical bathing aids and bath supplies; plus, it has instructions on giving that first bath, shopping checklists, and important safety warnings.

RUB-A-DUB-DUB, BABY'S IN THE TUB!

Most parents who buy (or are given) baby bathtubs end up using them only a handful of times. That's because these big plastic water holders typically accommodate babies to only about 6 months of age. And most babies just don't get very dirty that often—a warm washcloth can take care of most of the messes. But if you've got a baby who has a lot of spit-ups and/or big diaper messes, or is just learning to eat by pasting food all over himself, a contoured baby bathtub can help position your baby for bathing.

Baby bathtubs are very similar: They're huge, bulky, and will drench you if you try to move them once they're filled with water. They range from about $10 for a basic model to about $40 for a European style designed to mold to the contours of a baby's back. Some tubs also come with special features, such as a hanging hook, a rinsing pitcher, a water thermometer, or a shower hose attachment.

The best molded baby bathtubs have a nonslip, semireclined seating area, a plug in the base for easy draining, and thick sides for carrying the tub when it's filled with water. (Only a few inches of water will be enough to do the job). Some travel tubs are lightweight and fold in two for easy storage. Large tubs often have two ends—one for reclining newborns and the other for tots who are old enough to sit up. They can later be used for water play.

Fabric supports for use in the bathtub or sink are inexpensive baby-size wire frames shaped like lounge chairs, lined with a terry or absorbent fabric for the baby to recline on in the sink or tub. Once bathing is over, you set the bath support out to dry.

Foam bath supports are inexpensive thick slabs of foam shaped to fit into a baby bathtub to help hold the baby in place. Once a toddler becomes curious and starts pulling foam pieces off, though, they could be a choking hazard and should be discarded. Mildew causes a problem, so after a bath wring out the foam and put it in a warm, sunny place to dry. Both types of supports sell for under $10.

Your least expensive (and most practical) option is to wash your baby in the kitchen sink. A stainless sink that you can wipe down with a little bleach and hot water afterward will be more hygienic and easier to clean thoroughly than a plastic tub with a porous cushion or cloth hammock. Our recommendation is to bathe the baby in the sink lined with a folded bath towel, since most of your messes will be of the organic variety, although some babies have a knack for eliminating the minute their bottoms hit the water.

Another practical baby bathing option is to sit yourself down in warm water in your bathtub and have your partner hand over your baby to you. Then you can bring your knees up to support him.

> 66 I hadn't counted on how slippery my newborn would be when he was wet. I nearly dropped him the first time I gave him a bath! 99

Quick tips

After the first bath with soap or shampoo, check for any skin or scalp reactions. If you find that your child is sensitive to the particular cosmetic, try an unscented version.

If your baby heartily resists being bathed the traditional way, damp mop him while he's wrapped in a towel in your lap. If you then decide to use a tub, lower your baby, towel and all, into the tub.

Girls may be susceptible to vaginal infections if they sit in soapy water. Use a washcloth and/or cup of water to rinse soap or shampoo residue off a baby girl's bottom after the bath.

Remember that babies hate being quickly lowered down backward. It sets off a primitive reflex that makes them throw their arms up, gasp for air, and start screaming. They also react to sudden changes in temperature—especially when they're undressed. One advantage to this "whole body" style of baby bathing is that you can nurse your baby if he gets upset.

When to Buy

Can wait until after birth. Baby won't need a bath until his umbilical cord falls off and circumcision site heals—between 2 and 8 weeks after birth. Tubs designed to accommodate both infants and toddlers can usually be used up to 2 years of age.

Baby's first bath

Regardless of the type of bathing accoutrements you choose to collect for use
with your new baby, there's no need to try
keeping him immaculate. Babies really
don't need baths all *that* much—they
don't sweat, they don't crawl around, and
they just don't get very dirty. In fact, too
much cleaning will deplete your baby's
natural skin oils, and his skin may get
dry. Furthermore, temperature changes,
such as those caused by the cooling of
water as it evaporates off his wet skin,
may arouse wails of protest.

It will be easier on both you and your
newborn if you postpone bathing for as
long as possible—definitely until after
circumcision and umbilical-cord sites
have healed. And the best way to ensure

bath time is pleasant for the two of you is
to keep your baby covered as much as
you can before and after the bath and to
do it when the two of you are both alert
and not too hungry or tired.

Most parents choose to use a sink for
baby's first bathing experience. Once you
have a few inches of lukewarm water in
the sink and a folded bath towel in the
bottom, move the faucet out of the way
to ensure you don't accidentally bump
baby into it or turn on the water. Most
parents find that simply using their
hands to soap and rinse the baby works
better than trying to manage a washcloth.
If you want to, keep a measuring cup of
warm water on standby to pour over your
baby's body for rinsing. Remember,
though, to use only mildly warm water.

 # Checklist

Bathtub shopping

Here's what to look for when you go bathtub shopping:

✔ **Thick shell.** Made of thick, rigid material with smooth rims, so it won't
buckle or spill water when you lift it.

✔ **Safety features.** A gentle seat angle and slip-resistant surface to help hold
the baby in place. Some baths also come with thermometers; check that the
bathwater temperature stays safely between 90 and 100° F.

✔ **Baby comfort.** Scaled right for your baby, at a comfortable angle, and
without any rough plastic seams or other parts that could scratch tender skin.

✔ **Small is better.** Miniature body-shape tubs are easier to manage with newborns than large one-size-fits-all models. Get one that will fit into your kitchen
sink. (Toddlers can use a regular bathtub for bathing.)

✔ **Hook for hanging.** Handy for draining and storage.

✔ **Tight plug.** A leak-resistant plug on the base makes emptying easier.

✔ **Easy cleaning.** No nooks, crannies, or porous surfaces that could harbor
mildew or make cleaning difficult.

✔ **Folding feature.** Tubs that fold in half take up less room when stored. Just
make sure there are no seams that could pinch the baby's fingers, or gaps
that could leak.

Highs and lows of tubs

Highs. A baby bathtub can be a big help if you're trying to bathe a baby alone. The tub will help support the baby while you soap him down and rinse him.

Lows. A product with a limited life span. Usually, the tubs are awkward to carry, take up a lot of closet space when stored, and fabric or foam inserts may take a long time to dry. And tubs and bath seats sometimes lure parents into a false sense of security so that they turn their backs on their babies.

WARNING

Suctioned baby bath seats are dangerous!

Suctioned bath seats were designed to hold baby in a sitting position in a full-size bathtub. Suction cups on the base are supposed to hold the seat in place. The seat may have a safety belt. These seats have been associated with the deaths of more than 60 babies from drowning by giving parents a false sense of security that it is safe to leave the child unattended. Drowning occurs when the suction cups don't hold and the seat falls over, or the baby slips out of the seat and into the water. **Don't buy or use a suctioned bath seat.**

4moms' Cleanwater Infant Tub with Digital Thermometer

($40)

A step above most standard baby bathers, this molded tub fits onto the rims of a single or double sink, or into the regular bathtub. It has a special reservoir at one end of the tub that continually fills with water that flows into the main tub area like a junior spa. Clean water, monitored by a digital thermometer with a high-temperature alert, continuously circulates around the baby while dirty water exits through the tub's side drains. The blue tub comes with a white rinse cup that can be filled from the reservoir. The downside: It can't be filled with water like a standard baby bathtub.

Checklist

Bathing supplies shopping

Here's a list of what to look for when you go bath-product shopping:

✔ **Baby shampoos.** Try for no-sting shampoos, but there's no such thing as a completely no-sting shampoo. Even brands advertised as gentle contain strong chemicals, and it's still important to protect baby's eyes.

✔ **Plain soaps.** Use gentle soaps such as Lowilla or Aveeno. Avoid deodorant bars and liquid antibacterial soaps. The longer the soap's ingredient list, the more likely it is your baby will be allergic to something in it.

✔ **Diaper-rash cream.** If needed, a thin layer of either zinc-oxide-based ointment or one with vitamins A and D can help to treat diaper rash. (A lingering cherry-red rash in the diaper area could mean your baby has a yeast infection. Consult your child's pediatrician for advice.)

Bath time soaps and shampoos

When it comes to baby cosmetics, as little as possible is best. You can usually avoid using soap completely until the solid-food-mess stage makes it necessary. The same goes for shampoo: You only need it if your baby's hair smells, his scalp has major cradle-cap scales, or has sticky other messes that water alone can't handle. Otherwise, rinsing off with warm water or a soft washcloth will do the job.

Toddler bath-time accessories

Here is a list of other bath-time accessories to explore when your baby's old enough to enjoy bathing in a regular tub.

✔ **Spout guards.** Flexible vinyl spout guards are available in a variety of animal shapes to pad bathtub faucets so that babies don't get burned or hurt when they bump into them. Examples: Homegrown Kids' Spout Guards and Sassy's Supersoft Spout Guards.

✔ **Toy hammocks.** A suctioned hammock fastens onto the wall over the bathtub to hold bathtub toys. Example: Prince Lionheart Bathtub Hammock.

✔ **Bathtub toys.** Those that are the most fun give tots ways to experience what water does, such as pouring water through a sieve. Plastic household funnels, cups, and pitchers are a lot cheaper than commercial bathtub toy "kits" and work just as well.

✔ **Shampoo shields.** A stretchy foam shampoo shield fits around your tot's forehead to protect his eyes from shampoo, but an easier answer is to use a pair of tot-size swim goggles.

Avoid:

✗ **Bath soaks.** Don't buy bubble bath and/or bath oils. They strip the skin's protective oils, which can increase the risk of diaper rash or of vaginal infection for girls.

✗ **Baby powder.** According to the American Academy of Pediatrics, baby powder serves no medical purpose and doesn't help prevent diaper rash.

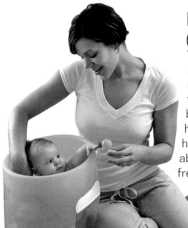

Prince Lionheart's WashPOD
($30)

This small translucent bucket (13¼ inches x 14¾ x 9 inches) for babies weighing 10 to 25 pounds allows even small babies to curl up in comfort with their backs supported. Its cylinder shape allows the baby to be immersed in water up to 2 inches below his armpits to keep him from getting chilled. Padded handles make toting and emptying the tub comfortable, and the shape of the tub leaves both hands free for washing the baby's body. An indicator mark shows the appropriate water level.

Downsides: The tub doesn't fit in the sink, and the WashPOD should never be left unattended with water inside, since a tot could fall in headfirst and not be able to right himself.

WARNING !

Baby oil and talcum powder

Baby oil and talcum powder can be deadly for your baby's lungs. If the baby swallows mineral oils, called hydrocarbons, found in baby oil, he can choke, causing him to inhale them, so that the oil coats his lungs, causing a serious lung problem, and possibly death. Suntan oil, makeup remover, bubble bath, and quick-dry nail polish can also kill. Some baby powders may contain talcum, closely related to the carcinogen asbestos, and may contain microscopic asbestos particles that can cause a rare form of pneumonia if the baby inhales the powder. Keep these products away from your baby.

SAFETY CONSIDERATIONS

The biggest danger of baby bathing is drowning, and babies can drown in less than an inch of water in only a few minutes. With or without a baby bathtub, you can't leave baby alone in even an inch of water. Have all bathing equipment ready before bathing. Don't answer the telephone; don't go to the door; don't stop to deal with another child or pet; don't leave your baby alone in the tub with another child. Stay right by your baby's side when he's in water or carry him with you.

Scalding is another danger. Water at temperatures that might feel comfortably warm to an adult's hand can be hot enough to burn your baby. Check the bath temperature with your wrist or elbow. And start and end by turning on the cold water to prevent burns and to cool down the metal faucet.

The largest (and most serious) recalls have been for suctioned baby bath seats when components have failed. For recalls of bathtubs and bathing equipment, go to www.recalls.gov and click on the Consumer Product Safety Commission's section (www.cpsc.gov) to search for "baby bathtubs" or the names and model numbers of specific tubs or bathing accessories. Baby powders, shampoos, and other baby skincare products are overseen by the FDA, and whose recalls can be found through www.recalls.org or www.fda.gov.

6

BOUNCERS

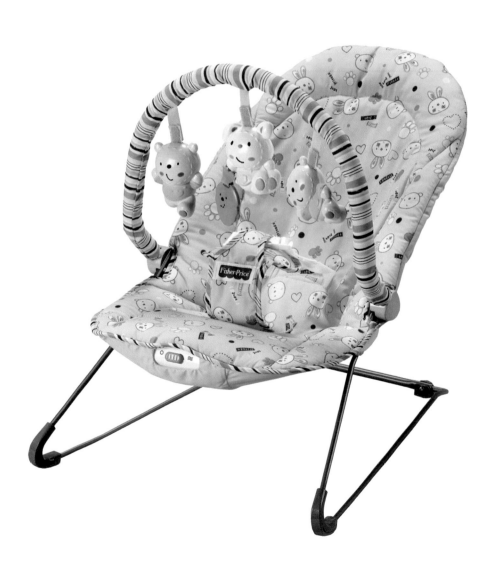

Some parents find their baby's bouncer indispensable, while others feel they're not worth the money or are even patently unsafe. One point to remember is that your baby will outgrow one rather quickly, since you ought to discontinue using one as soon as your baby is strong enough to sit up on her own, at around 5 to 6 months, or else she could vault herself out.

BOUNCING BABY BASICS

Bouncers are one of those entirely optional items that some parents swear by, while others swear they're just an unneeded extra that isn't worth the money, especially since they're only useful for the first half year, when a baby is unable to sit up on her own. Bouncers range from about $20 for a used or basic model up to $50 or more for all of the bells and whistles (rocking, vibration, light shows, and dangling toys). All models with music or motion use batteries, so consider battery expense as an operating cost. Bouncers are designed to hold baby in a comfortable semisitting position. Most jiggle in response to a baby's movement, and others jazz up baby motion by vibrating or rocking (back and forth or side to side). They may come with toy bars, and/or music and light features to help keep baby entertained.

Quality safety restraints are indispensable, as is a cover that can be removed and machine-washed, should baby find the bouncing a little too stimulating.

Some bouncers claim to be suitable for toddlers and even preschoolers; but usually once baby starts crawling, she may be resistant to being strapped down. And you'll definitely want a frame that's sturdy and won't bend under pressure.

A nonskid surface on the base of the frame is important to help prevent the bouncer from "walking" off a table or counter. Some bouncers that rock come with a "kickstand" to disable the rocking feature. Seats in the rocking mode may not be safe for babies who are strong enough to rock the seat forward and flip it over.

> **ʟʟ Our son is really gassy, and the seat seems to help him when we put him in it after meals. ʠʠ**

Before you decide to invest in a bouncer or keep one that has been given to you, make sure you really need it. If you have a baby swing and/or a reclining high chair, you already have something to strap the baby in to let her sit up and look around, so you may not need to buy a bouncer as well—unless you're seeking a specific function, such as a vibrating action that is soothing to some babies.

Consignment shops, eBay, yard sales, and other parents can be good sources for finding a cheap, or even a free, bouncer. But make sure that all of the parts are in perfect condition! The frame should be intact and not bent, the fabric pad should fit well, and the seat belt and buckle should work well and not be broken or frayed.

Highs & lows of bouncers

Highs. A baby seat is a handy place to hold your baby. It can provide stimulation while giving your arms a much-needed rest. The semi-upright position and vibration may help your baby digest food after feeding, which can be a big help if you've got a gassy baby. Jiggling, vibrations, or rocking can soothe in a way similar to a baby swing, without swallowing up as much floor space. Suspended toys or interesting sounds can be temporarily entertaining to the baby, but they don't take the place of carrying, rocking, or walking with your baby in your arms.

Lows. They're only useful for the short time before the baby can sit up. Some babies feel confined in them and work hard to wriggle out. Even with the safety belt firmly fastened, many a mom has left the room just for a second, only to return and find her little Houdini hanging out sideways. The sound effects intended to entertain the baby can sometimes be more irritating than pleasing. Bouncers have serious safety issues. (See warning, page 81.)

When to Buy

Buy one between months 1 and 4 if you discover your baby needs extra soothing or you want a place for your baby to sit to watch or play with you.

Fisher-Price's Soothe 'n Play Bouncer
($25)

The fabric hammock enfolds the baby. The removable, U-shaped toy bar has 3 detachable toys with rattles that can be changed around to offer variety. There's a T-shaped waist-and-between-the-legs strap to keep the baby inside. The seat pad is removable and machine washable. For babies from birth to 28 pounds. The vibration feature requires one D alkaline battery (not supplied). (Note: Fisher-Price often changes its bouncer names, so look for the most recent model on www.fisher-price.com.)

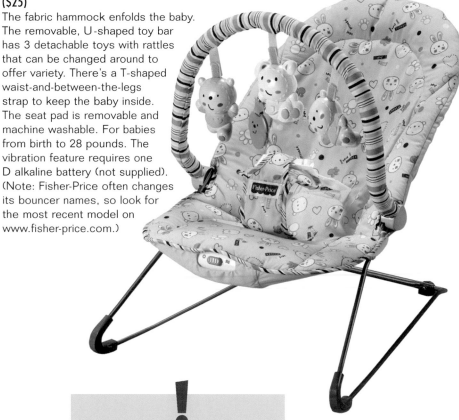

!

WARNING

Bouncing babies
Bouncers sometimes slip or walk off countertops and tables from babies' motions, resulting in serious head injuries, and frames can bend or break if parents try to carry the seat with the baby inside, toppling the baby to the floor.

"We liked our baby's reclining high chair much better than a bouncer. His bouncer had to sit on the floor or else it would be unsafe, while he seemed secure strapped into his high chair in a semireclining position; plus, we could roll him around the house and maintain eye contact with him.**"**

Summer Infant's Deluxe Soft Embrace Gund Puppy Bouncer

(\$60)

A soft haven for baby to sit and rest, this bouncer features a stable, wide base, a 3-position recline, and a cushioned head support for the baby. A U-shaped arch suspends 3 soft pastel puppies. Its battery-operated features include a choice of 5 melodies and 3 nature sounds as well as variable-speed vibration. The thickly padded seat cover is removable for washing. There's a T-shaped waist-and-between-the-legs strap to secure baby inside. From birth to 6 months or 25 pounds. Requires 3 AAA batteries (not supplied).

Checklist

Bouncer shopping

✔ **Stable frame.** Place your hand in the center of the seat to test how easily it tips sideways, forward, or backward. A sturdy frame that's larger than the seat indicates better stability.

✔ **Good seat belt.** Necessary to hold baby safely inside.

✔ **Recline options.** Extra reclining positions give some options for finding the most comfortable position for your baby.

✔ **Nonslip base.** Skid-resistant pads on the bottom of the frame to keep the baby from walking the seat off a table or countertop when she jiggles.

✔ **Seat comfort.** Colorful, deeply padded seat covers are a plus, but make sure they are removable and washable.

✔ **Toys.** Any toys and the bar holding them must be well secured, and any cords attaching the toys could pose a strangulation hazard if they are more than 7 inches long.

✔ **Quiet operation.** If the bouncer plays music, be sure you can turn the sound down or off.

✔ **Canopy.** If you plan to use the seat outdoors or under bright lights, you'll want a canopy to protect baby's eyes.

✔ **Entertaining extras.** Vibration, music, and rocking may help soothe a fussy baby. Buy an extra pack of batteries.

✔ **Folding option.** If you have limited space, look for a seat that can be folded and stored when not in use.

SAFETY CONSIDERATIONS

Repeatedly, babies have fallen from the seats, become entrapped in the straps, or the seats have walked off tables or counters from babies' motions, sometimes resulting in serious internal or head injuries.

Federal bouncer recalls by the Consumer Product Safety Commission (CPSC) are most often for broken parts, such as frame failures that cause the baby to fall out, or for ineffective restraints. To search for bouncer recalls, go to www.recalls.gov and search for "bouncers" or by brand or model under "Consumer Products."

The Juvenile Products Manufacturers Association (JPMA) along with the American Society of Testing and Materials (ASTM) have created a voluntary certification standard for infant bouncers. It requires manufacturers to use an independent testing laboratory to validate that their bouncers comply with the certification standard.

The standard addresses the bouncer's stability in resisting tip overs, the strength of the restraint system, slip resistance, structural integrity, the risk of collapsing or coming apart, and performance during a drop test. Note: Being certified does not mean that a bouncer is immune to recalls, and not being certified does not mean that a seat is unsafe.

Safety Checklist

Here are the safety precautions you need to take when you put your baby in a bouncer or infant seat.

✔ **Use harnesses.** Always use the safety belts and make sure they fit snugly around your child, to prevent serious injury or death from falling. Never leave your baby unattended in a bouncer or seat.

✔ **Use only on the floor.** Your baby's movements can cause the bouncer to walk across tables or counters. Place it on the floor to protect your baby from life-threatening head and body injuries should she and the seat go over the edge.

✔ **Follow age and ability guidelines.** Infant seats are only for babies who can't sit up on their own. Stop using the seat if your baby attempts to climb out. And don't use it when she reaches the manufacturer's stated weight limit, such as 18 pounds.

✔ **Keep off soft surfaces.** Don't place the bouncer on a bed, sofa, cushion, or other soft surface. Those could let the seat turn over, and your baby could suffocate.

✔ **Don't carry your baby in the seat.** The frame could break or buckle or you could trip, causing serious injury to your baby.

✔ **Keep away from cords.** Don't suspend strings, ribbons, or elastic over the seat or place it near window-blind cords, drapes with strings, phone cords, or anything that could strangle your baby.

✔ **Discard if broken.** A damaged or broken seat could be hazardous to your baby.

✔ **Do not use as a car seat.** Never substitute an infant seat for a car seat! Not only will it not protect your baby, it may injure her during a crash.

7

CAR SEATS, CAR BEDS & BOOSTER SEATS

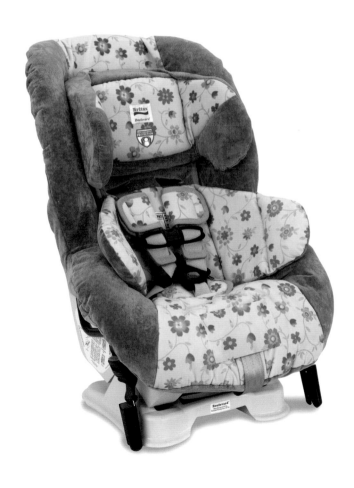

Call them car seats, car restraints, or safety seats—their jobs are essentially the same: to protect your precious cargo if there's a crash. This chapter helps you choose the best car seat for your baby. As with other baby-product categories, you'll find featured car seats and boosters chosen for their comfort, convenience, and safety features.

SAFE RIDING AT ANY SPEED

The National Highway Traffic Safety Administration (NHTSA) estimates that proper use of an approved child car seat could prevent up to 71 percent of deaths and 67 percent of injuries to babies and children from vehicle crashes. Yet many babies and children either don't ride in a car seat or aren't buckled in properly.

There is no one "best" or "safest" seat for your baby. With thousands of car models on the road and nearly 100 different car seat models in stores, ultimately the best seat for your baby is the model that is right for your baby's weight, height, and age; can be correctly installed in your vehicle; and is the one you are most likely to use properly every time you and your baby hit the road. Plus, it's the one that fits your budget.

All 50 states and the District of Columbia now have laws that require all babies and preschoolers (and in many states, children between 6 and 9 years of age) to be restrained in correctly installed car seats when they're riding in passenger vehicles.

Backseat *and* backward

Babies up to a year of age and 20 pounds in weight should ride in car seats that are fastened down in the backseat of the car and that face exactly the opposite of the normal direction people sit in cars. Their seats should face the rear of the car, rather than the hood. In fact, safety experts recommend that babies face rearward as long as possible, even after one year of age, as long as they're the right weight and length for the seat according to the seat manufacturer's guidelines.

By law, *all* rearward-facing babies must ride in the backseat of passenger vehicles instead of the front seat, to protect them from the serious dangers of ruptured metal, the hostile dashboard, and from being killed by a front passenger air bag when it explodes. For the same reason, children up to the age of 13 should ride in the backseat of passenger vehicles, not in the front.

Babies face rearward for important safety reasons: They have very heavy heads in comparison with the rest of their bodies; their skulls are soft; and their necks and spines aren't fully formed. A protective shell is needed to support babies' heads, necks, and bodies when the forces of a front crash are unleashed.

The impact of a crash results in hundreds of pounds of force being set in motion in less than a second. Your baby's car seat will help to spread that force across his body so that his head, neck, and spinal cord are protected and will reduce the likelihood of other injuries. A parent's arms, no matter how strong, can't offer that protection.

Making the right choice

As with baby products in other categories, your car seat choice shouldn't be based solely on the price of the seat. A higher-priced seat isn't guaranteed to be safer, to fit better in your car, or to be easier to install. A costlier seat may simply have extra convenience features and more finishing touches.

Generally, imports cost more than seats manufactured in the U.S., even though they have to pass identical safety tests. Seats sporting licensed characters or designer names generally cost about 10 percent more than very similar seats made by the identical manufacturer. The bottom line is: All car seats must pass

WARNING

Air bags and babies don't mix
Air bags are designed for adult passengers. Even though their deployment is more controlled now than in past years, they explode out of their housing with several hundred pounds of force when there's a crash. While rapid air-bag deployment is good for protecting properly restrained older children and full-grown adults, it can be life-threatening for babies and young children.

Car seats shouldn't wobble!
Always follow the directions in your vehicle owner's manual as well as those that come with the car seat to make sure your baby's seat is firmly fastened down in the car. After tightening the LATCH straps or adult seat belts as much as possible, tilt and push your baby's car seat to and fro and to both sides. A correctly installed car seat should not move more than one inch in any direction when you pull on the seat with a reasonable amount of force.

stringent U.S. safety tests, and even seats costing hundreds of dollars have had their share of recalls.

There are three types of car seats for newborns through the first year of life: rear-facing infant-only seats, convertible seats, and infant car beds for babies with special needs who can't safely sit in a semi-upright position.

Rear-facing infant-only seats often resemble small tubs and have slanted, padded seats with straps to hold the baby inside. A rigid U-shaped carry handle clicks into an upright position for toting the baby outside of the car. The handle folds down behind the seat when it's being used in the car. Most seats come with a separate base that can be installed in the car to allow the seat portion to be unlatched for carrying the baby or locking the seat into a specially adapted stroller frame.

Infant-only seats are designed to protect babies weighing between 5 and 20 pounds, and some newer models can support babies weighing 22 pounds or more. Parents often prefer infant-only seats as their first car seat purchase because they are compact, well-angled, and seem to fit newborns and young babies best. However, one-fourth of girls and three-fourths of boys outgrow these seats before they reach their first birthday, requiring the purchase of a different seating system.

Convertible seats are larger reclining ones, with 5-point harnesses, that can be used for a longer time. They face rearward for babies, and most can accommodate babies weighing 5 pounds and up. Then the seats can be turned to face forward in a more upright position for 20- to 40-pound toddlers (until about age 4). Parents choose these seats when they want to economize with a single car seat purchase to use from birth through the first few years. (Toddler-only seats that face forward and resemble convertible seats are also available for toddlers over one year of age.)

Infant car beds are small rectangular, fully reclined beds with harnesses to strap the baby inside and straps that fasten the bed to the car. They're designed to ride parallel to the car's seat back and are specifically for special-needs babies whose physical problems prevent them from sitting in a semi-upright position, or those who may stop breathing when seated at an angle in a regular baby car seat (positional apnea.)

High-back booster seats are for children over age one and supply 5-point harnesses for use until the child exceeds 40 pounds in weight (or sometimes heavier). Once the child exceeds the weight limit for using the harnesses, special slots in the sides of these seats are used with adult lap and shoulder belts, positioning them so that the shoulder belt crosses the child's collarbone and chest and the lap belt crosses the child's thighs rather than the vulnerable soft parts of his abdomen.

Belt-positioning boosters are raised seats for children past the toddler stage. They're designed to position adult shoulder and lap belts correctly on the child's body, and some have detachable backs, allowing the seat base alone to be used with the adult lap belts.

Some vans and SUVs offer **built-in car seats** as an optional purchase. These seats have definite drawbacks. They can't be moved from one vehicle to another, and you'll be stuck with the system even after your child outgrows the seat. Nor do they accommodate rear-facing babies. We recommend purchasing a removable seat.

Manufacturers also sell **portable harnesses and vests** that are supposed to be replacements for car restraints. These devices are not NHTSA approved and cannot be recommended as a safe alternative to car seats with rigid shells.

INSIDE CAR SEATS

The **shell** is a car seat's rigid outer frame—generally in beige, gray, pink, or blue. It's usually hollow, created by molding a special type of plastic that can flex under the pressure of crash forces without splitting.

The **inner liner** is the fabric and padding that create the comfortable upholstered place where the baby sits. While infant-only seats are likely to sport extra cushioning and have colorful pastel fabrics and fanciful patterns, liners of car seats for older toddlers and children tend to be more subdued, to blend in with the colors of car interiors.

The **padded liner** is shaped to fit into the seat and to allow various straps to thread through them from the back of the seat. Liners are held in place by elastic or by plastic fasteners, allowing the liner to be removed for cleaning. Most manufacturers recommend that only mild soap and water be used.

The type of **padding and foam** that manufacturers are allowed to use inside the seat is federally regulated and must meet standards for flame resistance and crash protection. But the thickness of the liner's cushioning, the types of fabrics, detailing such as ruffles, the sun shield, and extra body and head support pillows mark the difference between trendier, more expensive models and no-frills economy versions.

Harnesses

Forces that are unleashed during a crash depend on the characteristics of the vehicle you're driving, such as whether it's large or small; the speed your vehicle is going at the time of the crash; and the type of crash—head-on, rear-end, or sideways. Hundreds of pounds of force could be involved.

Harnesses of strong webbed material inside your baby's seat serve to distribute crash forces evenly over the strongest parts of your baby's body as he is forcefully thrown forward and then backward during the seconds following a crash.

Car seats for babies have either **3-point** or **5-point harnesses.** These terms indicate the number of straps that come through the seat's shell and fasten together to secure the baby.

While 3-point systems have only two shoulder straps and a between-the-legs crotch strap that buckle together, 5-point systems have those straps plus waist belts that secure each of the baby's hips. The 5-point design is thought to be the best for maintaining the baby's body position and for evenly distributing the forces of a crash across much of the baby's body and his hard thigh bones, rather than across his soft, vulnerable belly.

The height of the shoulder harnesses is adjusted by threading them through small slits, called **harness slots,** found at various heights in the seat's back. Seats typically offer 3 or 4 rows of slots. Some newer car seat models have a yoke that slides up and down behind the seat so the shoulder harnesses can be adjusted easily without having to go through a complicated process of threading through a new set of slots each time your baby grows an inch or two.

With infant-only seats, the shoulder-harness height should be at the baby's shoulders or one inch or less below them. For forward-facing convertibles or toddler seats, shoulder harnesses should be positioned level with the tot's shoulders or just above them.

Snug fit is important. You should be able to fit no more than one finger between the baby's chest and the straps that hold him in the seat. (Some models also have a strap or an adjuster knob at the front of the seat to tighten or loosen harness fit.)

A **harness clip** (or chest clip) is used to hold the two shoulder straps together so the baby won't be ejected from the seat during a crash. The clip is unfastened to put the baby in the seat, and then is locked to secure the straps while the baby is riding in the seat. The clip slides up or down the straps and should always be positioned at the level of the baby's armpit. (When you test seats, you'll discover that some clips are easy to operate, while others are fingernail breakers.)

Metal **tongues** from the shoulder and waist belts click into a **center buckle** attached to the between-the-legs strap. The buckle is made of metal, too, and usually has a plastic **push button** in the center for releasing the tongues when you're ready to remove your baby from the seat.

Anchoring the seat inside the car

Even when the straps of your baby's seat are correctly fastened around his body, the seat must also be securely anchored inside your car. Car seats can safely be fastened down using the vehicle's lap belts, but federal regulations require that newer cars and car seats also offer a LATCH system (Lower Anchors and Tethers for Children).

CHILD'S DESCRIPTION	SEAT TYPE/POSITION	
Low-birth-weight baby or newborn with physical disabilities	Infant car bed	
Baby and young toddler	Rear-facing infant-only seat	
	Convertible seat in the rear-facing position (See the same seat below in the forward-facing position)	
Toddlers and preschoolers (from approximately 1 to 4 years)	Convertible seat in the forward-facing position (See the same seat above in the rear-facing position)	

* Depending on model
** Go by child's weight

Car seats at a glance

Here's a quick overview of the types of car seats currently on the market and their general specifications. The baby weight and length ranges are only averages, since specific guidelines vary for different seat models. Check the specifications for each model as you shop.

PRODUCT DESCRIPTION	AGE	BABY WEIGHT RANGE	BABY HEIGHT LIMIT	PRICE RANGE
Small, rigid baby bed with harnesses and seat anchors	Birth to 1 month (or less)	To 9 pounds	19 inches	$80–$125
Deep bucket-style seat with a U-shaped carry handle. Most have bases that fasten into the car but with detachable seats for use outside the car.	Birth to 1 year of age	5–22 pounds or more*	28–30 inches	$40–$200
Tall seat with reclining feature, for rear-facing babies under 1 year of age (converts for use by toddlers)	Birth to 1 year	5–30 pounds or more*	36 inches	$55–$300
Tall seat converted from the reclining, rear-facing position to the upright, forward-facing position. Some seats offer recline options.	Approx. 1–4 years of age**	20–40 pounds*	27–49 inches (or more)*	$55–$300

Under this law, cars are required to have 2 pairs of U-shaped metal **anchors** built into the crease ("bight") where the cars' backseat cushions meet the seat back. Seats for babies and toddlers must also offer special fasteners, called **connectors,** in the back to fasten the seat to the LATCH anchors. (See the car seat illustration on page 96.)

Some experts feel that the middle of the rear seat is the safest place for babies' and children's car seats to be installed, since it offers an extra zone of protection on both sides of the seat in the event of a side crash.

Unfortunately, most vehicles offer LATCH anchors only on the sides of the car (not in the center), as that makes them more convenient to use. If your car doesn't have a fold-down armrest, you may want to try firmly installing your baby's car seat in the center of the backseat, following the instructions in your car's owner's manual and those that come with the car seat about how best to use the adult seat belts. But using the side LATCH anchors or adult belts is considered by most experts to be an acceptably safe option.

A **tether strap** or adjuster strap also comes with forward-facing toddler and convertible seats. It fastens onto special anchoring hardware attached to the car's frame. The **tether anchor** usually is secured to the ledge behind the backseat. The tethering system stabilizes the seat and helps to keep it from tipping forward during a crash.

Most vehicles manufactured after August 1999 come with anchoring hardware already installed, and those manufactured in the decade before that may have predrilled holes on the ledge behind the backseat, or on the floor behind the

CHILD'S DESCRIPTION	SEAT TYPE/POSITION	
Toddlers and preschoolers (from approximately 1 to 4 years)	Toddler-only seat	
	Combination toddler and high-back booster used with 5-point harness. (See the same seat below used without harness.)	
Young child	Combination toddler and high-back booster relying only on adult shoulder and lap belts without harness. (See the same seat above used with harness.)	

* Depending on model
** Go by child's weight

Car seats at a glance (Continued)

PRODUCT DESCRIPTION	AGE	BABY WEIGHT RANGE	BABY HEIGHT LIMIT	PRICE RANGE
Tall upright seat with 5-point harness, designed for use only in the forward-facing position with toddlers and preschoolers. Some seats offer recline options.	Approx. 1–5 years**	20–50 pounds (or more)*	19–57 inches*	$130–$450
Tall seat relies on a 5-point harness until child exceeds the seat's 30–40 pound weight limit, when adult belts are threaded through the shell.	Approx. 1–4 years using harnesses**	22–40 pounds (Some models available for children weighing up to 65 pounds)	36 inches	$40–$160
Boosters raise the child and position adult seat belts safely across the collarbone and hips. Some have removable seat backs that also allow seat base to serve as adult-belt positioner.	4–10 years of age*	30–100 pounds*	37–57 inches tall*	$40–$160

seats of station wagons, SUVs, or pickups, but without installed hardware. You can ask a car dealership to install the anchor hardware for you, and some will even do it free. For more information on tethers and tether anchors, refer to your vehicle's owners manual or contact the dealership.

Interior foam cushioning

Increasingly, manufacturers are using high-impact EPS (Expanded Polystyrene) or EPP (Expanded Polypropylene Particle) foam to line the car seat in the area surrounding the baby's head—and sometimes the whole interior. You can see the foam if you pull back the seat's padding. The material can be a white, firm foam like bicycle helmet liners, or a thin layer of dense, cushiony colored material like that sewn inside shoulder straps of some backpacks.

Either way, the foam is thought to improve the seat's ability to absorb crash forces and to soften the impact on a baby's body. Sometimes parents mistake the foam for packing material and attempt to remove it from the seat. It's protective and should be left in place. If the seat is in an accident, you may need to replace the seat, since some foam may lose its protective value after a crash. Contact the customer service department of the seat's manufacturer for instructions on what to do.

Side-impact protection

Increasingly, car seat manufacturers are paying attention to the importance of offering side-impact protection on car seats designed for infants and children, especially for vehicles equipped with side air bags in the rear passenger compartment.

Rear compartment side-impact air bags differ according to the vehicle. They vary in the area they cover, where they exit, and how far out they balloon when they deploy. Passenger vehicle manufacturers are currently paying special attention to how side-impact air bags could affect the safety of children in car seats, and so far, side air bags appear to be safe for children as long as they stay inside their car seats and don't lean out of their protective shells.

While most car seats for babies and children offer little or no side-impact protection, some have exaggerated side wings for the head area and deeper than usual seat sides that make the seats resemble old-fashioned wingback chairs. The one drawback is that overly deep wings in the head area may not be appreciated by your child if they obstruct his view out windows.

Getting the correct angle

The back of your baby's rear-facing seat needs to be angled between 30 and 45 degrees from a straight vertical line, or about halfway between straight up and lying flat. Angle indicators on the sides of most seats will help you find the correct position. Reclining the baby too far backward could increase the forces that his shoulders have to bear during a crash and might even increase the likelihood of his being ejected from the seat. On the other hand, leaning the seat too far forward may make his head flop down, potentially closing off his airway.

If your car has steeply angled backseat cushions that drop down toward the crease at the rear, it's all right to use a rolled-up towel or blanket or a length of a round firm foam (swimming noodle) under the car seat at the seat crease to help position your infant's car seat at the correct angle.

Q/A

Q We're planning our baby's first airplane trip to visit my parents. Do we need to buy an extra ticket for him and use his car seat on board?

The Federal Aviation Administration (FAA) and the American Academy of Pediatrics (AAP.org) recommend that babies and children under 4 be securely fastened in car safety seats in airplanes, with the seats fastened down by airplane seat belts. Doing so will help keep your baby safe during takeoff and landing or when there's turbulence. Your infant or convertible seat will need to be certified for use on airplanes, and airline personnel will require an "FAA approved" sticker on the seat's shell. Besides protecting your baby, the seat will be available for driving away from the airport even if your baggage is lost or the car-rental company runs out of car seats. Note: Most airlines offer discounts on seat tickets for babies less than 2 years of age.

WARNING

Avoid car seats with front shields Some car seats have shields that are raised to put the baby inside and lower to lock into place in front of the baby. Shoulder harnesses thread through the top of the shield, and a crotch strap underneath the shield locks into a buckle on the seat. These models give the erroneous impression that they're more protective than seats with the usual simple webbed harnesses, but that's not the case, particularly for small babies. Typically, the shield positions the harness straps too far away from a small baby's body, which might allow him to strike his face or neck on the shield during a crash, or even allow his body to be thrown from the seat. The American Academy of Pediatrics and the National Highway Traffic Safety Administration have both cautioned against using car seats with front shields, since seats with 5-point harnesses offer better protection.

If your baby flops to one side or the other because the car seat's seating area is too large, roll up a towel and bend it into a U-shape to keep his head in a forward-facing position. Just be sure not to place any padding between your baby's neck and head and the car seat's shoulder straps.

You can also place a rolled up U-shaped towel between your baby's legs and the between-the-legs strap to help him sit more upright, rather than slouching forward. But it's critical not to place padding behind his back, because doing so could compromise the ability of the seat to distribute crash forces evenly across your baby's body. A certified child passenger safety technician from a safety organization, the police department, fire department, or the hospital where your baby is delivered can help you to adjust the seat to best fit your baby's needs.

Car seat terms

Car seats are very technical, and trying to understand them can be quite a challenge for most parents. Here's a quick reference guide for some common car seat terms to help you get up to speed.

Buckle A metal fastener connected to the crotch belt that is used to lock all of the straps together in the center of the baby's body, just above the thighs.

LATCH connector Push-on or hook-on metal devices on straps that exit the top or back of the car seat and are designed to fasten the seat or its base to the car, using special anchors that come preinstalled between the backseat cushion and seat back in newer vehicles.

CRS Short for Child Restraint System—a car seat or bed designed to restrain, seat, or position children who weigh 50 pounds or less.

3-point harness system Found on the seats of some infant-only car seats. It consists of three straps: two adjustable ones that restrain the baby's left and right shoulders, plus a between-the-legs strap that usually holds the

buckle that fastens all three straps together.

5-point harness system Found on most models of infant-only car seats, on all convertible seats, toddler-only seats, and high-back boosters with harnesses. The number of points indicates the number of straps that exit the seat's shell: one adjustable strap for each shoulder; adjustable straps for each side of the waist; and one for between the legs, which usually holds the buckle to fasten all the harness components together.

Chest clip, harness clip, harness tie, or harness retainer clip A sliding plastic fastener resembling a large hair clip, designed to be positioned at the level of the baby's armpits to keep the two front shoulder straps together in order to prevent the baby's body from being ejected between the straps during a crash.

Harness slots Rows of slits in the back of the car seat shell, with corresponding upholstery holes, to allow harness straps to be routed into the seating area. They are used to adjust the height of shoulder harnesses and the closeness of the between-the-legs

Overview, rear-facing infant-only car seat base

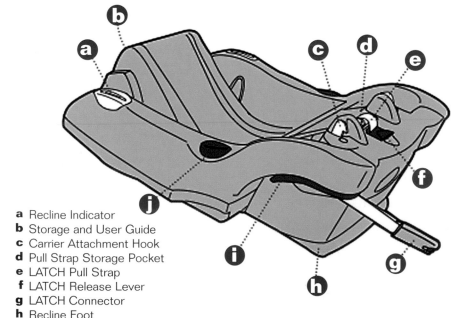

a Recline Indicator
b Storage and User Guide
c Carrier Attachment Hook
d Pull Strap Storage Pocket
e LATCH Pull Strap
f LATCH Release Lever
g LATCH Connector
h Recline Foot
i Shoulder Belt Lockoff
j Recline Button

Overview, rear-facing infant-only car seat

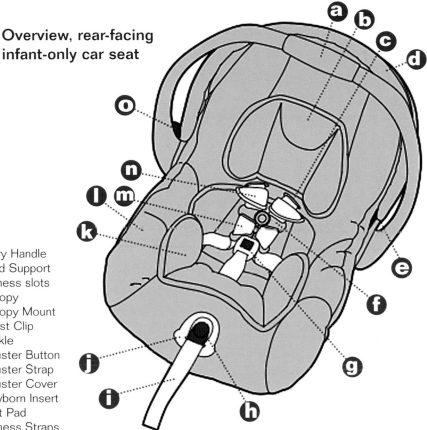

a Carry Handle
b Head Support
c Harness slots
d Canopy
e Canopy Mount
f Chest Clip
g Buckle
h Adjuster Button
i Adjuster Strap
j Adjuster Cover
k Newborn Insert
l Seat Pad
m Harness Straps
n Neck Pads
o Handle Button

Illustrations courtesy of Chicco

straps to fit babies as they grow. (Shoulder straps for infant-only seats should be threaded into the frame at or an inch below the baby's current shoulder level, and at or one inch above the baby's shoulders for forward-facing seats.)

Locking clip (belt-shortening clip or heavy-duty locking clip) A flat H-shaped metal piece, usually stored in the back of a baby's car seat, that cinches together the lap and shoulder portions of a retracting, single-piece adult shoulder-and-lap belt so the lap-belt portion can securely hold the child's seat in place.

Shell The molded, hard plastic outer body of the car seat.

Adjuster strap or Tether strap A straight or V-shaped, adjustable strap on the top of forward-facing convertible and toddler-only seats that fastens onto hardware attached inside the car (the "anchor point"). The anchor point is usually found on the rear window shelf of a car's passenger compartment, or on the floorboard of vans or station wagons behind the rear seats. When anchored and pulled tight, the tether stabilizes the seat to keep it from tipping forward during a crash.

INFANT CAR BED

Baby car beds are fully reclined, new-born-size padded rectangular shells that strap into the vehicle using adult seat belts' internal harnesses to hold the baby in place.

An infant car bed may be needed at first for a tiny baby, weighing less than 5 pounds, especially if he suffers from apnea (periods when breathing stops temporarily), bradycardia (slow heart-beats), or oxygen desaturation (lower than normal oxygen levels in the blood) and shows that he can't tolerate a semi-upright position in a car restraint.

The American Academy of Pediatrics recommends that all infants born earlier than 37 weeks gestational age be moni-tored for the above-mentioned conditions, while in a car seat, before they're allowed to leave the hospital, to check whether the baby will be affected by the sharp angle of semi-reclined infant car seats.

The baby's body should face sideways on the backseat of the car with his head in the center of the car and his feet toward one of the back doors.

When to Buy

After birth and before first car ride. For use only with low-birth-weight babies and those with developmental disabilities who weigh 9 pounds or less and who have breathing problems when they're placed in the semi-upright, steeply angled seat position of a rear-facing car seat.

Angel Guard's Infant Car Bed
($100)

An infant car bed is useful for only a very limited period of time and only for babies with special physical needs. The Angel Guard Infant Car Bed is specifically designed for transporting reclining babies weighing less than 5 pounds and until the baby reaches 9 pounds and 20 inches in length. The baby can ride on his back, stomach, or side, depending on his phys-ical needs.

The bed also provides a slight angle to raise the baby's head to facilitate breathing. There are shoulder straps and a crotch strap to hold him in place in a sudden crash. The shell is deeply padded, and slots on the side provide ventilation for continuous air circulation. The bed's rear strap secures to the vehicle with a lap belt. (The bed is not to be used in aircraft.)

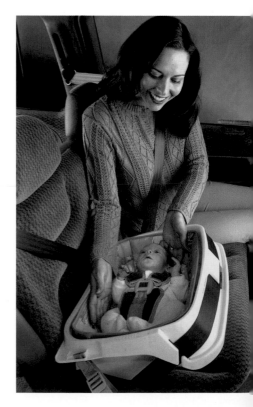

REAR-FACING INFANT-ONLY CAR SEAT

All babies have to ride in the backseat and face the rear of the car until they reach one year of age. Rear-facing infant-only seats are specifically designed to protect infants weighing 5 to 20 pounds, but more recent models can protect babies weighing up to 22 or even 30 pounds.

They're shaped like small tubs and have deeply slanted, padded seats and a pivoting U-shaped handle on top to allow an adult to carry the baby outside the car or for the seat to be locked into a specially adapted stroller or wheeled frame.

Infant seats usually come in two parts: a detachable seat and a belt-secured base.

The base is designed to be used like a docking station so the seat can be removed without having to undo the LATCH belts or adult belts that are holding the base down. (All infant-only seats are equally safe being fastened into the car without their bases).

Some strollers have special adapters to carry specific brands of infant-only seats, and with an extra base the seat can be moved back and forth between different vehicles.

Even though most rear-facing seats are designed to fit into the toddler-seat section of grocery carts, that's not considered safe,

since the seat could topple over with the baby inside or even fall out of the cart.

Avoid:

✗ Recalled or used seat. Don't buy a used infant seat unless you're certain it hasn't been recalled and that it's never been in a crash.

✗ Difficult to install or use. If the seat is hard to position and install and it's hard to put your baby inside and take him out, you're less likely to use it safely.

Highs & lows of infant seats

Highs. They fit small babies better in the early months than larger convertible seats do. Bases, which fasten down separately from car seats, allow the seats to be easily removed from the car for carrying or locking the seat into specially adapted strollers or wheeled frames for rolling around. Most come with canopies to provide shading from sun glare inside and outside the vehicle. You may be able to save money by purchasing a "travel system" that combines a color-coordinated car seat and stroller. (Travel systems are discussed starting on page 287 in the stroller chapter.)

Lows. It is recommended that all babies under a year of age ride facing rearward, but some rear-facing infant-only car restraints aren't designed to protect babies weighing more than 20 to 23 pounds, which means you'll have to buy another seat in 7 to 9 months. Although carrying your baby around in the seat may seem convenient, the seats are heavy, and unless you're prepared to heft 20 to 30

When to Buy

Last months of pregnancy to before baby's first car ride. Use from birth to 1 year of age or 20 pounds for the rear-facing position, whichever comes first. (Always follow the manufacturer's weight guidelines for your specific car seat model.)

pounds at an angle after bending over to unlock the seat and lift the seat and baby out without injuring your back, you may decide it's simpler to remove your baby from the seat and carry him in your arms. From an ergonomic standpoint, the handles of infant-only seats are seldom comfortable for carrying the baby for very long. Whether you try to support the seat in the crook of your elbow or tote it with both hands in front of you, you're likely to bruise your carrying arm or thigh. Safety issues include hardware and handle failures and seats detaching accidentally from their bases when they're not properly clicked into them.

 # Checklist

Rear-facing infant-only car seat shopping

Here's what to look for when you shop for a rear-facing, infant-only car seat.

✔**Good car fit.** Before you buy, check how it fits, in the reclined position, in the backseat of your car. It's hard to tell by simply eyeballing the seat.

✔**5-point harnesses.** Models with straps for the baby's waist as well as the shoulders and crotch offer more security than 3-point versions that omit the waist belts.

✔**Higher weight range.** Seats that safely carry larger babies are a good value. A model that can restrain a 22-pound (or even heavier) baby could save you from having to purchase another seat before your baby reaches his first birthday.

✔**Comfortable handle.** A carry handle shaped for carrying comfort and with dense foam cushioning will make toting the car seat less of a strain. (But don't expect to be able to do that for more than a few minutes at a time!)

✔**Canopy.** A generous, adjustable sunshade will help to keep your baby protected from glare and bright sunlight.

✔**Base.** Most seats come with a separate base to lock the seat in place using your car's LATCH anchors, or by threading adult seat belts through the base. Get a base that allows you to adjust the angle that the seat reclines, to adapt it to the slope of your car's backseat, and consider buying an extra base if you have more than one vehicle.

✔**Clear directions.** Directions should be clear and easy to follow. Check both the directions that come with the car seat and the car seat installation guide in your vehicle's owner's manual.

✔**Brand-new.** This ensures you'll be getting the advantage of the latest car seat technology, a seat hasn't been on a recall list, and one that has never withstood a crash.

Baby Trend's Flex-Loc Baby Seat
($90)

Highly rated for its performance in crash tests, this seat with a 5-point harness system is rated for babies from 5 to 22 pounds. Harnesses adjust easily without having to remove straps from the rear of the seat. The seat offers EPS foam protection for the baby's head, and the crotch belt is adjustable for smaller babies. "Flex-Loc" refers to the flexible straps at the base of the seat and the rigid locking connectors that fasten to the anchors in car LATCH systems. The comfortable rubber grip on the triangle-shaped top of the carry handle makes it easier to tote than some other models. The seat pad is removable for washing. The seat's stay-in-car base adjusts to 4 positions, and there is a level indicator to show proper seat angle. Extra bases are available to allow the seat to be transferred to other vehicles. The seat can be carried by mainstream strollers such as Baby Trend by using special adapters.

Chicco's KeyFit 30 Infant Car Seat
($160)

For babies weighing from 4 to 30 pounds, the KeyFit for infants has a 5-point harness with 3 adjustments for shoulder strap heights. It has a cushioned washable seat pad and infant insert. Energy-absorbing EPS foam lines the interior of the shell. Deep side wings provide enhanced side-impact protection. The seat's cushioned carry handle can be left in any locked position in the car. The removable canopy has a vinyl sun visor that folds down for glare protection. A squeeze-release handle releases the base and its spring-assisted leveling foot offers multiple seat angles with an angle indicator. The seat is compatible with several models of Chicco strollers.

CONVERTIBLE SEATS

Convertible car seats are erect, tall-backed children's restraints that do just what their name implies. They convert from seats that protect rear-facing babies (weighing 5 pounds up to 20–30 pounds or more) to seats that can be turned to face forward and upright for toddlers (up to 40 pounds or nearly 4 years of age, depending upon individual seats' requirements).

Some models, such as the Britax Marathon, are designed for children from birth up to 65 pounds. The unique Alpha-Omega Elite from the Cosco division of the Dorel Juvenile Group can be used as a convertible car seat from birth up to 40 pounds and as a belt-positioning booster seat for children up to 100 pounds. Unfortunately, the Alpha-Omega Elite is huge and cumbersome and gets poor marks from parents.

Newer seats have a tether strap fastened to the back of their shells, which hooks onto a tether anchor on the back shelf of newer-model cars. The strap helps to stabilize the seat in the forward-facing position and to control its forward and sideways movements during a crash.

Avoid:

✗ **Poor fit with your car.** Some vehicle seat belts and backseat shapes simply aren't compatible with some car seats. And some car seats are just too large for smaller-sized vehicles.

✗ **A gigantic one-size-fits-all seat.** As economical as they may sound, the giant seats that adapt for children at every stage are usually awkward and cumbersome and do a poor job of supporting newborns.

✗ **Recalled or used seat.** Don't buy a used convertible seat unless you're certain it hasn't been recalled or in a serious crash.

Highs & lows of convertible seats

Highs. Since the seats adapt to both infants and toddlers, you're basically getting two seats in one, and you may not have to buy a second seat before your baby's first birthday.

Lows. The hefty size of some models, and the amount of room they take up in the rear-facing reclined position, may make them unsuitable for use in your car. Some models don't adapt well to small babies. Models with front shields are not thought to be safe for small babies.

WARNING

Don't leave a baby alone in a car
Don't leave your baby inside the vehicle unattended. In warm weather, temperatures can soar to deadly heat levels as much as 20 degrees hotter than outside in only a few minutes, and your baby is extremely vulnerable to heat stroke. Your child could also be taken during a car theft or kidnapped from the vehicle. Hide a spare key on the car's frame in case you lock yourself out while your baby is still inside.

✔ **Checklist**

Convertible car seat shopping

Here's what to look for when you shop for a rear-facing infant-only car seat.

✔**Good car fit.** Try out a variety of seats to find the best fit for your particular vehicle. A convertible reclined in the rear-facing position can eat up a lot of car space, and it may bump into one of the front seats. If you have a small car or a truck with a small rear seating area, try the seat in the reclined position in your backseat before you buy. (Or at least make sure the store has a liberal return policy if you later discover problems when you install the seat.)

✔**Good fit for a newborn.** Look for the lowest weight range the seat will support. For a smaller than normal baby, such as one weighing less than 7 pounds, the seat's harnesses, and especially the between-the-leg strap, may not fit well.

✔**Extra harness slots and moveable crotch strap.** A low shoulder harness slot position will ensure that your small baby can be safely strapped in. Make sure there are several positions for the crotch belt, especially if your baby's small.

✔**Infant head and body supports.** Removable infant head and body cushions will help stabilize your infant's head and body so that he doesn't slump and so his head faces forward.

✔**EPS or EPP foam lining.** Shock-absorbing material embedded in the seat's shell beneath the padding surrounds your baby's head or both head and body to help protect him during a crash.

✔**Side wings.** Side protection is a serious issue, and having wings on both sides of your baby's head, as well as reinforced car seat sides, could help to protect him during a side collision.

✔**Extra width and length.** If you or your baby's dad is above average in height or weight, and your baby is predicted to be above the 50th percentile on the standard growth charts, then a roomier, taller seat may work best, especially in the winter when outerwear will expand his dimensions.

✔**Heavier weight limits.** It makes sense to buy a seat that allows for extra poundage, but check that it can still recline in your backseat.

✔**Easy-to-use LATCH fasteners.** LATCH fasteners should be easy to lock and unlock in case you need to trade cars.

When to Buy

Last months of pregnancy to before baby's first car ride. Use from birth to 1 year of age (20 pounds) for the rear-facing position; approximately age 1 to 4 years (20 to 40 pounds) in the forward-facing position. (Always follow the manufacturer's weight guidelines for your specific car seat model.)

Britax's Roundabout
($220)

Highly rated by consumer organizations for crash-test performance and ease of use, the Roundabout reclines and faces rearward for babies weighing 5 to 35 pounds and sits erect and forward for toddlers weighing 20 to 40 pounds (or until about 4 years of age). It features EPS impact foam surrounding the child's head and torso, plus thick cushioning in the seating area. The seat back offers 3 height-adjustment slots for the shoulder straps of its 5-point harness and built-in hinged latches (lock-offs) for securing the seat when adult retracting seat belts are used. The harness buckle is padded for baby comfort. A harness-adjuster strap in the front of the seat allows for tightening or loosening the harness. It has push-button-release LATCH fasteners. The upholstery fabric is available in a variety of patterns (Puma shown) and can be hand washed and line dried. It comes with a tether strap for use in the front-facing position.

Sunshine Kids' Radian80
($280)

The Radian80 is designed to be rear-facing from 5 to 33 pounds and forward-facing up to 80 pounds using a 5-point harness. The seat uses a unique steel alloy frame with 4-panel EPS foam side-impact protection and its energy-absorbing SafetStop harness system. The seat offers more shoulder room inside than most convertibles, yet it's narrow enough to fit 3 seats in your backseat. The seat includes full body support cushions for infants that convert into adjustable head cushions for older babies and children. It weighs 23 pounds and can be folded flat and carried using padded shoulder straps. Available in 4 color combinations.

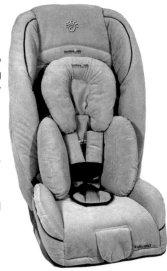

TODDLER-ONLY CAR SEAT

Toddler-only seats resemble convertible seats, but they're designed only to hold tots who are the right age and weight for sitting up and facing forward. Unlike convertible seats, they don't hold babies under one year of age.

Highs & lows of toddler-only seats

Highs. They're designed specifically for the needs of toddlers, and some offer reclining positions and extra side-padding around the head area for napping comfort.

Lows. An extra expense. Not usable for babies under one year of age, and will have to be replaced by a booster seat within a few years.

Graco's Toddler Safeseat
($130)

The Toddler Safeseat has a 5-point harness system and is designed for forward-facing toddlers and children weighing between 20 and 40 pounds or about from age 1 to 4. (It cannot be used in the rear-facing position.) The seat and side arms have thickly cushioned upholstery. It offers multiple recline positions that can be adjusted while the child is inside. Wings for the head area and deep sides are designed to offer side-impact protection. It comes with a headrest, extra body cushioning, and cup and snack holders that are removable. An easy-to-use belt path can be used to anchor the seat with adult seat belts if the LATCH system isn't used. And there's a belt lock-off to secure the adult lap belt that holds

In the child'd first 1 to 3 years. Used for babies and toddlers of 20 to 40 pounds, in the forward-facing position (only). (Always follow the manufacturer's weight guidelines for your specific car seat model.)

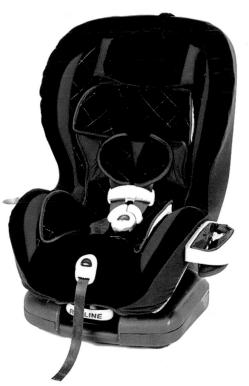

the seat down. The harness system's buckle features a front adjustment strap to make buckling and unbuckling easier.

BOOSTER SEATS

Children under 8 years of age shouldn't use just a car's regular adult shoulder and lap belts. The lap belts are likely to slide across the child's vulnerable, soft abdomen, potentially causing internal injuries during a crash; and shoulder belts may come too close to the child's neck.

As the names imply, boosters give children a boost so they can see out the windows better. Car booster seats work well with adult seat belts to safely secure children in cars, but should never be confused with the rigid molded-plastic booster seats that strap onto chairs as substitutes for high chairs.

Booster seats come in several varieties. Combination toddler/high-back booster seats with removable 5-point harnesses can be used by children weighing less than 30 to 40 pounds who still need chest, waist, and between-the-leg harnesses. High-back and backless models are designed simply to position adult shoulder and lap belts. Once the child weighs more, the harness system can be removed and slots in the seats can be used to correctly position adult lap belts across the child's pelvis and thighs and the shoulder belt across the child's collarbone, not across his vulnerable neck.

To offer your child maximum protection from whiplash, backless boosters and the seat-only portion of boosters with removable backs shouldn't be used if the top of your child's ears is higher than your vehicle's backseat or its head restraint.

Highs & lows of booster seats

Highs. Children's bodies are the wrong size for adult seat belts, but boosters help to place lap and shoulder belts in the safest position for restraining a child in the seat during a crash. The seats also allow a child's legs to bend at the knee, which is more comfortable than having them straight out on auto seats built for adults.

Lows. Some boosters perform poorly when it comes to managing adult belts and are not particularly comfortable. Their belt-positioning mode may allow a child to move sideways or out of position, which could be hazardous during a crash, especially if the rear passenger compartment is equipped with side-impact air bags.

When to Buy

In the child's first to eighth year. Used for children of 30 to 40 pounds, up to 80 to 100 pounds (depending on model) or approximately 4 to 8 years. (Always follow the manufacturer's weight guidelines for your specific car seat model.)

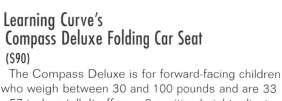

Learning Curve's
Compass Deluxe Folding Car Seat
($90)

The Compass Deluxe is for forward-facing children who weigh between 30 and 100 pounds and are 33 to 57 inches tall. It offers a 6-position height adjustment, so the seat grows with your child. Extra seat width is designed to fit larger children. The seat's energy-absorbing EPS foam headrest with elongated side wings provides improved side-impact protection. Flip-up cushioned armrests make entering and exiting easier for the child. The thick triple-layer padding makes the seat comfortable even for long trips. Narrow rails on the seat's base enable the seat to fit even in a vehicle's small bucket seats. There are retractable cup holders on both sides, and a convenient built-in carry handle for transporting the seat with an optional zippered carry case. Compass models come in a range of prices and offer a variety of fabric patterns, some with frankly "boy" or "girl" looks.

Britax's Monarch Booster Car Seat
($150)

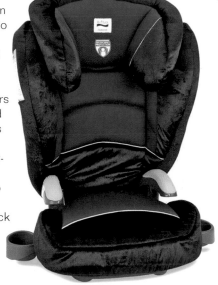

This high-back booster accommodates children weighing from 30 to 100 pounds who are 38 to 60 inches tall. It is designed to be used as an adult-seat-belt positioner only. Deep head and side wings are padded with EPS foam to protect the child's head, shoulders, and torso in the event of a crash. The seat features 3 layers of soft cushioning, plus it has wide, cushioned side wings. Color-coded adult-seat-belt guides help with installation. The headrest and shoulder-belt positioner can be raised and lowered with one hand to adjust to the child's height. Armrests can be spread wider apart to accommodate a larger child, and there are retractable cup holders on both sides. The back is removable to convert the seat into a backless booster. The seat's fabric cover is removable and washable. It is available in a variety of color combinations.

Car seat recalls

Recalls for car seats by manufacturers is a voluntary process monitored and overseen by the National Highway Traffic Safety Administration (NHTSA), a division of the U.S. Department of Transportation. The primary reasons car seats are recalled are they failed to pass federal safety standards, including crash-test performance; the materials used to manufacture the seat don't comply with federal standards, such as flammability requirements; or there are missing or malfunctioning parts.

Manufacturers of recalled seats may offer replacement units or repair kits to make the seats safe to use. At one time or another, nearly all major manufacturers of car seats have faced recalls. There's no need to avoid versions of the seat that have not been recalled. Even though the seat carries the same model name, it may not be in the specific series of model numbers or manufacture dates of the recalled versions.

The Consumer Product Safety Commission (**CPSC, www.cpsc.gov**) handles safety of car seats when they're being used outside of vehicles, such as at home, being used as a baby carrier, or used in a stroller or wheeled car seat frame. The best place to search for recalls from either NHTSA or CPSC on the Internet is www.recalls.gov. Simply enter the manufacturer's name, model name, and number of the car seat you are researching under each agency's Web link provided by the site.

NHTSA's Web site (**www.nhtsa.dot.gov**) also offers a locator for child passenger-seat inspection stations by state or Zip code. Its annual "Child Safety Ease of Use

Ratings" grades car seats in every category—for labels, instructions, installing features, and ease of installing the child, as well as forms for registering a used car seat with the manufacturer. Although most seats earn an A, some seats get B's and C's when they perform poorly on these criteria.

Parents can file complaints about defects and problems with car seats and boosters on the NHTSA site, and some car seat complaints are available for viewing. But viewable records are spotty, and it appears that only complaints written as letters on paper are offered, and some "paperless" e-mails don't show up.

Car seats also have a voluntary certification program overseen by the Juvenile Products Manufacturers Association (JPMA) and American Society of Testing and Materials (ASTM) that covers safety issues for hand-held infant carriers in different categories. You may find a JPMA certification sticker on the seat or on its packaging if the manufacturer elects to display it.

Additional sources for car seat safety information

Several nonprofit organizations offer reliable car seat information. (Note: A listing of Internet sources for car seat information can also be found in Chapter 23, *Web Resources*, starting on page 338.)

Consumer Reports (*Consumer Reports magazine* and **www.consumer-reports.org**) offers impartial ratings and repair histories for new and used vehicles, and also publishes ratings for car restraint crash-test performance nearly every year.

The American Academy of Pediatrics (www.aap.org) publishes an annual, "Car Safety Seats: A Guide for Families," that details various seat types and models and their weight requirements. SafetyBeltSafe U.S.A. (www.carseat.org) is an excellent source for information on car seat safety and choosing and correctly installing car seats. The technical section and glossary are particularly informative. SeatCheck (www.seatcheck.org) has a locator for Child Passenger Safety (CPS) technicians by state, city, and Zip code. If you're having trouble finding a car seat that works in the backseat of your particular vehicle, Car Seat Data (www.carseatdata.org) posts information on the compatibility between specific car models and car seats, based on parents' and car seat technicians' ratings.

Safe use tips

Surprisingly, safety surveys show that approximately 80 percent of all parents don't install or use their babies' car seats correctly. Here are tips for helping your baby stay safe while riding in the car.

Keep the baby out of the front seat. If you're holding your baby, your body will sandwich around him, crushing him into the hard dashboard or the seat in front of you with many more pounds of force than just the weight of your body. If your car has a front seat air bag on the passenger side, it will strike him with hundreds of pounds of killer force whether you are holding him or he's sitting in his car seat when an air bag deploys.

Avoid older seats. Know the history of a car seat before you buy it. The seat's shell may have invisible weaknesses from a crash—frayed straps and harnesses can be an indicator that the seat has been in an accident. And the instruction booklet that contains directions for installing the seat could be missing. Car seats that are more than 6 years old shouldn't be used at all—look for a sticker with the date of manufacture on the seat's shell.

Install your infant's seat facing rearward. Face your baby's car seat toward the rear if he's less than a year old, so he's looking toward the car's rear window, not forward toward the front windshield, and keep him rear-facing as long as he doesn't exceed the manufacturer's recommended weight and height limits. This will help to protect your baby's vulnerable head, neck, and spine during a frontal collision.

Firmly anchor the seat. Follow the car seat's instruction and your vehicle's owner's manual about how to anchor the car seat using adult seat belts or the metal U-shaped LATCH anchors that come in newer-model vehicles. Instructions will tell you how much "give" is safe—usually about one inch in any direction.

Angle correctly. Vehicle seats differ on how deeply angled or curved they are. If your baby's rear-facing car seat is leaning too far forward, it may intensify the forces of a crash on his body. If it rides angled too far back, it may cause the seat to tip backward in a crash. Rear-facing seats usually have an angle indicator on the side to help you judge if the seat is angled correctly. If the seat simply won't sit at the right angle, you may need to change car seats or to use a folded-up towel or a portion of a firm foam tube (swimming noodle) under the seat to attain the correct pitch.

Always adjust the harnesses. Choose the right height for your baby's shoulder straps—to one inch below the baby's shoulders in an infant-only seat and at shoulder level or one inch above in forward-facing seats. There should be room for no more than one of your fingers between the belt and your baby's chest.

Use the harness clip. The harness clip (or "chest buckle") that holds the baby's shoulder straps together must always be latched while your baby's in the seat. It should be at armpit level, not near, the baby's waist or too close to his neck.

Be careful with padding. Avoid placing any padding inside the seat that could come between the baby and the seat's harnesses, unless the pads and accessories are supplied by the specific car seat's manufacturer. Extra padding could split the belts apart, affecting your baby's safety or allowing him to be ejected during a crash.

Keep loose and hard objects out of the backseat. Don't insert a front tray or allow hard toys in front of your baby's car seat. Keep groceries, suitcases, and all heavy objects out of the backseat. They could become flying projectiles during a crash.

Don't keep your baby in a seat that's designed for babies heavier/lighter, taller/shorter than recommended by the manufacturer. And keep your child's needs in mind. Don't use a restraint with a harness with a 45-pounder when the harness should be removed at 40 pounds; don't try to adapt a car seat with equipment that doesn't belong to the seat, such as repairing broken parts with substitute parts; and don't use the seat as an adult-belt positioner if your child is still in the weight range for harnesses.

Be conscious of side air bags. Not all cars have side air bags in the rear passenger compartment. If your car does, be sure to read the instructions about the safe placement of a car seat in the owner's manual for your vehicle, and train your children to stay upright in the seat and to keep their hands and bodies inside the seat.

SAFETY CONSIDERATIONS

Strict government regulations control how babies' and children's car seats are made, such as the height of seat backs (to protect children's necks and spines), the amount of pressure needed to unlatch the seats' buckles (to keep toddlers from releasing them), and the type of impact-absorbing foam used.

The location of warning labels on the seats and their precise wording are also prescribed. Car seat installation instructions must also meet exacting requirements, and seats must provide a permanent place to store the instructions.

Car seats also have to go through mock crashes in sled tests, using a variety of weighted baby- and child-size dummies wired to reveal crash pressures. The tests simulate two cars hitting head-on while each is traveling at 30 miles per hour and a car crashing into a brick wall at the same speed. Tests' results must show that the dummies' heads and bodies were well protected by the seats. Most car seat manufacturers hire engineers and laboratories to ensure that their car seat designs not only meet but exceed federal safety standards.

8

CLOTHING & SHOES

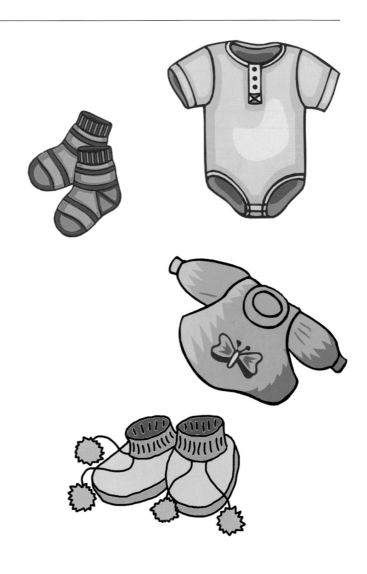

Your baby will arrive in her birthday suit, but from there on out, it's up to you to supply her with outer trappings. Whether you go for basic tee-shirt-and-diaper combos or choose to make a pint-size fashion statement is completely up to you. All your baby really asks of you is to be kept comfortable and protected from the elements. This chapter will help you weigh all your head-to-toe options and includes tips on how to launder baby clothes and choose shoes. It also discusses flammability and other clothing safety issues.

DUDS FOR THE DIAPER SET

Strolling through the baby clothing section of stores is sure to evoke ooohs and aaahs from even the most cynical shoppers. They're so soft! So cute! So tiny! And nothing (besides your first sonogram) will make your baby feel more real than folding miniature shirts and gowns into a drawer.

There's no need to go overboard on goo-goo Gucci designer outfits (unless you want to and can afford it). A hardy supply of tee shirts, footed sleepers, and a few gowns will do for those early months when you and your baby are getting used to each other. Most parents also like to have at least one or two newborn-size show-off outfits in a little-girl or little-boy mode for photo ops.

One thing to remember as you start to shop and price baby clothes is that your baby is going to outgrow them with lightning speed—no matter how costly or cute they are. Most babies nearly double their weight within the first four months. Unless your baby is tiny because she arrived sooner than expected, all teensy shirts, sweaters, and gowns in the newborn size will soon be useless. (More about getting the right size later.)

Cotton knits are usually the preferred fabric for everyday baby wear. Babies wet and soil clothes with alarming frequency, and cotton is more absorbent than synthetics. Manufacturers size garments larger on purpose because cotton shrinks and becomes denser (and also softer) with repeated laundering. Cotton/polyester and all-synthetic clothes are more affordable, less likely to wrinkle, and more likely to sport brighter patterns. On the downside, they're usually less breathable and tend to hold onto stains more than natural fabrics do.

Your baby's point of view

Before you start shopping for your baby's unique look, we'd like to issue a minority report from the baby side. If your baby could talk, she'd let you know that she'd much prefer to go naked and be up against your skin all the time if she could. She'd tell you that she hates being dressed and undressed. Suddenly being exposed to drafts is scary and makes her think she's falling. Pulling a shirt down over her face is downright painful and makes her think you're trying to suffocate her. Her feet are more sensitive than her

---

Quick tip

Remember, you are going to be changing between 10 and 14 diapers a day! Buy baby clothes that are easy to get on and off. The easier the diaper change, the happier you'll be.

---

hands, and socks or booties can help her feel more secure. She'd also let you know that her new skin is hypersensitive to touch. She can feel the least amount of roughness and scratchiness from clothes, and her skin may turn red from rubbing or break out in a rash from chemicals and perfumes used to wash her clothes. Exercise care in what you put next to your baby's skin!

The temperature factor

The number one purpose for clothes when your baby is new is to help keep her warm and protect her from the elements. When you dress your newborn, keep indoor and outdoor temperatures in mind. At best, your newborn's body has a very primitive heating-and-cooling system. Babies lose as much as 50 percent of their body heat from the neck up, which is why nurses pop little caps on them as soon as they arrive.

Your baby will need more warmth at first. After all, she's used to floating in amniotic fluid that's nearly 100 degrees. If your baby is feeling chilled, her skin will become mottled and there may be a slightly bluish cast to her skin and lips. Her jaw may tremble, and she may become more active, moving her arms and legs closer to her body in an attempt to get warm. If she's exposed to wind, a primitive reflex may cause her to gasp as though she were drowning. In some

---

When to Buy

Stock up on a small collection of newborn-size clothing before baby arrives, and then plan to purchase larger sizes after birth, since your baby will grow very rapidly. Booties and socks will be useful until your baby starts to crawl and walk (6 to 15 months), then a pair of soft-soled shoes can help to protect toes and feet.

Clothing Basics

TYPE OF GARMENT	DESCRIPTION	NUMBER OF PIECES	COMMENT
Bibs	Small, washable shirt protectors with easy-open neck closures	3–4	Babies constantly drool and spit up, so use them to protect clothing
Booties	Soft knitted baby shoes with ties or elastic at the ankle to help keep them on a baby's feet. (See "socks" below)	1–2 pairs	They offer extra warmth for your baby's feet, especially outdoors or in chilly places
Caps	A close-fitting knitted hat for winter. For summer: a brimmed hat with a neckband to hold it on and a flap to cover the back of the baby's neck for sun protection.	At least 2	Most babies hate wearing hats, but head coverings can help keep a baby from losing heat in the cold and protect from glare and sunburn in warm weather. (Expect to lose them often.)
Fabric diapers	Thick, soft refolded terry or flannel panels	At least 2 dozen, even if you plan to use disposables; and 4 dozen if you'll always use fabric diapers, not throwaways	Useful if you run out of disposables, they make great milksops, and they can protect your shoulder from spit-ups. Always carry 1 or 2 in your diaper bag.
Footed sleepers	Stretchy pajama suits with long sleeves and covered feet	2–5	Use in winter to keep your baby warm overnight. Avoid exposed metal zippers, and metal snaps. Inspect for loose strings that could tightly wrap around and pinch fingers, toes, or a penis.

TYPE OF GARMENT	DESCRIPTION	NUMBER OF PIECES	COMMENT
Nightgowns	Full-length all cotton or cotton-poly blends with an open or gently elasticized hem	2–5	Use in fall and spring to keep baby's legs covered at night. Fold-over cuffs for the hands keep your baby's fingernails from scratching her cheeks. Avoid gowns that have string ties.
Onesies	All-cotton knit shirts that have wide neck openings and snap at the crotch	6 or more (or 6 tee shirts)	Choose long sleeves for winter, short sleeves for summer in 3-month or 6-month sizes
Shoes	Soft-soled and flexible—in leather, suede, or durable fabric with Velcro or elastic closures	Several pairs as your baby starts to crawl	Soft-soled shoes help protect your baby's toes from carpet burn when she starts to crawl and from injury when she's learning to walk. Avoid shoes with high sides or inflexible soles when walking begins—they will interfere with balance.
Sleep sack	A baby sleeping bag with armholes, made from fleece or quilting for cold weather	1 or 2	Use instead of a crib blanket and sheet in cold weather. Buy 6-month size with shielded zipper front, or snaps for access to the diaper area. Avoid appliqués that are scratchy on the inside.

TYPE OF GARMENT	DESCRIPTION	NUMBER OF PIECES	COMMENT
Snowsuit	The suit should have insulation, a hood, legs, and a zipper from crotch to ankles for diapering	1 or 2 (for cold weather)	Buy one plenty big enough to easily take your baby through her first winter. For a late-winter baby, a sleep sack (see above) may suffice. Use only garments that can adapt to the shoulder and crotch straps in car seats.
Socks	Cotton knit with soft cuffs, preferably with elastic to keep them on the feet	6 or more pair for starters	Booties may be warmer, but socks stay on better. Tiny socks get lost easily, and washing machines tend to eat them. Fold down one cuff of the pair over the other to keep the two together, or stuff them all in a zippered lingerie bag.
Sweaters	Choose soft, well-knitted cardigans that close in front with a zipper or snaps. Use for winter warmth or in buildings with air-conditioning.	At least 2	Buy the 6-month size and roll up the sleeves. Sweaters should be washable and not have scratchy lace or appliqués. Avoid loose knits that could capture tiny fingers.
Tee shirts	All-cotton baby tees that snap on the side, or have wide necks that slip over the head	5–12 (depending on how often you'll be doing the laundry)	Quickly outgrown. Buy 2 in newborn size but get the rest in 3-month size. Choose short sleeves for summer and long sleeves for winter.

cases, if a baby seems too sluggish to nurse actively, undressing her a little will awaken her and get her to nurse better. (Note: For the first half year, babies' feet are almost always cooler than the rest of their bodies.)

If it's cool or drafty in your home, a nightgown or footed sleeper, a cap on her head and socks on her feet will help maintain her body temperature. After a few weeks, her body will mature enough so that she'll feel comfortable in approximately the same temperature zone as you. If it's cold outside, your baby will also need a cap and a "bunting" that resembles a sleeping bag with sleeves, and possibly a hood.

It's also important to avoid overheating your baby by bundling her up too much or exposing her to high temperatures. Babies' bodies don't sweat to cool down, and being overheated can make them very ill or even kill them, especially if they're already ill and running a fever. Babies have died from heatstroke when left in hot cars at temperatures that wouldn't harm an adult.

Baby-clothing basics

How many shirts, gowns, and other clothing items to stock up on will depend a lot on how easy it is for you to do laundry. Babies mess up and wet on shirts and other clothes several times a day. If you don't have a washer or dryer at home, you'll definitely want to buy more baby clothes, so you can wait longer than a day before you have to haul a load off to your mom's or the self-service laundry.

Experienced parents often wait to stock up on clothes until after their babies arrive. That makes it easier to judge what you need and how much. (Note: If you have a preemie or a low-birth-weight baby, tiny clothes are sometimes hard to find. You might try browsing Internet specialty stores such as www.preemie-clothes.com and www.preemiesleepers-.com.)

Getting the right size for your baby

Baby clothing sizes are all over the board! While some brands reflect most babies' actual sizes, others run big or small. There are no uniform standards that manufacturers and brands follow and no uniform standard for newborn, 3-, 6-, 9-, or 12-month (or larger) sizes. And if you've got a girl or boy who's in the 90th percentile for her age, or a petite preemie, you'll have to adjust age recommendations for fit. Since babies grow so rapidly, it makes sense to bump your baby's clothing up a size or two (if you're sure they won't swallow her) when you're purchasing new clothes.

In some cases, clothing marked the same size from the same brand may vary in actual size. Sometimes all-cotton garments are larger than those made from synthetic materials because cotton shrinks with washing. Or it could be that the clothing company has outsourced its garment making to different factories, so the same product in the same-style packaging may have variations in sizing.

While prepackaged clothes often have baby weight and length guidelines listed on the back of the package to help in finding the right size, folded and hanging clothing in stores may have to be eyeballed to tell what size to buy. Some baby-clothing stores have size charts at the customer service counter, so it's worth asking.

If you want to take advantage of sales or to stock up in advance, a quick source for predicting your baby's future height and weight is to print out growth charts that are available online for both boy and girl babies at www.cdc.gov/growthcharts. You can use the chart to help you to project how your baby's weight and length will change month by month for the first 36 months.

Remember, though, that your baby's clothing needs will change by seasons, too. For example, if you come across a great buy in winter wear and your baby will arrive in late summer or early fall, you'll probably need a 12-month size to take her through the year. But if your baby is expected mid-winter, then the 6-month size will do.

WARNING

Baby clothes can burn!
The U.S. Consumer Product Safety Commission (CPSC) recommends that parents avoid using loose-fitting, all-cotton garments for babies' and children's pajamas, because they ignite rapidly if they're exposed to a flame. It requires that clothing labeled as sleepwear be flame resistant. Form-fitting clothing is considered safest. Newborns are not likely to wander near flames, but if you or someone in your household smokes, you use a woodstove or kerosene heaters, or you have open-flame stovetop units, consider flame-retardant sleepwear and clothing.

 # Checklist

Baby clothes shopping

Here are a few things to look for when shopping for baby clothes.

✔ **Quality fabrics and construction.** Absorbent and able to withstand multiple washings without fraying, unraveling, or shrinking. While some shirts and gowns may be thick, well sewn, and generous in sizing, others may be flimsy, have loose threads, and be smaller than normal. Open the packages to make sure what you're getting.

✔ **Washability.** All baby clothes should be machine washable and fade resistant.

✔ **Comfort features.** Wide or stretchy necks or front closures make dressing the baby easier. Zippers should be plastic, rather than metal, and have protective plackets to keep them from scratching skin.

✔ **Soft elastic.** Elastic should have a lot of give so it won't constrict baby's wrists or waist, and it should be soft to the touch, without scratchy seams or stitching.

✔ **Snap-open crotches.** Pants and footed sleepers (one-piece pajamas) should have snap closures for quick access to the diaper area. Gowns should offer easy diaper access.

✔ **Flexible cuffs.** Pants or shirts with easy-to-roll-up cuffs will make room for your baby to grow.

Highs & lows of baby clothing and shoes

Highs. Clothes and shoes designed with babies in mind can help keep your baby cozy and comfortable. The best qualities are softness, quality construction, ease in putting on or taking off, washability, and well-finished seams and details. Color and patterns can be visually intriguing to babies. Warm winter outfits, booties, caps, and socks can help keep baby warm.

Lows. Clothes that are stiff or scratchy can be uncomfortable to babies and irritate their skin. Dresses interfere with crawling. Clothing that is flimsy or can't stand up to frequent washing is a waste of money. Metal zippers and snaps can scratch, cut, or cause skin reactions. Small objects sewn onto clothing, such as ribbons, flowers, or decorative objects, can be ingested and cause choking. Loose strings can badly pinch fingers, toes, or baby's penis, and hood strings are a strangulation hazard.

Avoid:

✗ **Tight or scratchy elastic at wrists, around the waist or legs.** Could irritate baby's skin or leave marks.

✗ **Turtleneck shirts.** Will be a challenge to pull on and off.

✗ **Tiny, sharp metal-backed snaps.** Could scratch baby's skin or cause an allergic skin reaction.

✗ **Unshielded metal zippers.** Could scratch or catch baby's skin.

✗ **Appliqués.** Inside liners and stitching are scratchy.

✗ **Drawstring hoods.** Could catch on something in the crib or playground and strangle the baby.

✗ **Pull-down pants.** Not having snap access to the diaper area can be a hassle.

✗ **Small bows or buttons.** Your baby can remove and choke on them.

✗ **Bulky winter outerwear.** Unless they are adapted to car-seat harnesses, they may interfere with the holding power of the seat.

✗ **Anything requiring dry cleaning.** The garments may be outgrown by the time you pick them up, and they may be returned with chemical residues that can harm your baby.

CENTS SENSE

Buy multipacks. 3- or 4-packs of tee shirts or socks are cheaper than individual units.

Shop discount stores. You may be able to buy shirts, gowns, and other items at a great saving. Just be sure you're getting quality garments and not poorly made ones.

Buy one to two sizes larger. Your baby will be growing rapidly over the next few months. Go up one to two sizes, and select garments with sleeves or cuffs that can be rolled up when your baby is small and unfolded as she grows.

Go used. Beg and borrow baby clothes from friends who no longer need them, and shop thrift and consignment stores to get great bargains. (Some stains are to be expected, but you can easily handle that. See our laundering tips below.)

Watch for end-of-season sales. Most department and baby-apparel stores periodically put clothes on sale. You may be able to find high-quality garments at half the price when they go on sale.

Shop Internet auctions. You may luck out and get stacks of previously owned baby clothes for a steal.

Return (or exchange) impractical clothing gifts. Exchange baby clothes that aren't practical and comfortable or that require dry-cleaning—or ask for a refund so you can buy more appropriate duds.

Make your own. Most fabric shops offer easy-to-make baby patterns. Consider sewing your own bibs, nightgowns, or toddler overalls. While ready-made corduroy or quilted overalls for crawlers are expensive to buy, they're simple to make and can help protect your baby's knees from carpet burn.

Laundering tips

When you've got a baby in the house, you can be certain that you'll be washing piles of soiled shirts, onesies, pants, and gowns. Typically, babies run through several changes a day when they burp down the front of tee shirts and when onesies get damp from diaper overflows.

Special "baby" detergents aren't needed for laundering your baby's duds. These tend to cost more, and powdered versions can clog up fibers in baby clothes, making them less absorbent. Perfumed detergents can irritate a baby's nose or cause skin reactions.

For these reasons, we recommend using a liquid, fragrance-free detergent and that you avoid both liquid and sheet-style fabric softeners. Milk is a great thing for growing babies, but it tends to set in and stain the baby shirts and gowns (as well as your own clothes), and urine can stain,

> **"** Newborn outfits aren't worth the money. Your baby will only wear them a couple of times. My baby stayed in gowns and little one-piece pajamas for the first three months. I especially liked the gowns because they allowed her to curl up her legs like when she was in the womb. **"**

too, especially if you take a few days to get around to doing the laundry.

Here are our suggestions for handling stains.

Blot. Blot the stain with a napkin or paper towel to absorb as much of the liquid as you can. This will make it easier to get the residue out during washing.

Presoak. Soak the stained item in cold water as quickly as possible to keep milk from drying and flaking. A half-teaspoon of household ammonia and peroxide stirred into water may help to lift the stains, and some parents find that color-safe (non-chlorine) bleaches work well. The best place to do this is directly in the washing machine or in the kitchen sink.

Follow directions. Read the laundering tag that comes on the garment. Regular bleach should not be used on garments made from polyester or other synthetic materials, but the newer non-chlorine bleach products may work.

Treat before washing. Rub some liquid laundry detergent into the stain with your finger or a toothbrush and let it sit for a few minutes before laundering. Oxygen-based cleaners and soaks may help, but run an extra rinse cycle in the washing machine to make sure there are no chemical residues.

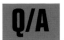

Q **We've decided not to find out the sex of our baby, but to wait and be surprised. Any suggestions for neutral baby clothing that could go either way?**

Whites, pastel yellows, pale turquoises, and greens all work well. And baby girls and boys both look good in stripes. Remember, too, that you don't need to stock up beforehand. The stores will still be open after your baby arrives, and shopping then will make for a fun outing.

Q **What do you suggest for our newborn's first, take-home outfit?**

We recommend a soft one-piece stretch sleeper with attached feet and snaps between the legs, in a newborn size. This will keep your baby's feet and body warm and make it easy to strap her into the car seat. Top the sleeper with a small jacket or a sweater in a tight weave that won't capture your baby's tiny fingers. A simple skullcap will help keep her from losing heat, but bonnets with ties or elasticized straps will set off your baby's sucking reflex and drive her nuts. Be sure to bring along a blanket and put it over her after she's strapped in the car seat, since you don't want it to interfere with the seat's harness straps. All clothing should be washed in a fragrance-free detergent to remove sizing and chemicals before putting them on your baby. (If this is your first baby, expect to feel awkward dressing her at first. A nurse may offer to help you.)

Q **My best friend is expecting her first baby, and I'd like to buy some clothes for her baby shower. Have you any suggestions about what to get?**

The more practical, the better! We'd suggest several footed sleepers and gowns that could go either "boy" or "girl" (in case the sonogram is wrong!). For colors, select pastels in gentle patterns. Some onesies (tee shirts that snap at the crotch) and one or two long nightgowns with gently elasticized hems to keep them from riding up over the baby's knees are also useful. Consider buying just a few of the clothing items in the newborn size, and the rest in the 3-month size so the baby can wear them longer. A matching pair of booties and a cap will complete a gift ensemble. For a fun touch, clip each piece of clothing on a length of thick, bright yarn, knotted on each end, to make an imaginary clothesline. Line the gift box with baby-themed tissue paper and carefully fold each item so that the clothes can be drawn out one at a time.

Choosing baby shoes and socks

Soft-soled shoes may help protect your baby's toes from getting red and sore from rug burn when she starts to crawl. Shoes made from leather with Velcro-style closures work well, as do those made with sturdy fabrics with ankle ties to keep your baby from pulling them off easily.

First steps aren't a signal to go out and buy shoes with high sides that resemble combat boots, those with artificial arches, or baby versions of track shoes. Babies are naturally flat-footed and they use their toes and foot muscles along with their sensation of the ground beneath them to help them learn how to balance upright. Barefoot is the best way to go, unless it's cold, there are rough surfaces, or she tries ambulating outside where extra foot protection is needed.

The best shoes for new walkers are those with flexible soles and soft leather booties with easy-on Velcro or elastic closures. Shoes with nonslip soles can snag on carpeting and cause the baby to trip; and stiff, slippery-soled shoes may make it all too easy for your baby to slip and fall.

Be sure to inspect shoes frequently to make sure your baby's big toe isn't getting squeezed in the front of the shoe, and examine your baby's feet every time you take shoes off to be sure there's no red-

WARNING

Avoid soaking clothes in buckets

Soaking buckets can be dangerous. Toddlers can drown in buckets or containers, even if they're only partially filled. Their heads are proportionately much heavier than their bodies, and they don't have the strength to right themselves if they fall in headfirst. Typically, drowning happens when babies drop objects into the bucket and then reach down to retrieve them.

ness from chafing or pressure points.

Socks should be absorbent cotton knits that are a little longer than your baby's feet. If they're too tight, they could cause her toes to curl and affect muscle action and gait. The seams should be smooth, with no rough edges that could rub or chafe baby's feet.

Each time you put socks on your baby, turn them inside out to make sure there are no loose threads that can get wrapped around her toes and cut off circulation. Buy new socks, rather than using hand-me-downs, since older socks tend to shrink and get tighter over time, causing toe seams to become more uncomfortable.

SAFETY CONSIDERATIONS

Hundreds of items of baby clothing have been recalled by the U.S. Consumer Product Safety Commission (CPSC) over the years. Usually, recalled items have fasteners, buttons, ribbons, or other small parts that come loose and could choke a baby if they're swallowed. Loose-fitting sleepwear for babies over 9 months of age, such as nightgowns and pajamas, are also recalled if they fail flammability standards.

Hooded clothing for children can be recalled if it uses tie strings that could catch on something and lead to strangulation. If you'd like to learn more about clothing recalls or flammability issues, you can do a search from CPSC's site (www.cpsc.gov). Recalls can also be accessed from www.recalls.gov by entering keywords such as "recalls," "baby clothing," and the year you would like to search under the CPSC listing.

9

CRIBS, MATTRESSES & BEDDING

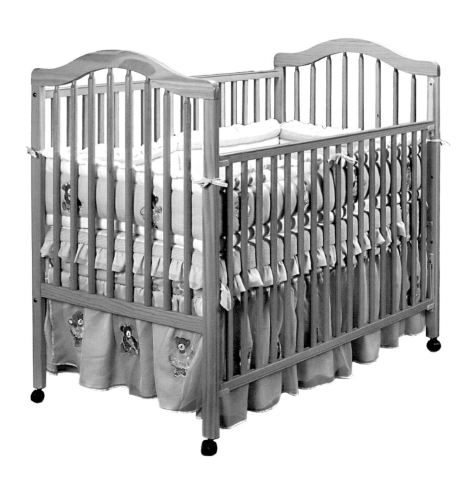

A crib is one of the first pieces of major baby equipment you'll probably invest in. Although cribs come in lots of different furniture designs and finishes, all standard cribs are identical when it comes to their inside dimensions—thanks to federal regulations. Here's everything you need to know about bedding down your baby, from cribs and mattresses to sheets and blankets, plus lots of important information about crib safety and SIDS issues.

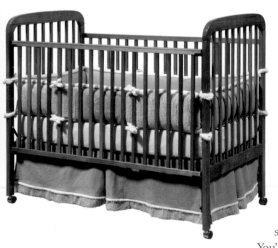

GETTING A BEAD ON BABY BEDS

It goes without saying that full-size cribs are the rectangular baby beds with bars on 2 or 4 sides that are sold in virtually every baby store. When it comes to choosing the best crib, it's important to remember that your baby will probably spend more time in his crib than any-where else, so sleeping comfort and safety are important.

You'll have to admit it's a little daunting to stroll through the crib section of a big-box baby store. Except for changes in wood finishes or painted colors or a few styling touches on each end, the 25 cribs in the row are apt to look almost identical.

Stringent federal safety regulations have been established to address the thousands of crib-related accidents that have occurred over the past dozen years. Because of these accidents, the interior dimensions of all standard cribs are required to be the same so that mattresses fit flush against all sides.

All bars must be no more than $2^{3/8}$ inches apart to keep babies' bodies from slipping through, leaving their heads caught inside. There can be no less than 26 inches between the tallest part of the crib and the mattress support when it's in its highest position, to help prevent babies from falling out. Regulations also limit the size of crib elements that stick up out of the end boards (protrusions), to help protect babies from getting their clothing or pacifier strings tied around their necks caught on them, which could lead to strangulation. (Find out more on crib safety issues starting on page 144.)

When to Buy

Purchase your baby's crib and mattress during the second or third trimester of pregnancy, or postpone and use a portable crib or bedside bassinet or sleeper until the baby starts to roll over and pull up—around 4 to 6 months—then move him to a larger bed.

What you get for the money

Bottom-of-the-line cribs are priced between $100 and $150. The only problem is that the least expensive cribs will probably feel cheap, too, with rough or careless wood finishing, a chalky or peeling painted surface, thick flat slats, flimsy mattress supports and hardware, plus the cribs' frames may be a bit rattly when given a good shaking.

Most mainstream cribs fall in the $200 to $350 price range. In this arena are better-finished cribs in natural wood colors or smooth, rich painted colors, with an easy-to-operate drop side on at least one side, thicker metal hardware and mattress supports, and an overall feeling of sturdiness when given the jiggle test.

Sometimes costing a few hundred more are convertibles—cribs with parts that can be screwed into other furniture configurations after the crib stage is over. Then above $350 and going as high as $1,000 (or more) are imported cribs, some of which have deep-colored wood stains, silky smooth finishing, and heavily detailed headboards and end boards worthy of a millionaire's home (and bank account).

The trouble with convertibles

Convertible cribs—otherwise known as 2-in-1s, 3-in-1s, 4-in-1s, and even 5-in-1s—are all the rage right now. On the surface, they appear to be an economical purchase: With one buy, you get not only a crib but the components for a toddler bed, and possibly a love seat, a daybed, and a frame for a full-size bed made by combining the crib's end boards.

Here's what the numbers mean. A 2-in-1 converts into a toddler bed using the baby's mattress, once the crib sides are removed. A 3-in-1 reconfigures into a daybed, and the sides of the crib can be dismantled and screwed together to make a full-size headboard and footboard. Four-in-1s offer not only the crib and toddler-bed options, but can also be screwed together into a daybed or configured into a full-size headboard and footboard. Finally, 5-in-1s come with components that let them morph from a crib to a toddler bed, to a daybed, a love seat, or a full-size headboard and foot-board.

The more "in-ones" the better—right? Not exactly.

It's a case of convertibles being so "practical" that they're impractical! A 2-in-1 with a toddler bed conversion can come in handy for transitioning your toddler into a new sleeping arrangement once he tries climbing over the side of his crib, but most convertibles, including 2-in-1s, don't offer a lowering side, as standard cribs do. So you'll be bending over quite a bit to pick up or lay down a hefty sleeping baby, and when he's already asleep, it's deadweight going down.

Daybeds for 3-in-1s and up look exactly like what they really are: a crib with one side taken off. Most have an annoying wooden ledge in the front that can bruise small legs, and they're so deep that it takes a heap of pillows to make them even moderately serviceable, since even the hip-to-back-of-knee dimension of tall adults can't reach from front to back of a crib's mattress width.

As for the full-size headboard and end board option, a full-size bed will eat up all the space in your child's bedroom. If you're thinking "guest room," most adults sleep on nothing smaller than a queen-size bed these days.

Putting together a furniture ensemble for your child's room once the baby stage is ended makes much more sense. Then you can match furniture finishes, including a desk for doing homework, shelves for storing books and toys, twin beds, a night-stand, and possibly an armoire, all coordinated, rather than having an awkward and cumbersome furniture puzzle that will likely end up in the attic, being auctioned on eBay, or put out for your next yard sale.

Why pay more? A sturdy, mid-price crib with at least one easy-to-lower side will be the most serviceable and economical choice over the long haul (and the least amount of trouble). No matter what crib you buy, it's likely the mattress will be sold separately, so you'll need to add that cost into the equation. (Mattresses are discussed starting on page 139.)

How to assess a crib

There are subtle differences among cribs that aren't immediately apparent to the naked eye, and knowing how to spot them can help you make the best possible crib decision. Here are the important things to notice.

Type of wood. Cribs can be constructed of soft woods, such as pine, that are more likely to crack and dent; from composition materials, such as molded plastic combined with wood, that are virtually impossible to tell from all-wood versions; and they can be made purely from hardwoods, such as birch, oak, ash, or beech, that are superior because of their hardness and durability. In addition, the metal screws, which hold the crib's frame together and fasten the mattress support hardware to the frame, are far less likely to pull out of a hardwood frame. Asian wood is now being used for many cribs. Although the wood is likely hardwood, there's no way to tell for sure. The basic rule of thumb is that the heavier the crib frame, the denser the wood and the thicker the hardware.

Wood finish. Painted cribs come in a variety of colors from pale whites and creamy pastels to barnyard reds and even black. Most parents prefer natural or stained wood finishes. Wood finishes that are pale are less likely to show scratches and dents than darker cherry and mahogany stains. In some cases, painted cribs and darker stains are used by manufacturers to cover up flaws found in less expensive cuts of wood or composition materials used in end boards.

Hardware and construction. It pays to "take a look under the hood" and check the quality of all the parts that hold the crib together. The critical pieces of hardware in the crib are the screws and brackets that hold the sides and ends together; the components in the sides and the frame that allow the sides to raise and lower, often made of white molded nylon; the metal parts that fasten the mattress support to the frame; metal stabilizer bars that run the length of the crib from one end board to the other to stabilize the crib's frame; and the wheels or casters on the bottoms of the legs, which need to be sturdy and lockable.

Side-lowering mechanisms. While some cribs, particularly convertibles, don't have sides that can lower at all, standard mainstream cribs, sometimes called single cribs, usually have at least one side that can be lowered by a simple lift-and-knee-press action. The side will lock into place when it's raised to its highest position. Try out the side-lowering mechanisms to make sure they're easy for you to operate but will be impossible for a tot to work from either inside or outside the crib.

Bar finishing. Crib slats, sometimes called bars or spindles, have top and bottom railings. Unfortunately, teething babies like to pull themselves up by the slats to gnaw on the wood railings that run across the top of the sides. Look for rounded plastic covers, called teething rails, on the crib's top rails, which discourage chewing. They should be well secured, so your baby can't pull them off, and fitted all the way to the end of the

railing, with no sharp or loose edges that could cut or capture your baby's fingers. And there should be no rough, splintery, or exposed wood where the teething rail ends.

End-board design. Crib end boards can be smooth and plain, or they may be carved and have posts or wooden cornice-like configurations that stick out over the edge of the top of the ends. Avoid cribs with scrollwork, overhanging edges, knobs, protrusions, or decorative posts at the end that could hang your baby if a shirt, the neck of a nightgown, or a pacifier ribbon tied around the baby's neck got caught on them.

Underside storage drawer. Storage drawers that slide or roll out from under the crib can be useful, but a drawer could run up the price of the crib by as much as $100. Check out the drawer's quality, particularly the strength of the floor and how easily the drawer slides in and out from under the crib, before you pay extra for one.

Assembling the crib

Cribs come in long slender boxes. You can expect the assembling process with screws and bolts to take about an hour, and it takes two people to do it. Be forewarned that installing the lowering side can be a hassle. Plan to assemble the crib where it will stay. Once it's together, it will be too large to go through the doorway. For safety's sake, follow the directions very carefully.

Checklist

Crib shopping

Look for the following features when you shop for a crib:

✔ **JPMA certified.** A "JPMA Certified" sticker shows that the brand passes voluntary safety tests beyond federal safety regulations.

✔ **One (or no) drop side.** An easy-to-lower crib side simplifies putting your baby in and taking him out, especially in that stage before he can stand up on his own. The action should be a simple lift-and-knee-press maneuver that you can easily do, but a toddler inside or outside the crib can't.

✔ **Smooth finish.** All surfaces smooth and splinter-free.

✔ **Solid structure.** Frame doesn't rattle when shaken. Bars are well fastened on top and bottom and won't twist or move. (Glue residue spilled out onto the wood and uncovered nail or staple holes are signs of poor craftsmanship.)

✔ **Sturdy mattress support.** Some mattress supports can be raised to a variety of heights. More important is the sturdiness of the support and the hardware that fastens the support to the crib's frame. Check the hardware underneath that fastens the mattress support to the crib corners, to make sure it is strong and thick.

✔ **Locking wheels.** If the crib has wheels, they should be lockable to prevent a baby's motion from "walking" the crib.

✔ **Assembly option.** Paying to have the store assemble the crib in your baby's nursery may be worth the money. It will save you an hour or two of intense labor; plus, it will enable you to inspect the crib for flaws or dents on the spot.

Avoid:

✗ **Used cribs.** Older-model cribs, heirloom cradles, and bassinets can be hazardous! Deadly problems: weakened screw holes; broken hardware; loosened or widely spaced bars; varnish or paint containing lead; poorly fitting, mushy, or mildewed mattresses; and protruding knobs or wide cutouts that strangle by capturing clothing or small heads.

✗ **Ornate models.** Avoid cribs with scrollwork, overhanging edges, knobs, protrusions, or finials that could be safety hazards.

✗ **Crib-mattress combos.** Cribs are *not* usually sold with the mattress unless the crib is an unusual shape (round, for example). Be cautious about buying a "crib-and-mattress store special" unless you're sure the mattress is of good quality and sufficiently firm. (See mattress discussion beginning on page 139.)

✗ **Flimsy teething rails.** Avoid a crib with a plastic teething rail that can be pulled loose to expose rough, splintery wood underneath or one that has exposed sharp edges.

✗ **Puffy quilts, pillows, and bumper bedding ensembles.** They're beautiful, they're fashionable, they're costly—and they're *deadly*. Don't let an overeager salesperson talk you into buying these accoutrements. They've figured in numerous baby suffocations and should never be used inside a crib.

Highs & lows of cribs

Highs. The biggest advantage of buying a crib, rather than other types of baby beds, is that cribs are governed by stringent federal regulations, which means they are constantly being monitored for flaws and recalled when baby injuries and near misses start showing up. In addition, certain crib models are also covered by voluntary JPMA certification standards, so crib models sporting a "JPMA Certified" sticker are from manufacturers who have chosen to have their cribs tested for additional safety and durability compliance.

Lows. Full-size cribs are so large they can't fit through most doorways. Newborns and young babies don't need all that room. Poorly functioning older cribs and newer models with poor craftsmanship can be hazardous, and sometimes fatal injuries occur.

Keeping baby safe for sleep

Once you've set up your baby's crib and he's ready to be put down for sleep, there are some important practices you should remember to protect your baby from crib and sleep hazards. These suggestions from the Consumer Product Safety Commission (www.cpsc.gov) are for putting babies to sleep who are less than 12 months old.

✔ **On the back.** Place baby on his back on a firm, tight-fitting mattress in a crib that meets current safety standards.

✔ **No soft items.** Remove pillows, quilts, comforters, sheepskins, pillow-like stuffed toys, and other soft products from the crib.

✔ **Tuck blanket to underarm level.** If using a blanket, put baby face-up in the lower half of the crib with his feet a few inches from the crib's end panel. Then tuck a thin blanket at least 2 inches under the mattress on 3 sides, reaching only as far as the baby's chest.

✔ **Keep head uncovered.** Make sure your baby's head remains uncovered during sleep.

✔ **Avoid waterbeds and other soft surfaces.** Do not put baby to sleep on a waterbed, sofa, soft mattress, futon, pillow, couch cushion, or other soft surface.

✔ **No low-hanging objects.** Keep low-hanging objects away from the crib—that is, cords from window blinds, drapes, wall hangings, etc.— and ensure that mobiles and toys are at least 10 to 12 inches away from baby's face. Remove the mobile from the crib entirely when your baby begins to pull up.

Q/A

Q We ordered our baby's crib from the Internet when my wife was 6 months pregnant. We left it in the box for 2 months, and now we're putting it together in the baby's room. It's a piece of junk! There are lots of flaws in the wood, and the side doesn't work right. There's rough wood in places and glue residue where the bars fasten in. We want to ship it back, but customer service for the company says it's too late to return it. What should we do?

The malfunctioning crib side could be a life-threatening safety hazard for your baby, so that may be your strongest bargaining chip for getting your money refunded. You could try writing to the president of the company that manufactured the crib, listing the specific problems that you're having. (Enclose a duplicate copy of your online order and detail the crib's flaws.) Close-up pictures will help, too. You could also contact the consumer service line for the attorney general's office in your state to get advice, since the e-tailer is doing business in your state. Most states have lemon laws that apply not only to cars but also to other consumer products.

Explain to the manufacturer that you need to have the problem resolved, mention the safety issue, and refuse to take an exchange for the same model crib because of the problem. As a last resort, mention your hesitancy to sue the company using state lemon laws or to post negative reviews of the e-tailer on the 25 major parenting and consumer sites you are compiling. Tell the company that if it isn't willing to be reasonable, you feel you'll be forced to take action.

Q I've read online that SIDS deaths could be related to poisonous gases from the toxic materials used to make crib mattresses nonflammable. Is there any truth to that claim?

The jury is still out. Most of the studies of SIDS deaths that relate to levels of toxic gases that arise from chemical reactions between mattress materials and baby urine or molds are still very tentative and not based on large numbers or clear science. But the radical reduction in the sheer numbers of baby deaths from SIDS when babies are placed on their backs instead of face-down on mattresses does appear to confirm that breathing has something to do with the problem. Current scientific thought is that, at least in some cases, the baby's rebreathing of his own exhaled carbon dioxide may be the cause. Other theories suggest unusual heart rhythms or brain-signaling abnormalities. But the definitive answer for what causes SIDS is yet to be found.

Q My baby hates sleeping on his back, plus his head seems to be getting flat in the back. Is it safe to place him on his side sometimes?

Not according to the Consumer Product Safety Commission and the American Academy of Pediatrics. Recent studies appear to show that the SIDS risk is roughly equal whether the baby sleeps on his stomach or side but is greatly reduced if the baby sleeps on his back. Plan periodic "tummy time" sessions throughout the day. Put your baby on your lap or lie down on a blanket with him, along with a few appealing toys, and give him a chance to practice raising his head and to experience some eye-to-eye contact.

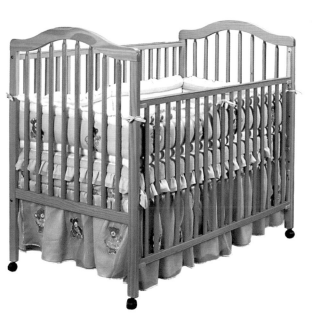

Storkcraft's Sandra Crib
($100)

Storkcraft is a Canadian firm, and its cribs conform to Canada's more stringent crib-safety standards. This simple crib design in a natural shade has locking castors, a one-piece mattress support that adjusts to 3 positions, and an easy-to-use one-handed side release for one side. (Note: Comes without mattress, bedding, or dust ruffle.)

Delta Children's Products' Normandy 3-in-1 Crib
($190)

This traditionally styled, JPMA-certified crib has arched end panels and smoothly rounded bars on all sides. There's a 3-position mattress support and one child-resistant drop side that can be released with one hand. The crib has 4 locking casters and the assembly of the crib is simple, requiring no tools. The crib can later be converted into a toddler bed. Stabilizer bars underneath help to strengthen the crib's frame. Available in different wood finishes. The manufacturer offers a limited 1-year warranty on defective parts. (Note: Comes without mattress, bedding, or dust ruffle.)

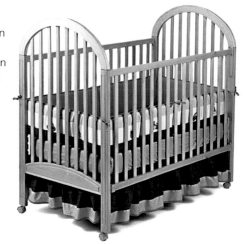

Million Dollar Baby's Da Vinci Alpha Crib — Oak

($225)
A dark-stained hardwood crib with rounded bars on all sides. It has a 4-level mattress support system and locking casters on the base. It features a smoothly gliding side-lowering system with a lift-and-knee-press action. (Note: Comes without mattress, bedding, or dust ruffle.)

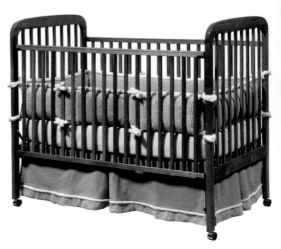

CHOOSING NURSERY FURNITURE

Choosing furniture and coordinating it with wallpaper or wall paintings, lamps, curtains, and other nursery trappings that would feel right at home in the pages of *Metropolitan Living* can be a great pastime during that l-o-n-g wait while you're growing your baby inside. Remember, though, that any nursery setup is scheduled to become obsolete in about two years when your baby turns into a rambunctious little tot with an entirely different set of furniture needs and visual interests.

Manufacturers and sales people like to talk parents into buying not just a crib but an entire coordinated bedroom suite—say, in pastel green with gentle meadow flowers painted on every piece of furniture, or some other coordinated design. Included in the suite might be a matching armoire and a chest with a diaper-changing platform on top, and possibly other pieces.

Although your friends and in-laws will all be gaga over the room, it's important

to remind yourself that your baby couldn't care less. All he *really* will want from you is to be nursed, rocked, soothed, and talked to.

If you do decide to purchase matching furniture pieces, it's important to give each one a thorough inspection. We've found that many armoires and chests that are made to coordinate with cribs are poorly constructed pieces that are simply stapled and glued together and ornamented with painted facades intended to coordinate with specific cribs offered by the crib manufacturer.

Soft, inexpensive woods may be used, with a thin fiberboard backing stapled on that is likely to warp over time. A foldout changing table on top of the chest may cause it to be unstable, or it may have hinges with screws that are likely to pull out of the furniture base from the weight of the baby.

Nursery furniture safety precautions

✔ **Drawer pulls.** Look for flush drawer pulls rather than protruding knobs, since babies can get hurt falling into them.

✔ **Drawer stops.** Drawers should have stops to keep them from being pulled out by a tot and falling on him.

✔ **Sturdy construction.** Inspect the insides of drawers and the backings of chests and armoires to assess their quality. Note if there are uneven staples or glue beads—signs of careless work.

✔ **Smooth finish.** Painted and wood-stained finishes should be smooth and have perfectly even coverage, with no roughness or areas with thin finishes.

✔ **Stable changing-table surface.** The changing area should offer adequate protection from baby falls, such as rails on all sides. If the changing table accessory is attached to the top of a chest, it should be well affixed by multiple screws. Try pushing down on the changer in its folded-out position to see if adding extra weight could cause the chest to tip over. The pad for the changer should be thick and smooth for easy wipedowns, and the retaining belt should be high quality, with a buckle that's easy to lock and release. (See page 161 for more information about changing tables.)

✔ **Add stability.** Fasten shelves and chests to the wall using straps or L-shaped hooks (available from hardware stores) so that these heavy pieces of furniture can't fall over on your toddler if he tries to climb them like a ladder.

Lead dangers in old furniture

You may be able to save money by purchasing quality furniture somewhere else besides a baby store, with an eye for using it later in the den or other places in your home. Antique or thrift stores are sometimes great places to find quality pieces that you can leave "as is" or refinish to go with your baby's room décor.

If you decide to use antique furniture in your baby's room, make sure it isn't finished with lead-containing lacquer or paint, since that poses a serious poison risk for babies (and their parents).

Furniture with a clear finish, and extremely old pieces aren't likely to be a problem, but those manufactured from the 1900s onward may have finishes that contain lead. Steer clear of old pieces with deteriorating finishes that are cracked, chipped, peeling, flaking, or have material that rubs off on your hands. Old varnish that's cloudy could contain lead, which was often mixed with varnish to produce a deeper, richer color. Finishes with an "alligator" crackling pattern that rubs off on your hands probably contain lead. (Don't try to refinish the pieces yourself, since the dust you stir up in the house or track in from the garage could affect both you and your baby.)

WARNING

Don't use an antique crib
The Consumer Product Safety Commission estimates there are 32 deaths per year in crib-associated accidents, and most of the deaths happened with older, used models. Old cribs made before CPSC and industry safety standards were enacted can entrap, strangle, or suffocate children. Old cribs with more than 2 3/8 inches between crib slats, with corner posts, or with cutouts on the headboard or footboard present suffocation and strangulation hazards. Those with missing or broken parts are also hazardous. Destroy old cribs and those with missing or broken parts, and never try to repair them yourself. Instead, purchase a crib that meets current safety standards.

Keeping your toddler in bed

Once your baby can pull to a stand inside his crib, he's likely to attempt climbing out by getting a leg up and over the bars. If he succeeds, it could mean a nasty head blow when he falls to the floor. In addition, some rambunctious tots like to use their cribs like trampolines, or to walk the crib by pushing and pulling inside so it bangs against the bedroom wall.

Here are some safety tips for keeping your baby safely secure in his crib.

✔ **Check the height of the mattress support.** While some cribs offer only one mattress height, others have mattress supports (otherwise known as springs) that adjust to different heights. The rim of the support fastens to the crib frame using brackets with S-shaped hooks, or other types of hardware, to allow the mattress height to be changed. (For maximum safety, except for a newborn, we suggest keeping the mattress at the lowest possible position.)

✔ **Take out the toys.** Remove the crib mobile once your baby gets up on all fours. The mobile could strangle a baby who becomes entangled in it. Enterprising climbers can use stuffed animals and toys for a boost over the rail.

✔ **Give the hardware a once-over.** A toddler can give a crib quite a workout. Check all screws, bars, and joints to make sure nothing is loose. Tighten any loose screws. But don't try to fix a broken crib. Doing so could be deadly. Completely dismantle and stop using a crib with any missing bars or malfunctioning hardware or side-lowering mechanisms. Either buy a new crib or move your tot to a toddler-size bed that uses a crib mattress.

WARNING
Pacifier danger!
Babies have accidentally hanged themselves when strings or ribbons tying pacifiers around their necks have gotten caught on crib or play yard components. Never tie a pacifier around your baby's neck.

✔ **Create a safety zone around the crib.** Move any furniture, including the chest or changing table, well out of your tot's reach from inside the crib, away from the window, and out of reach of drapery or blind cords. Watch out for wall hangings, the baby monitor, lamps, or other "reachables" that could be pulled over (or inside) the crib.

✔ **Pad the landing.** Put a soft rug or couch cushions on the floor underneath the crib in case your baby topples out.

✔ **Change beds.** If you find your baby is trying to climb out, it's time to take him out of the crib and move him to a low toddler bed. Until you can obtain one, place the crib mattress on the floor, since a fall from the height of the crib bars could cause head injuries. You may want to position a safety gate at his door so he doesn't get into trouble while you're sleeping.

CRIB MATTRESSES

Your baby will be sleeping on a crib mattress for 2 to 3 years—and maybe a couple more if you buy a 2-in-1 crib that converts to a pint-size toddler bed with the same dimensions as the crib. Since you'll be paying between $30 and $230 for a mattress, it's useful to learn all you can about their inner workings to make sure you get the best value for your money.

Although stores always display cribs with mattresses in them, they aren't included in the price of the crib. In some stores, salespeople are trained to immediately walk you to their mattress displays while you're still excited about choosing a crib for your baby and to bump you up to the most expensive model in the store.

It may surprise you that crib mattresses with famous mattress brand names usually aren't made by those companies at all. The brand name of the mattress has just been licensed to an entirely different company, and the name used as a way of appealing to shopping parents. The advantage of the brand name is that the mattress is likely to be constructed using top-grade materials, or it wouldn't be allowed to carry the famous name.

Claims that drive up mattress prices

Having a quality mattress is important, but there's no need to pay extra because of a sales pitch that your baby needs extra cushioning, more coils for back support, antibacterial protection, or a lifetime warranty. At best, these "deluxe" features are just sales ploys.

The claim that a mattress has antibacterial qualities simply means that a germ-killing chemical has been used to help destroy bacteria on the surface of the mattress, but research has shown that the results are minimal over the long haul. If a mattress claims to be nonallergenic or hypoallergenic, that merely means it's made of foam, instead of cotton and other fibers that could attract dust mites, which can cause allergic reactions.

And when it comes to a 10-year or lifetime warranty, read the fine print. You may find lots of loopholes that allow the manufacturer to get off the hook, including a sliding discount on the purchase of another mattress, rather than an actual replacement guarantee for a unit that breaks or splits open from toddler wear and tear.

The single most important consideration is mattress firmness. Babies' bodies are quite flexible. It's the adults who tote babies around who need the cushioning. Experts agree that the firmest possible mattress is best—one that adults might not feel comfortable sleeping on. Firmness helps prevent suffocation pockets created by a mushy surface that could surround the baby's face and cause him to suffocate.

It's what's inside that counts

There are basically two types of crib mattresses: innerspring and foam. The coverings on crib mattresses (called ticking) come in a variety of colors and materials, such as quilted, moisture-resistant fabric, laminated vinyl with nylon, or a combination of fabric and vinyl.

Ticking on baby mattresses needs to be thick and moisture-and stain-resistant. The best coverings are made from triple-laminated material, meaning the ticking is sewn from three thick layers of material heat-welded together, with nylon threads sandwiched between the layers.

As with cribs, federal regulations enforced by the U.S. Consumer Product Safety Commission mandate that all mattresses for standard rectangular cribs be a uniform length and width so that they will fit flush against crib sides and corners. That's to prevent the baby's throat from being compressed by the edge of the mattress should he lie over a sharply defined edge. Special-size cribs, such as round models, have to furnish appropriate mattresses with the crib.

Some mattresses may be thinner than others, with the maximum required depth being 6 inches. Once you get home with both the crib and the mattress, give the mattress the 2-finger test when it's inside the crib. No gap between the crib's frame and the mattress side should be wide enough for you to insert 2 fingers. If you find wide gaps, measure the interior of the crib as well as the mattress to see which is at fault, in order to return the offending product. The interior of the crib should measure 28 5/8 inches wide x 52 3/4 inches long, while the mattress should measure no more than 1 inch less.

How the mattress's cover is stitched together can be important. The binding around the edges of the mattress should be durable and double-stitched to prevent ripping and tearing.

Air vents—small metal-lined holes along the side of the mattress or pocket-style openings at both ends—allow the insides of the mattress to "breathe," and they also help to keep the seams from splitting when a toddler jumps up and down on the mattress. Higher-quality mattresses have woven bindings, such as strips of nylon tape to hold the seams together, rather than thin strips of vinyl.

Seams on higher-quality mattresses are also tightly double-stitched so they won't come loose.

Watch out for flimsy mattresses like the ones that are sold with cribs as a single unit and put on sale as "loss leaders" to draw parents into the store. You may discover that these poorer-quality mattresses have small metal grommets with holes in the center fastened onto the sides of the mattress, which can pose a choking hazard if a curious tot plucks them off and swallows them.

Quality, waterproof mattress pads that you can pull off and launder will help to protect the mattress from baby wetness and odors. To clean the mattress, wipe it down from time to time with a damp washcloth containing a few squirts of mild soap, such antibacterial hand soap. Rinse completely with a second moist cloth, then blot dry with paper towels. Never use harsh chemicals to clean the mattress, such as bleach or household cleaners. And don't attempt to dry the mattress with a hair dryer. It will melt the protective vinyl coating on the surface. Frequently flip the mattress over and rotate it end to end, too, to prevent sagging from constant use.

> **"Our son, Jared, drove us crazy! He would wake up at dawn, jam his crib back and forth until he walked it to the wall, and bang over and over until we came in to get him. Finally we put the crib on a rug and put the wheels inside circular holders, which we got in a hardware store, so we could have some peace. "**

Innerspring mattresses

Innerspring crib mattresses are like miniature adult ones. Underneath the ticking are thick layers of padding, a series of metal coils, and thick metal wires to support the mattress rim. As with mattresses for adults, better crib innersprings generally have more coils than less-expensive versions, and the coils in higher-quality models are generally made from steel.

Poorer-quality mattresses will have as few as 80 coils, while top-of-the-line models will offer 280 coils or more. Since mattress dimensions stay the same, additional coils create a firmer, less yielding mattress. But babies weigh only up to about 36 pounds while using the mattress, versus adults weighing 3 to 5 times that amount, so a huge spring count drives up the price but not the functional performance of a baby mattress. Claims that lots of coils will last longer than a good quality foam mattress simply aren't true. With only a few years of use and a lightweight sleeper, almost all mattresses except the truly flimsy ones will hold up sufficiently well as long as they're firm.

Mid- to upper-price mattresses will also offer additional girding to keep them uniformly firm from the center out to the edges and corners. Border rods, vertical steel bars, and frame bars are part of the internal support of higher-quality mattresses. Border rods run the perimeter of the mattress so if your child stands at the edge of the crib mattress it won't sink down but will remain firm. Interior steel vertical or X-frame bars help maintain an even, flat surface throughout the entire mattress.

WARNING

Crib suffocation dangers

Each year about 40 babies suffocate or strangle in their cribs when they become trapped between broken crib parts or in cribs with older, unsafe designs. Soft bedding such as quilts, comforters, or pillows can suffocate a baby. As many as 3,000 infants die each year from Sudden Infant Death Syndrome (SIDS), and up to a third of crib-related baby deaths are thought to be related to suffocating on soft bedding. The Consumer Product Safety Commission (CPSC) recommends that a baby under 12 months be put to sleep in a crib on his or her back, with no soft bedding. Adult sheets should never be used in a crib because they don't fit properly and pose a strangulation and suffocation risk to babies.

Highs & lows of innerspring

Highs. The main advantage of an innerspring mattress is that it offers variable support to different parts of your baby's body as he grows and gains weight.
Lows. The biggest drawback of innersprings is that they're substantially heavier and less flexible than foam mattresses, and that makes sheet changing—which you'll be doing once, possibly three times a day—more of a backbreaking hassle than with a foam mattress. Some innersprings sag in the middle after half a year or more of use. Plus, innersprings tempt toddlers to use them like trampolines, which could make your baby more vulnerable to falls and injuries when he hits the bars.

Foam mattresses

Foam mattresses come in a variety of prices and grades. The higher the quality of foam, the heavier they're likely to weigh and the denser they are.

Most foam mattresses are constructed from a single slab of foam, but higher-quality versions offer more than one density in the same mattress—a firm surface where baby sleeps and a tough, non-springy edge to reinforce the outer edges.

While a high-quality foam mattress will be hard and dense, poorer-grade versions will be lighter weight and squishy when you squeeze them. Foam mattresses vary in the quality of coverings, too. Quality mattresses will have thick ticking that's hard to pinch between your thumb and forefinger, while a poorer-grade version will have only a single layer of vinyl for a covering, one that can be easily pinched, and it will have vinyl rather than woven seam bindings, and possibly no venting.

There are two quick tests for the denseness of a foam mattress. One is to stand the mattress on end and lean on it with the top edge braced under your armpits. A less dense mattress will bow into a curve under the weight of your arms, but an adequately dense mattress won't. The second test is to press your palms together with the mattress in between. A dense mattress will stay put without compressing inward, while a less-dense mattress will change shape under the pressure of your hands.

Highs & lows of foam mattresses

Highs. Quality foam mattresses can be really firm, almost like a brick, and that's a good thing. You don't want a mattress so soft that it could create an unsafe pocket around your baby's face and cut off his air supply. Foam mattresses are lighter weight, making sheet changing easier; plus, they have squared-off corners that help keep fitted sheets in place.

Lows. Poorer-grade foam mattresses can compress and sag in the area where your baby lies, which could form a suffocation pocket if your baby happens to turn facedown. Some foam versions have only a single layer of vinyl ticking that's poorly bound on the sides, which can lead to tears and stretching. (Stick with a name-brand manufacturer with dense, quality foam and reinforced upholstery and bindings.)

WARNING

Never put these inside a crib!
Don't put a heating pad or hot-water bottle inside your baby's crib in an attempt to soothe him. Either of these items can cause severe burns, since your baby's skin is far more sensitive than an adult's (or even a child's) skin. Also, never use a thin plastic bag—such as those used for garbage or dry-cleaning—as a mattress protector. They could suffocate your baby.

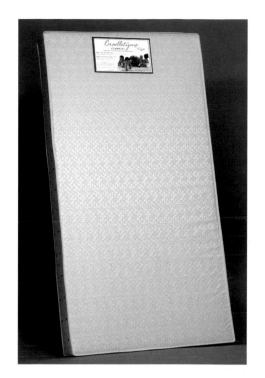

Colgate's Classica 1 Foam Mattress

($100)

The Classica 1 is 5 inches deep and extra firm, as well as extremely lightweight (6 pounds versus 30 pounds for a heavyweight innerspring mattress). It has a waterproof triple-laminate cover for moisture protection and durability.

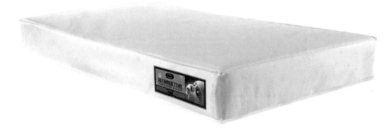

Simmons' Baby Series 300 Innerspring Mattress

($100)

This 6-inch-thick innerspring features 104 interlocking coils with strong tempered-steel components. Its reinforced borders effectively resist tears and rips, and there is a firm layer of foam on each side edge for long-lasting durability. Square corners allow a better sheet fit. The "no-flip" design means that the mattress is designed to stay in a single position for the life of the mattress. The vinyl ticking is hypoallergenic. The mattress comes with a limited 15-year warranty.

Checklist

Baby-bedding shopping

Now that you've chosen your baby's crib and mattress, next comes sheets, blankets, and other bedding. Expect your baby to wet the bed several times a day. Here's a list of bedding items to have on hand. You may need more if you don't have easy access to a washer and dryer; but remember, you can always buy more later on.

✔ **Crib mattress protector.** 2 (or more) hypoallergenic, absorbent, or waterproof crib mattress pads. Make sure the corners of the pads are elasticized to fit snugly around the mattress and not bunch on top of it.

✔ **Crib sheets.** 5 (or more) fitted crib sheets with strong elastic to go around the mattress. Crib-size sheets are available where cribs are sold and online from a variety of outlets, including www.sheetworld.com. They come in flannel, jersey knit, and cotton in a variety of colors and patterns. (Unfitted sheets are more likely to bunch around the baby and could lead to suffocation.)

✔ **Blankets.** 3 to 4 thin blankets that should be tucked at least 2 inches under the mattress on 3 sides and then folded to fit under the baby's underarms (not under his chin).

✔ **Sleep sacks.** 2 to 3 of these small sleeping bags, which can be sleeveless or with sleeves and have snaps or plastic zippers for easy access to the diaper area. They come in different weights for winter and summer for use in place of blankets. (See more about sleep sacks in the clothing chapter, page 112.)

Safety standards for cribs

Rigorous federal safety standards are overseen by the Consumer Product Safety Commission (CPSC). There is also a voluntary certification program overseen by the American Society of Testing and Materials (ASTM) and the Juvenile Products Manufacturers Association (JPMA). To be certified, crib brands must undergo extra testing for sturdiness. Certified cribs will usually have a "JPMA Certified" sticker somewhere on the frame.

Certified cribs carry an extra margin of safety because of extra testing, but being certified isn't an absolute guarantee of safety. For example, some certified cribs have undergone federal recalls because of loose bars or component failures. Also, paying a lot for a crib is no guarantee that you'll be getting better safety or durability. Costly cribs may have a solid feel of quality to them, but could still be recalled because of serious flaws inside—lowering hardware or other product failures.

If you're concerned about crib recalls, we suggest going to www.recalls.gov and entering the word "cribs," or search a specific crib model and brand there under consumer products. You can also report crib safety problems directly to the Consumer Product Safety Commission on its Internet site, www.CPSC.gov, or by using its toll-free hotline at 1-800-638-CPSC.

The baby-safe crib

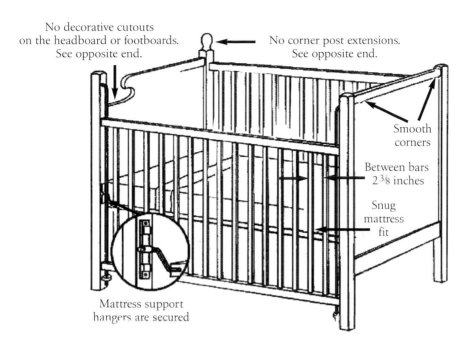

No decorative cutouts on the headboard or footboards. See opposite end.

No corner post extensions. See opposite end.

Smooth corners

Between bars 2 ⅜ inches

Snug mattress fit

Mattress support hangers are secured

SAFETY CONSIDERATIONS

Crib-related accidents are the most frequent cause of baby-product-related deaths. Each year, about 50 babies suffocate or strangle when they become trapped between broken crib parts or in cribs with unsafe designs. Usually the culprit is older-model cribs with loose or broken bars or frames, malfunctioning mattress supports, or gaps between the mattress and the side of the crib's frame—all of which can capture babies' vulnerable necks and compress their airways, causing them to suffocate.

Suffocation from crib bedding or mattress covers is also responsible for numerous crib-related deaths. This can happen when babies' faces, noses, and mouths become buried in soft bedding, such as pillows, quilts, comforters, air mattresses, beanbag chairs, or sheepskins. Some babies have even died while sleeping on their backs, when their faces became covered by soft bedding. (See: "Keeping baby safe for sleep" on page 133).

Sudden Infant Death Syndrome (SIDS), sometimes called cot death or crib death, is the other major cause of baby deaths related to cribs and sleeping, and it's linked to more than 2,000 baby deaths per year. Otherwise healthy babies are found lifeless after having been put down to sleep. SIDS is more likely to affect babies less than 6 months of age. The causes of SIDS are still not fully understood. Fortunately, placing babies to sleep on their backs instead of their stomachs has been associated with a dramatic decrease in SIDS deaths. (See more about SIDS in the Q & A section on page 134.)

10

DIAPERS, DIAPER PAILS & CHANGING TABLES

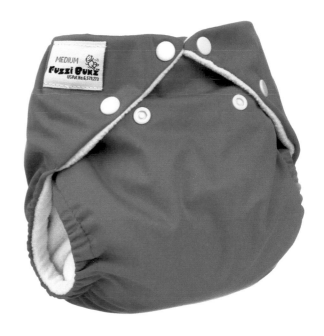

Until the glorious day that your child is potty trained (at around age 3), she will go through about 9,000 diaper changes. At an average of two minutes per change, that's 300 total hours of diaper duty! Here are tips for picking diapers, a diaper pail, and a changing table.

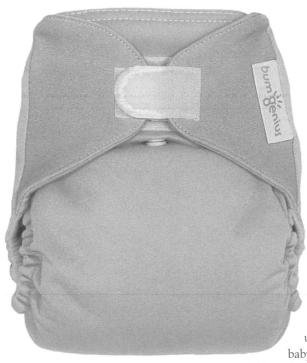

THE PRINCESS AND THE PEE

A diaper will be the key feature of your baby's wardrobe—and sometimes her only outfit—for about the first three years of her life. Typically, your baby will use about 60 diapers per week in the early months. That rate will gradually slow down as your baby's digestive system matures, and eventually your child will be able to use a potty or the toilet but may need training pants or pull-up pants at night.

The majority of parents opt for disposable diapers for the convenience and the time and mess they save. And if you plan to use a childcare center, disposables may be required. The downside to disposables is the cost outlay over time, which can top $2,000.

Cloth reusables are the least expensive option by far, since a few dozen can last for years and be handed down. However, the initial investment can be upward of $700 for a supply of cloth diapers, covers, and inserts. Some parents also prefer the soft texture and the more natural feel of fabric. And they believe that recycling diapers is kinder to local landfills and to trees (though it's not any kinder to water and energy supplies).

Other parents take a middle road between disposables and reusables by putting their babies in fabric diapers at home and reusables when they go out, or by using fabric in the daytime and using disposables at night for the absorbency and leak control they offer.

A few cities still offer diaper services, although they're a dying breed. Surprisingly, diaper services that deliver clean fabric diapers to your door can cost less over the total time a baby needs them than disposables do.

Whichever option you choose—all disposables, disposables plus reusables, all reusables, or a diaper service—is purely an individual choice and, as you'll discover, every option has both advantages and disadvantages.

When to Buy

Late pregnancy through 30 months. Disposable diaper sizes are based on baby weight, and they're numbered from 0 or N for newborns through size 6 for babies weighing 30 pounds or more.

Getting the right size

Disposables are sized by baby weight, starting with preemie and newborn sizes, and going up to size 6 for toddlers. As your baby gets heavier, the diapers get larger, and you may pay the same price for a package that contains fewer diapers than you got when buying smaller sizes. As your baby matures, however, she'll also wet less often and need fewer diapers per day than a newborn would.

Even though disposables offer a lot of size options, it's not a case of one size fits all, even within the weight categories specified by manufacturers. When you read the backs of disposables packages, you'll notice that there is a lot of overlap in sizes—a 16-pounder could wear either a size 1 or 2, a 23-pounder either a size 3 or 4.

Added to that, babies at every age differ in their length and girth and in the size of their hips and thighs. Wetting patterns differ, too—some babies might be considered light wetters, while others are classified as heavy wetters. So the ultimate disposable solution is to experiment until you find what works at any given time in your baby's diapering career.

Dealing with leaking

Leaking is a universal problem for all diapers—fabric or reusables. Nighttime leaking is especially common since babies sleep on their backs and wetness works its way up the back of the diaper and soaks the baby's clothes and sheets. Most disposables can handle the first wetting or two, but typically they start to fail after they've become saturated by multiple wettings.

The best solution for leaking is to change your baby more often, even in the night, or to use an overnight disposable or absorbent insert designed to help contain the wetness. How the diaper is fitted on your baby can make a difference with leaking, too.

Here are some solutions to try.

✔**Shift the diaper position.** Raise the front of the diaper or lower it below your baby's belly button to see if a different diaper position helps.

✔**Reposition the tabs.** Fasten the tabs lower down on the diaper so that they meet as nearly as possible.

✔**Reposition the leg bands.** Try pulling the elastic leg bands further out on your baby's leg to offer a better seal.

✔**Change son's position.** Positioning a boy's penis so it's pointing down each time you change him can help to put the wetness where the diaper is most absorbent.

✔**Change diapers just before bedtime.** Put a fresh diaper on just before putting your baby down for the night.

✔**Try a different diaper size.** Many parents find that the leaking problem stops when they change to a different size diaper within a brand. Try the next size up, especially at night, and fasten the tabs closer together.

✔**Fold down the front and back.** Sometimes folding down the diaper's waistband, especially if the diaper's a little big, can help capture wetness inside.

✔**Use the top of the brand.** The top diaper line of the big manufacturers may deliver better fit, such as elastic in the back, and may also offer more absorbency than a mid-price version.

✔**Use an absorbent insert.** Some stores sell diaper inserts that help increase moisture absorption.

✔**Change brands.** You may find that a different diaper brand fits your baby better and is better at preventing leaks, particularly diapers designed specifically for nighttime use.

Diapering a breastfed baby

Breastfed babies' poop tends to be liquidy, and the baby may hold a BM in for a day or two, followed by a big gusher that can seep out of leg holes and up your baby's back. A well-fitted diaper that fits snugly around your baby's butt and thighs will help keep BMs inside. The diaper should also be well centered from front to back with no gaps above the baby's rump to prevent the baby's "shooters" from squeezing up and out.

ALL ABOUT DISPOSABLES

Disposable diapers continue to improve every year, mostly because of the steep competition between Kimberly-Clark (Huggies) and Proctor & Gamble (Pampers and Luvs)—the two giant disposable-diaper makers. The absorbency, fit, and ease of fastening and removing these leading brands keep getting better. (And they've become more expensive over time, too.)

At the time of this writing, disposables typically cost between 25 and 30 cents each with store brands, such as Wal-Mart's White Cloud, CVS's Explorers, Target's store brand, and Costco's Kirkland Signature being the most economical. The highest-priced diapers are the top-of-the-line offerings from Huggies (including Huggies Supreme) and Pampers Premiums, priced 30 to 35 cents each or more.

The extra cost of these name brands translates into softer outer covers, better peel-and-restick closures, and soft, stretchy elastic waistbands and leg holes. They also come imprinted with cute licensed designs, like Disney prints on Huggies and Sesame Street on Pampers that probably won't matter all that much to your baby, but at least they'll help sleep-deprived new moms and dads know where the diaper's front is.

It's smart to sample widely among both mainstream and store brands to find what works best for you and your baby. If your baby is prone to rashes or is hard to fit, then premium diapers may be the best way to go.

Some parents find that one brand works best with young babies but may not perform as well with toddlers or during the night, when leaking is more of a problem. Diaper manufacturers have addressed this by producing extra-absorbent diapers to help your baby make it through to morning.

Diapers that claim to be more environmentally friendly than mainstream and store brands because they degrade more readily, or which are advertised as chlorine and fragrance-free (such as the Seventh Generation brand), generally cost more. Still, as with other brands, there may be problems with fit, absorbency, and tabs that don't stick and unstick as readily as parents might prefer.

When it comes to the biodegradable claim, landfills aren't composting facilities, and nothing degrades very well there. Any environmental advantage of disposables depends more on the resources of water and energy required to manufacture them. The use of recycled materials in making the diapers is the most environmentally friendly focus.

No matter what brand you start out with or that other moms recommend, it doesn't pay to stick slavishly to a single brand if it doesn't continue to perform for you and your baby or if you discover that a lesser-known brand works just as well. And you should be prepared to change brands at various stages in your baby's growth as her weight and body dimensions change if you encounter fitting problems.

Highs & lows of disposables

Highs. They're the most convenient of all options and tend to fit babies better than one-size-fits-all diapers. Their absorbency truly does wick dampness away from a baby's bottom, which may mean fewer diaper-rash breakouts (although some babies have skin reactions to certain diaper brands). Newer diapers are specially designed to prevent leaks around the legs and waist.

Lows. They're the most expensive option. They can develop quite an odor when piles of them stack up waiting for garbage day. They use trees and account for about 2 percent of landfill use, so if you have environmental concerns, you may elect to recycle by using cloth diapers. There's always the possibility of running out of disposables in the middle of the night. And last but not least, some enterprising toddlers master how to rip them off for running around the neighborhood in the buff.

Checklist

Quick disposables shopping

Here are some practical tips for helping you save money when you shop for disposables.

✔ **Shop ahead.** Save money by stocking up on diapers in large packages if you're sure your baby will stay the same size for a while. The quickest way to estimate your baby's growth is to refer to your pediatrician's growth chart for your baby. You can also printout a growth chart for predicting your baby's size changes from this National Center for Health Statistics site: www.cdc.gov/growthcharts.

✔ **Watch your baby's weight.** Weight, not age, determines proper sizing. If your baby is really close to the high end of the weight category, go for the larger size.

✔ **Check the package weight.** You can't open packages of diapers in the store to give them a feel, but as a general rule, the better quality the diaper, the heavier the package. If you're trying out new brands, use the scale in the produce department to compare, being sure you're weighing packages with the same number of diapers.

✔ **Be specific.** If you're sending someone out for diapers, specify not just brand but type. There's a big difference between Pampers Premium and Pampers Baby Dry, for instance, even though they're the same brand and may have a similar price.

✔ **Use money savers.** Sign up on company Web sites or subscribe to free baby magazines online to receive coupons in the mail or in your inbox. Buy by the case from large discount chains, such as Sam's Club, and stock up if you see a sale. But watch out—your baby may outgrow the size before you run out!

✔ **Consider a compromise.** There's no need for your baby to be either all-disposable or all-reusable. If you have a washing machine and dryer, consider disposables for out-of-house use and fabric diapers for at-home use.

FABRIC REUSABLES

Fabric diapers are a good choice if you want to economize by laundering your own, and you can save hundreds of dollars by recycling diapers over and over instead of buying the disposable variety. You may also prefer the soft texture and more natural feel of fabric and find it kinder to landfills and to trees (though not any kinder to water and energy supplies).

Standard old-fashioned diapers are the least expensive and are usually packaged by the dozen for under $15. These diapers are simply a single large square of absorbent fabric. The package gives instructions about how to fold the cloth in order to concentrate absorbency in the middle of the diaper where it's most needed. Usually the final fold resembles a triangle with one point at each side of the baby. The third point is drawn up between the legs. All three points are pinned together in the center of the diaper.

Prefolded diapers are rectangular, with thicker fabric folds sewn into the center to maximize absorbency where it's needed. Not only are they handy if your baby is a disposable user and you run out of supplies at night, but they're also great for throwing over your shoulder or putting on your lap to absorb burps and leaks. They're priced about $2 each and are usually packaged by the dozen.

Reusable diehards report that the types of reusables you find in big-box baby stores aren't worth the money, but specialty diapers you find online are. For example, organic or hemp prefolds that are extremely soft and absorbent cost about $5.50 each. (Hemp fleece is a blend of cotton and hemp that is very soft and considered by many to be the most absorbent.)

Modern diaper systems feature outer pants with elasticized legs, snaps or Velcro-type closures, that offer an effective waterproof barrier while still letting the diaper breathe. Fitted diapers often come in a variety of baby sizes and are hour-glass-shaped to reduce chafing and bulkiness between the baby's legs. They are priced between $15 and $17 each, and sometimes more. All-in-one diapers that combine both diapers and covers are priced between $12 and $23 each. Pocket diapers use absorbent, washable inserts to help handle wetness. Some diapering brands to look for online are BumGenius, Bummi Super Whisper Wraps, Fuzzi Bunz, Kooshies, Wonderoos, and Mother-Ease.

Moisture-protecting outer pants vary in price, too, from inexpensive grocery-store brands with snaps for under $5 each up to $8 to $12 pants that feature a breathable poly/nylon cover. You can pay from $12 to $17 for fleece covers and $18 to $22 for wool versions.

A new trend in cloth diapering is "WAHM" diapers, which stands for Work-At-Home-Mom diapers. These are diapers made by moms with their own at-home businesses, and some can be true works of art. Because they aren't mass-produced, the diapers have a much more limited supply, which is why some brands, such as Baby Moon, are highly sought after, coveted, and sometimes available only through auction (even when they've been used). If you want to get into collecting homemade diapers, try www.diaperpin.com, an online cloth-diaper directory.

How many to buy

The number of diapers and outer pants you buy depends upon how often you plan to do laundry. You're likely to do it every day or every other day to keep on top of the dirty-diaper pile. (And note, they take longer than baby clothes to dry.)

Quick tip

Nix sewn-on plastic outer pants
The thicker the reusable, the longer it will take to dry. On our do-not-buy list are diapers sewn together with vinyl (non-breathable) outer pants. They don't launder well, which allows them to harbor bacteria and detergent residues; plus, they take forever to dry.

If you plan to launder diapers, consider investing in a high-efficiency front-loading machine—the largest you can afford for your space. The machine will cost upward of $800 but will clean diapers better while using 40 to 50 percent less water and 50 to 65 percent less energy than a conventional top loader, repaying your investment over time.

Typically, a baby will use between 8 and 12 diapers per day, and newborns even more. With a supply of 24 diapers and 4 to 5 diaper covers, you will need to launder diapers every other day. And if you can afford it, the ideal supply would be 3 to 4 dozen to spread out your washing times and to have plenty on hand for milksops, too.

The only caveat is that you need to be sure that the diapers you invest in are the ones you want to use for the next three years. The only way to know the brand to use is to sample widely among different types and brands to find what fits your baby best, absorbs the most, chafes the least, and launders well.

Cents Sense

✔ **Sample around.** Before you commit to a cloth diapering system, try one or two diapers from different companies. Many cloth diaper companies will send out a sample diaper and cover for free or at a steep discount if you're considering their brand.

✔ **Buy on an as-needed basis.** Rather than stocking up, start out with a dozen diapers with 4 to 5 covers and plan to order more as needed.

✔ **Consider used diapers.** To make sure they're clean, stain- and odor-free, soak them in boiling hot water in a stain-resistant container in which you have dissolved about half a cup of dishwasher (not dishwashing) detergent. Use gloves to handle the diapers. Then give them thor-

---

 # Checklist

Reusables shopping

Here are some practical tips for helping you save money when you shop for reusables.

✔ **Soft, absorbent material.** Most cloth diapers are made of cotton knit terry or thick flannel.

✔ **Fit.** What fits right and doesn't leak for one baby is another's up-and-out-the-back blowout. You may have to try a few brands before you find one that fits your baby well.

✔ **Customizable absorbency.** Lets you customize absorbency by how you place or fold them. You add an absorbent panel for nighttime to help save baby's pajamas and sheets.

✔ **Adjustable sizing.** To extend the life of a cloth diaper, look for Velcro, Aplix, or snap closures (or ones that use good old-fashioned diaper pins) that allow you to adjust the waist size.

Q/A

Q I have big problems with changing the diaper of my energetic nine-month-old son! He absolutely hates being on his back and wants to crawl away. So far, I've had to hold him down by force (which makes him cry a lot), and I feel so bad each time. What can I do?

This is not unusual—as babies get more mobile, they can't stand to lie still! Here are a few suggestions: Be fast and have everything ready to go. For a diaper that's just wet, you may be able to change it while he's standing up. Use bribery—let your baby play with things that are usually off-limits: your cell phone, intriguing toys, a flashlight, and so on. (Busy hands can't play with poop.) Try posting pictures of family members on the wall by the table to capture your baby's attention. Be goofy—sing silly songs, make raspberries or other noises, make funny faces, nibble his toes, etc. And if all else fails, try a new venue, like changing your baby wherever you can capture him and using a towel for a pad.

ough laundering several times in extra-hot water using an oxygen-based cleaner, with a 1-cup white vinegar rinse in the next-to-last cycle, and dry them in the sunshine to ensure they're completely sanitized.

Highs & lows of reusables

Highs. After your initial investment, you can expect to save several thousand dollars during your baby's diapering career, compared to the cost of disposables. Plus, you'll never run out as long as you keep your washing machine chugging along. They'll still be around to use again with your next baby.

Lows. They're not very portable and can be smeary and stinky. They're more labor-intensive because they need laundering. They require a hefty up-front investment to get started, and they can be stained by BMs. Even top-of-the-line diaper fabrics don't absorb wetness as readily as disposables, nor do they have an outside damp-ness barrier to protect your clothing and furniture. So a supply of waterproof outer pants will be needed—preferably made of breathable materials that won't turn your baby's bottom into a hothouse for bacteria. If not well laundered, they are associated with more diaper rash than disposables (although some babies have allergic skin reactions to the chemicals and plastics used in disposables). A broken washing machine or a power outage can be disastrous.

> **"For our second baby, I decided to test every brand there was and settled on a generic brand from a big discount chain. Okay, so they're not as cute or plush, but they still do the job. I have to admit I feel cheap hauling them into daycare, since I'm probably the only parent who puts her baby in them. We save several hundred dollars that way."**

CLOTH DIAPERS

bumGenius 2 Diapers
($18)

Parents offer high praise for these well-designed, highly adaptable pocket diapers that excel in fit, function, and ease of use. Snaps and stretchy tabs enable the diaper to change sizes for babies from 8 to 35 pounds. The suede-cloth inner lining wicks moisture into an absorbent insert to help keep baby's bottom dry. Stretch tabs similar to disposables' give a snug fit without exerting too much pressure on the baby's thigh. The hook-and-loop closures help make waist fitting more accurate and comfortable. The silky-soft outer fabric helps avoid wicking moisture to the outside, even when adapted to fitting babies of different sizes. The leg and back areas have super-stretchy elastic. They come with an absorbent cotton insert for the pocket (but smaller babies may need a smaller insert).

Fuzzi Bunz
($13–$18)

This is a pocket diaper with a waterproof outer layer and a very soft microfleece interior. Its elasticized sides help to contain messes. There are over 30 choices for colors of the outer layer. Multiple snaps help the diaper's waist and legs to widen as your baby grows. The diapers come in six sizes from XS to fit preemie and smaller-than-usual babies up through XL for extra-large and potty-training toddlers. Each diaper comes with a microterry insert, but you may need to purchase extra inserts if your baby is a heavy wetter and needs extra absorbency, especially through the night.

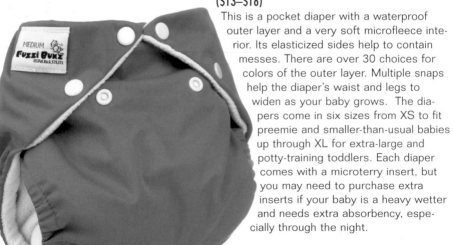

DIAPER SERVICES

Diaper services flourished in decades past, but they've become increasingly rare due to the competition from disposables. Diaper services are more popular in certain geographic locations than others. California, Colorado, Oregon, and Washington are big diaper-service states, but there are no services in Alabama, South Carolina, or Maryland, for instance. (To see if there's service in your state, check the list of providers with the National Association of Diaper Services, www.diapernet.com.)

Here's how a diaper service works: You choose the style of diapers you want to use; then a supply of diapers, and only those, are allotted to your baby—so there's no risk of contamination from another baby. Once or twice a week, a truck pulls up and takes away the soiled diapers that you've stored in a mesh bag inside a pail furnished by the service. In their place, the service leaves neatly wrapped stacks of clean diapers laundered at extremely hot temperatures that can't be matched by home machines. Most diaper services let you sign up for as long or short a time as you wish.

Highs & lows of diaper services

Highs. Your baby gets soft, clean diapers (and is less likely to have diaper rash than if you launder your own). You don't have the hassles of constant washing. And surprisingly, using a diaper service is still substantially cheaper than buying disposables.

Lows. The service costs more than doing your own laundering. Service may not be available in your area. You may risk running out of diapers before your next delivery. Old-fashioned diaper pins can prick babies' skin, and both pins and small diaper clips can be choking hazards for babies.

DIAPER PAILS

If you're breastfeeding, your baby's dirty diapers actually won't smell bad—not right away, anyway. But after those diapers sit for a while, they can work up quite a stench. Add formula feedings and, later, solid foods to the mix, and between trash-pickup days or trips to the dump to dispose of disposables or lugging reusables down to the washing machine, the diaper odor may bring tears to your eyes.

Because of the risk of contamination and the odor, you don't want to throw your dirty diapers in with the regular household trash (or laundry), and you don't want to use a regular trash can with a lid, because to throw the diapers away you'll have to pick up the lid, releasing evil fumes every time. Thus, the invention of diaper pails!

What you get for the money

Diaper pails are plastic trashcans with toddler-resistant lids that let you stuff rolled-up disposables inside without seeing, smelling, or touching its filthy friends already buried inside. Other pails are designed specifically for soaking or storing fabric diapers before laundry time and may have special compartments where deodorizer tablets can be placed to help cover up the stink.

Most pails are in the $15 to $40 price range, though Safety 1st makes a model that's only $9.95 and is basically a trash can with a tight seal.

Laundering reusables

While disposables are simply rolled up and thrown into the garbage pail, fabric diapers, especially those with poop stains, clean better if they're not allowed to dry, which can cause stains to set.

Most parents find that soaking the diapers until they're ready to be put in the washing machine works best. A diaper pail must have a locking lid to prevent children from accessing the deodorant disk or drowning headfirst in the water.

Here are your options for preparing and laundering fabric diapers.

✔ **Liquid Pail Method.** Fill half the pail with cold water and add ¼ cup of either baking soda, vinegar, or washing soda to help control odors and stains. (Never soak diapers in bleach, detergent, or soap. It will cause the fibers to wear out and fray.)

✔ **Poop solutions.** Throw wet diapers and diapers with poop from a breastfed baby directly into the pail for soaking. For formula-fed babies, shake the stool into the toilet and flush it before soaking the diaper.

✔ **Dry pail method.** If you don't want to deal with hauling around a heavy pail of sloshing liquid, try spraying a solution of baking soda and water directly on the soiled diaper, or sprinkle baking soda between layers of diapers and store them in a dry pail that contains a deodorizer tablet. Make sure the tablet is secured in a holder that locks so that toddlers and children can't get to it.

✔ **Machine laundering.** Select the heavy-duty cycle on your machine and wash diapers separately from clothing, using very hot water and a nonallergenic, fragrance-free liquid detergent. Powdered detergents aren't recommended because they are usually per-

fumed, which can irritate your baby's nose and skin, and they don't rinse out well. (Make sure to close any Velcro-style closures so they don't collect lint or catch on other diapers.)

✔ **No fabric softeners or bleach.** Don't use fabric softener liquid in the wash or a fabric-softening sheet in the dryer—both can irritate your baby's nose and skin, and they may coat the fibers of the diaper, making it less absorbent. Bleach can deteriorate the diaper, causing it to fray and wear out.

PAILS FOR DISPOSABLES

Highs & lows of diaper pails

Highs. Anything that keeps diaper odor contained is a good thing.

Lows. Some pails have narrow openings that make it hard to stuff toddler-size diapers inside. The cutting blades and other sharp hardware inside some pails that use continuous bag liners could be a hazard if your baby gets her hands inside the lid. A pail that soaks diapers in water is a drowning risk if the lid can be pried open by a tot. Deodorizer tablets can also be caustic. No matter how great the pail, you will have to clean it and air it out at least once a month.

When to Buy

From birth for as long as your baby uses diapers—usually 24 to 36 months of age.

Checklist

Diaper pail shopping

Here are some basic features to look for when you shop for a diaper pail.

✔ **Locking lid.** The lid should be easy for you to open (with a dirty diaper in one hand) but make it hard for your tot to access the inside of the pail.

✔ **Affordable liners.** If you're buying a pail for disposables, check out the price of the refill liners when comparing one model with another.

✔ **Odor control.** The "phew!" factor is huge. Check out the manufacturer's promises for sealing off the smell and/or covering it up.

✔ **Foot operation.** A foot-release lid is a handy option.

✔ **Safe deodorizing system.** Deodorizer tablets should be locked safely into a compartment that a baby can't access (and ingest).

✔ **Large capacity.** Look for a pail with a large mouth and plenty of room to accommodate the growing number of your baby's diapers, especially for weeks when trash day falls on a holiday.

Avoid:

✗ **Small mouth.** If it's hard to stuff diapers into the pail, they'll just pile up on top.

✗ **Flimsy deodorizer compartment.** Test it, to be sure a curious toddler can't open it.

✗ **Too-easy access.** The concept is to keep diapers in and exploring toddlers out.

✗ **Sharp hardware.** Check inside the pail's lid to make sure there are no exposed blades or sharp hardware that could hurt a small child's fingers.

Quick tip
Expensive plastic liners

The biggest expense of specialized diaper pails for disposables isn't the up-front cost of the pail itself but the cost of the plastic liners that get thrown away with the diapers. Most come in toilet-paper-type rolls and are where manufacturers and retailers make most of their money.

Learning Curve's The First Years Clean Air Odor-Free Diaper Disposal

($13–$18)

This 20-inch-tall pail has a built-in quiet fan and a carbon filter to trap and eliminate diaper odors. The self-sealing pail uses standard kitchen trash bags rather than expensive special refills, but the unit requires four D-cell batteries (not supplied) and filter cartridges that last about 90 days before needing to be replaced. The unit holds approximately 40 newborn's diapers.

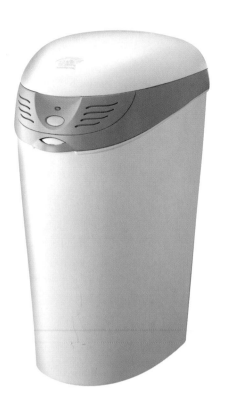

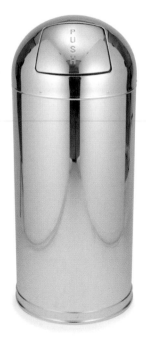

Rubbermaid's Commercial Products Marshal 15-Gallon Dome Top Steel Waste Container

($250)

If capacity, versatility, and durability are what you're after, nothing beats a heavy-gauge galvanized steel trash can with a push-in opening and a plastic liner. The can takes regular trash bags, and it's made to take a beating without absorbing odors. The push top offers simple one-handed disposal while keeping the stink inside. The steel is easy to clean—if spraying it with a bleach solution doesn't work, it can be hosed down. And after baby is potty trained, you have a retro-look kitchen trash can that can take years, if not decades, of wear.

CHANGING TABLES AND PADS

Once you bring baby home, you'll immediately need a place to change her. The least expensive of all changing options is a folded towel or sheet placed on the bed or floor. Your baby will be busy looking at you and/or being outraged at the indignity of a cold bottom, and won't notice a bit that she's not on a designer table.

Moving up from this option is a simple folding changing pad for under $10—like those that come in diaper bags—that can be used on the floor or on a bed, or stuffed in a backpack or purse. The pads don't offer safety straps and can't be fastened down, so they need to be used on a surface where your baby can't roll off. (And you may get tired of bending over or squatting.)

A contoured changing pad ($15–$30) is designed to be placed on a low chest, dresser, or other flat surface. Most come with screws to attach the pad to the back of a chest or dresser. Usually, they come with small, flimsy vinyl belts for keeping babies in place. The pads are a great space-saving option, but make sure to always keep a hand on your baby in case the belt doesn't work or she tries to roll over or scramble out.

Some manufacturers have created wooden, foldout toppers that can be bought separately or come attached to wooden nursery chests. They're priced from $60 to $100. Most come with a changing pad and waist belt. Once the baby outgrows diapering, the top can easily be removed. Lightweight molded-plastic changers, such as the Rail Rider ($32) that fit across the bars of standard-size cribs are also available.

Finally, a dedicated changing table is a somewhat expensive rectangular-shaped table designed just for diapering that positions the baby waist high for parents' convenience. On top of the table is a cushioned pad and a waist belt to keep the baby from falling off the table. Most have guardrails on two or all sides to help protect from falls.

These freestanding furniture units can be had for as little as $89 for a no-frills model, or as much as $700 to $2,000 or more for a "designer" piece made of solid hardwood, wrought iron, or even stainless steel. Mid-price models are constructed of wood or rattan with storage shelves or drawers underneath the baby's platform.

Highs & lows of changing tables

Highs. They raise the baby to a comfortable height for changing. You can place them wherever it's convenient, or have one for each floor in your home. They come with a waist belt to hold the baby in place. Railings on the sides will help prevent your baby from rolling over and falling out.

Lows. They're the most expensive option. Babies are injured when they squirm and roll overboard, falling headfirst to the floor. Using a restraining belt is important, but it can get in the way of diapering. Open shelves underneath may be an invitation to toddlers to pull things out onto the floor.

When to Buy

Late pregnancy through the first three years. Follow manufacturer's age and weight guidelines.

✔ Checklist

Changing table shopping

Here are some basic features to look for when you shop for a changing table.

✔ **Sturdy.** Jiggle a changing-table floor model. It should feel solid, not wobbly. Screws are preferable to staples for holding it together (but you'll likely have to assemble the table yourself).

✔ **High sides.** The table should have 3- to 4-inch railings on all sides to help prevent your baby from falling out.

✔ **Safety belt.** The belt on the pad should be sturdy and the buckle easy to use and adjust.

✔ **Wipe-clean changing pad.** No nooks or crannies to harbor bacteria.

✔ **Open shelves.** Open shelves make reaching for diapers easier so you don't have to turn your back on your baby. (But they'll also make it easy for your tot to pull everything down when she's wandering around on the floor!)

Avoid:

✗ **Flimsy materials.** Rattan is generally less sturdy than solid wood, and it also may have sharp edges.

✗ **Poor finishing.** Wood should be smooth, with no splintering.

✗ **Low or no railings.** The railings are an important backup to prevent falls, along with the restraining belt.

✗ **Flimsy changing pad and belt.** Seams may tear, and the belt will be useless if it can't hold down a squirming baby.

Child Craft's Dressing Table

($140–$245)

Available in a natural wood finish, this dressing table has sleek lines with open shelves and high railings on all sides. It comes with a changing pad, security strap and buckle, and three lined baskets for storing diapers, clothing, or baby toys. (Child Craft makes changing tables in a variety of finishes and features, some with pull-out drawers.)

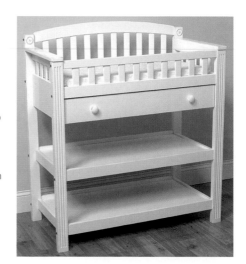

Simplicity's Aspen Changing Table
($80–$100)

Available in a natural hard-wood finish, this dressing table has rounded bars on three sides and a high rim all around to prevent baby fallout. There are two roomy shelves underneath for storing clothing or toys. It comes with a pad and safety belt.

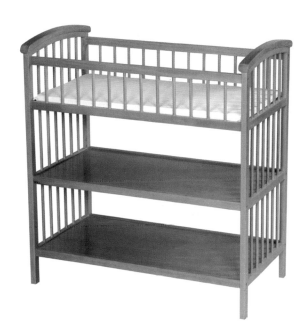

SAFETY CONSIDERATIONS

The most common diapering hazards are babies choking on pieces of disposable diapers; their drowning in diaper pails; and serious head injuries from falling off of diaper tables. Recalls for product hazards—involving diapers, diaper pails, and diaper-changing tables—are under the aegis of the U.S. Consumer Product Safety Commission (CPSC). You can look for recalls of these items by going to www.recalls.gov and searching for the product on the CPSC site.

JPMA's certification seal is available to manufacturers of changing tables who voluntarily submit their product designs for testing. Requirements for certification address the warnings that come with the table and the sturdiness and safety of its components. Certified products will display "JPMA Certified" somewhere on the product.

Only four small manufacturers had elected to opt in to the program as of this writing, so simply because a table is not certified does not indicate it is unsafe, nor does being certified mean that a product won't be subject to a recall at some point because of dangerous product flaws.

11

DIAPER BAGS

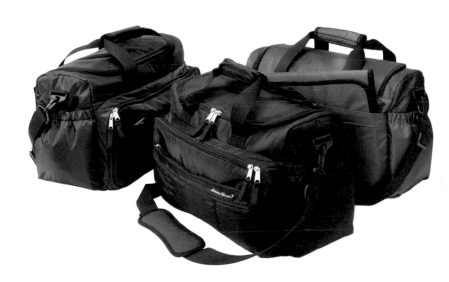

You don't need a special bag to carry diapers. An ordinary tote bag or purse will work just fine. But a designated diaper bag—whether made to resemble a roomy pocketbook, a sleek attaché case, or a sporty backpack—will help you carry all the baby booty you'll need when you're away from home. There are thousands of bags on the market. This chapter reviews all their best features to help you pick the one that's perfect for your needs.

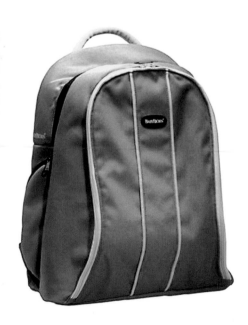

THE BEST BAG DEPENDS ON YOUR LIFESTYLE

IF you plan to walk a lot and wear the baby in a soft carrier, consider a combination backpack-style diaper bag, especially if you live in an area that's not stroller-friendly and you plan to tote the baby in a soft carrier. This will leave your hands free, and it will feel better to have extra weight balanced evenly on your back, rather than toting a heavy diaper bag on one side of your body.

IF you plan to get a lot of mileage out of your stroller, be sure that your diaper bag will fit in your stroller's storage compartment. Some companies offer attachable stroller bags as accessories, but they're usually stiff and small, and not as serviceable as regular bags. They are often more expensive, too. (Note: For safety's sake, don't hook the diaper bag or shopping bags over stroller handlebars that aren't for that purpose. Doing so can cause the stroller to tip over backward, and your baby could get hurt.)

IF it's a girl, but Dad hates pink, be aware that there are now messenger bags, tool-belt-style bags, and bags that look like briefcases to appease a more masculine aesthetic. If you think a manly bag might be the extra encouragement Dad needs to take the baby on an outing when you need a nap, then we say it's money well spent!

IF you know you're going to go back to work and continue breastfeeding, you'll need a specially designed bag for toting the pump and storing filled bottles. So plan your diaper bag around your pump needs. Most pump bags offer extra space for bottles and accessories. Some moms simply leave the pump in its case at work and use a separate insulated bag for toting bottles back and forth. (For more information on breast pumps see page 19.)

IF you see a lot of car trips in baby's future, consider getting more than one small diaper bag instead of one big one. You can leave one in the back of the car for restocking as needed, and have another, lighter one to carry along with you. This also means you'll always have backup supplies in case you forget something or end up staying away from home longer than you'd planned.

IF you plan airplane trips with your baby you may need a roomier bag that also has an insulated compartment for bottles and snacks, and plenty of room for clothes, extra diapers, and toys, too. A pair of wheels on the bottom might be useful if you don't want to bear the weight on your shoulders during long airport treks.

When to Buy

During pregnancy if you find one that's comfortable and durable, or after pregnancy if you prefer to wait and see if you receive a usable bag as a gift.

Quick tips

Until the glorious day that there's a dipe-and-wipe vending machine in every restroom, keep a few spare diapers, wipes, and small sealable bags in your car, your stroller, your purse—anywhere and everywhere you can think of—so you don't get stranded with a poopy baby and no resources.

What you get for the money

On the lowest price end of the diaper-bag spectrum (not counting the free promotional one full of baby-product samples most hospitals give away) are small and simple vinyl or polyester-blend bags that have a bottle holder, a simple vinyl-covered changing pad, and possibly an extra zippered pocket for storage. One of these could be had from a large discount store for under $20. Lands' End makes a bag called the Little Tripper that sells for $19.50 and has space for all the basics.

In the midrange are diaper backpacks and messenger-style bags, which typically retail for between $25 and $50, with name brands selling for between $80 and $125.

The price of a bag goes up as you add features, go to a larger size, or get better material and a designer name brand (all the way up to a Mia Bossi or Gucci). Those bags will serve as a true style statement worthy of appearing on the front of *Star* magazine, as will a $1,200 custom-made leatherwork of diaper-toting art.

Only you know if a designer bag is worth the extra money to you (and your image), but do keep in mind that the bag will quickly get stained inside and out, scuffed around the outer corners, and may end up sitting on the wet floor of public bathroom stalls when there's no hook and you've got a baby in your arms. In other words, don't invest in any bag you couldn't stand to see ruined over the process of several years of heavy-duty use.

Six strategies for selecting a good diaper bag

Buying a diaper bag is a lot like shopping for a purse—it just happens to be a very big one with specialized features. The most practical choice is a bag that sits comfortably enough on your shoulder that you can use it hands-free. It should hold enough baby stuff without being too big, too awkward, or too heavy; and it needs a go-anywhere look that coordinates (or at least doesn't clash horribly) with most of your wardrobe. Pay only for features you'll use—insulated storage for six bottles makes sense only if you plan a lot of long trips.

Here are our tips for finding the right bag:
1. Do research online.
Reading reviews by parents on sites like Amazon.com or epinions.com can help you research what's out there. It will let you take a look at brands you may not have considered, and learn from other buyers' mistakes.
2. Don't buy online (unless you know exactly which bag you want).
It's hard to get a sense of a bag's size,

Quick tips

When flying on a commercial airline with a baby, always pack your diaper bag under the assumption that the airline will lose your luggage and that you'll miss your connection in the middle of the night. Make sure you carry with you at least 24 hours' worth of supplies just in case, and enough for at least 20 diaper changes if you're traveling internationally. Don't forget a clean change of clothes for you if your baby spits up on your front while you're in flight. (It happens all the time!)

weight, fabric, feel, and color from a written description or an online picture. If the bag arrives and it's not quite right, you may find yourself leaving it at home or trying to find the time to repackage it and mail it back in the midst of all your other baby stresses.

3. Be wary of too many compartments. Lots of pockets can help you get organized . . . or they may have you frantically shaking the bag upside down while baby screams for his favorite pacifier. Look for bags that let you easily view what's inside every pocket.

4. Stain resistance is key. Diapering is often a messy business, so it doesn't make sense to pick something just because it's stylish unless it can also be hosed down inside and out. Even the most chic bags are destined to be put down in a puddle of mystery fluid on the ladies-room floor, get spit-up on, and have straps gummed by your small teether.

5. Be conscious of back strain. A diaper bag is light with nothing in it; but add lots of accessories, plus the weight of the baby, and you may be risking a muscle pull. Consider getting the smallest bag that meets your needs, or get a backpack-style bag with a carry handle at the top so you can tote it like a purse or distribute the weight on your shoulders and leave your hands free.

6. Access and closure. The mouth should open wide enough to let you peer in to search for items. It should also close tightly so everything won't get dumped out when your car makes a sudden stop or when you try to stuff the bag under an airplane seat. A fold-over flap won't work. Although zippered closures seal off the interior, some zippers can scratch the back of your hand

when you reach inside. Magnetic closures can sometimes work, but they could affect the magnetic strips on your charge cards, and they should be strong and hit the mark every time without your having to grope and squeeze.

Avoid:

✗ **Hard-to-clean or flimsy fabrics.** They'll stain and wear out quickly.

✗ **Loud prints.** If it screams "baby!" or makes you cringe, don't buy it.

✗ **Uncomfortable parts.** Sharp edges or seams that could chafe you or your baby.

✗ **Flimsiness.** Straps or construction that won't last.

✗ **Bad zippers.** Cheap zippers with hard-to-find plackets that can tear or break.

✗ **Too much going on.** Too many separated compartments and small pockets make things hard to find.

Highs & lows of diaper bags

Highs. They let you carry all of your baby supplies in one satchel to help with out-of-home diapering and feeding chores. Well-designed bags help to reduce the "fumble factor"—groping for small items buried inside.

Lows. They can be cumbersome and heavy, and sometimes get in the way when you're trying to carry your baby at the same time. Some are poorly constructed, flimsy, and stain or simply wear out before baby graduates from diapers.

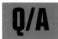

Q Should I buy a diaper bag while I'm pregnant, or wait until the baby's born?

We would suggest waiting until the baby's born, because you just may get a bag as a gift or get one free from the hospital that you actually like. You may also want to wait until you buy or register for a stroller so you can pick a bag that you're sure will fit in its storage compartment. If you do buy before baby's born, keep the bag's tags and receipts in case you find something better and wish to return it.

Q I want to buy my husband a "daddy bag" as a gift. What should I look for that he would enjoy using?

Daddy diaper bags are the biggest new thing. Dads don't have any particular, specific diaper-bag needs (except, perhaps, for extra space for milk since they can't make their own). But you may find that Dad's more willing to take Junior for an excursion if being draped in a cutesy bag doesn't have to be part of the deal. Some sites specialize in dad bags, such as www.dadgear.com.

DIAPER BAGS

BABYBJÖRN's Diaper Backpack Active
($70)

This durable, machine-washable backpack stands upright on its own. It has a U-shaped zip-down front, as well as a deep inside zippered storage area so you can separate messies from food. The insulated bottle carrier and cell phone pocket are on the outside for easy reach. Cushioned shoulder straps have nonslip surfacing underneath, and there's also a padded carry handle. Soft changing pad is included. Measures 17 inches high by 14 inches wide and 6 inches deep. Available in a variety of color combinations.

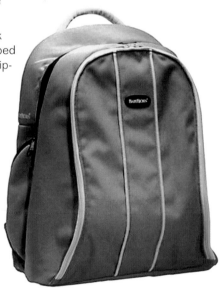

Eddie Bauer's Diaper Overnight Case
($55)

This roomy, utilitarian bag (16.5 inches wide by 11 high by 6 deep) features a padded shoulder strap with clips that unlatch for attaching the bag to rolling luggage or a stroller. The bag's gender-neutral colors—black, green (shown), or navy—work with just about anyone's style. The bag comes with a built-in changing pad, insulated side pockets, and lots of waterproof zippered compartments. On the downside, some parents report the changing pad, while handy, isn't big enough for large babies.

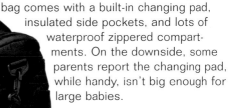

Diaper Dude's Camouflage Bag
($110)

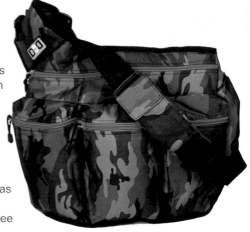

This bag (16" x 14") may be marketed to dads, but plenty of moms also like this bag's ergonomic across-the-chest design and well-padded, adjustable shoulder strap with cell phone holder. The durable, woven nylon bag offers numerous zippered pockets and elasticized bottle pouches. A variety of other Diaper Dude models are available in blacks, browns, and conservative prints as well as colorful "Diaper Diva" designs better suited to feminine sensibilities. (See www.diaperdude.com.)

✔ Checklist

Diaper bag shopping

Here are some basic features to look for when you shop for a diaper bag.

✔ **Sturdy upholstery.** Will resist moisture, dirt, and wear. Dense, moisture-resistant nylon weaves and thick canvas last better than thin cotton quilting or lightweight fabrics.

✔ **Moisture-proof interior.** Will make it easy to keep clean (and odor-free) after contact with milk or soiled diapers.

✔ **Handle comfort.** Carry handles and shoulder straps short enough so the bag won't drag if you're carrying it with one hand. Check underarm carrying comfort, too.

✔ **Lightweight.** Too many pockets and sections can weigh the bag down and make it harder to find lost items.

✔ **See-through pouches.** Clear or see-through-mesh pouches and dividers inside help you spot what you're looking for.

✔ **Zippered closure.** Closing the bag with a zipper helps prevent spills and keeps small hands out of mischief. Just be sure it's a "soft" zipper that won't scratch your hand every time you reach inside.

✔ **Reinforcements.** Reinforced stitching or other heavy-duty reinforcements where handles and straps join the body of the bag.

✔ **Style.** Pick a style that works well in a variety of situations.

✔ **Great alternatives.** Backpack and messenger-style diaper bags with padded straps and a center carry handle allow multiple carrying options, including hands-free.

Storksak's Emily
($170)

This comfortable, soft U-shape shoulder bag comes with an adjustable shoulder strap. It has a zippered top opening and two insulated zippered pockets on the sides to keep fluids warm or cold, plus a cell phone pocket. The padded changing mat is removable, and the inner lining can be wiped clean. A matching detachable inner bag holds wipes or makeup. Available in other colors, including black and pewter.

Mommy's Helper/McKenzie Kids' Diaper Bag Essentials
($20)

Here's all you need to convert your favorite purse or backpack into a diaper bag. The kit includes 5 items: an insulated bottle holder; a padded changing pad that folds to compact travel size; a dirty-duds bag for separating out soiled clothes or diapers; a toiletry bag for diapers, wipes, etc.; and an accessory bag for keeping baby's pacifier clean and close at hand.

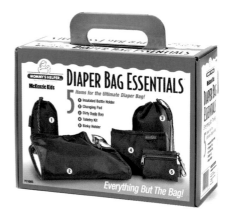

12

EXERCISERS & WALKERS

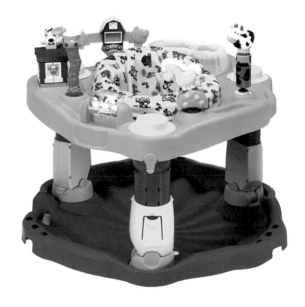

Stationary activity centers, called exercisers for short, are designed for babies who can sit up but aren't quite ready to walk. They're round with a rotating baby seat in the center and toys attached on all sides. Walkers are similar devices for pre-walking tots, but with wheels on their bases. This chapter gives you the information to choose the best and safest design for your baby.

WHEELS OF THE BABE GO ROUND 'N' ROUND

Baby activity centers, also called exercisers, are circular play centers with rotating seats surrounded by trays and toys attached to a frame. The best designs present baby with a circle of age-appropriate, interesting toys—like buttons to push and rotating noisemakers or spring-action toys that respond to hand motions. The worst have an overwhelming array of huge toys that make it hard to even see the baby.

The legs of most exercisers adjust to different heights, and some offer seat adjustments as well. Some models have a rounded base that allows a rocking motion—but if you pick one of these make sure it also has flip-down tabs so you can keep the unit from "walking" when the baby is very active or have it motionless while you feed her.

Walkers resemble activity centers in that they have legs, a tray, and a suspended seat. The big difference is that activity centers are stationary but walkers come with a set of wheels that let baby propel herself across the floor, which can present serious baby safety problems that we discuss later.

When to Buy

Wait until your baby has adequate neck and back strength to sit up on her own—between 5 and 8 months—before buying an exerciser, and then use it sparingly. Manufacturers typically recommend between 15 and 26 pounds for use and maximum height of 32 inches. Walkers aren't recommended, for safety reasons.

✔ **Checklist**

Exerciser shopping

Exercisers range in price from less than $30 for no-name imports to more than $100 for tricked-out, top-of-the-line brand-name models such as Graco's Baby Einstein. Here are the important features to look for in an exerciser, and what to avoid.

✔ **Certified.** A "JPMA Certified" sticker on the frame or carton indicates that the exerciser complies with rigorous voluntary safety standards.

✔ **The right size.** Don't use the exerciser until your baby can sit up and hold her head up for long periods of time. Stop using it once your baby exceeds the manufacturer's recommended weight limit.

✔ **Adjustable seat height.** At the least, the exerciser seat should offer height adjustment options to ensure that your baby's feet touch the bottom.

✔ **Washable surfaces.** A fabric seat removable for washing and easy to wipe down.

✔ **Plush seat padding.** A well-padded seat with back support for baby comfort.

✔ **Seat rotates smoothly.** Spin the seat around in the store to make sure it rotates with minimal effort.

✔ **The right size for your home.** Figure out how much floor space an exerciser will take up before you buy one.

✔ **Springy motions.** Look for a spring action that will reward your baby for flexing her thighs and calves.

✔ **Rocker lock-off.** Flip-down latches on units with rocker bases, to stop the rocking.

✔ **Fun toys!** Make sure the toys are the right size for your baby's hands, short enough so they won't block your baby's view and close enough so that she can reach them.

Avoid:

✗ **Sharp plastic seams.** Injection-molded plastic exercisers can have sharp seams or protrusions. While you're assembling the exerciser, sand or file down any you find.

✗ **Loose toy fasteners.** Babies have been injured when screwed-on toys worked loose, exposing sharp screws underneath. Make sure the toys on the exerciser are sturdy and can't be pulled off.

✗ **Uncomfortable leg holes.** Leg holes that are higher than the seat can cut off your baby's circulation, and rough seams can scratch her skin.

✗ **Flimsy imports.** A cheap exerciser from a little-known manufacturer may be more of a safety hazard than a bargain.

Quick tips

Buying a used exerciser. You may be able to find a bargain in a gently used exerciser at a yard sale or thrift store, or as a hand-me-down. But before you put your baby inside, check to make sure everything is in perfect working order and that the product hasn't undergone any recalls.

Exerciser alternatives. Babies need lots of practice pulling up and crawling—not just sitting up and pushing with their legs. Consider investing the $40 (or more) you'd spend on an exerciser on an appealing set of hand-sized toys that will prompt your baby to stretch and use her whole body to reach for them.

WARNING

Don't overdo upright sitting!
Spending too much time in an exerciser or walker (more than 30 minutes per day) can put a strain on your baby's back and trunk muscles and rob her of the vigorous crawling and pulling-up exercises she needs for balance and walking strength later. And if your baby has motor problems, a walker may force her leg and trunk movements into abnormal motor patterns that could be hard to break.

Highs & lows of exercisers

Highs. They let a lively baby stretch her legs in a safe place while parents work nearby or simply take a breather. Babies can sit and be entertained temporarily with toys in easy reach of small arms and hands, but that can't be tossed overboard. Toys requiring a variety of finger and hand motions can help the baby to practice eye–hand coordination.

Lows. For their price, exercisers have a very limited span of usefulness, and even then, they should used sparingly; so they could be considered large, costly entertainers at best. Some models have downright garish color schemes that verge on being eyesores, most eat up a lot of floor space, and a few play annoying music. Even though "stationary" exercisers don't have wheels, some babies can rock them so vigorously that the units "walk" across the floor, which could cause the baby to move close enough to touch a hot stove or allow both baby and exerciser to tumble down an unguarded staircase.

STATIONARY EXERCISERS

Evenflo's Ultrasaucer line
($55–$120)

Evenflo invented, and continues to improve, its Exersaucer line. The product is made in three levels of luxury, from the Deluxe with just a few toys to the Ultrasaucer with a whole cockpit of entertainment themes (jungle, underwater, circus, etc.) and designs and color schemes that change each year. Even the most basic models offer adjustable legs, seat adjustments, and a wide selection of toys scaled to toddler hand sizes. Moving up in price brings more toys and battery-operated sound and light features. A mid-range model should provide plenty that's entertaining. (For safety's sake, we suggest never leaving the baby alone with the product, though.)

"We were given an exerciser for our baby when he was five months old. We tried putting him in it, and he hated it. But we tried again two months later and he loved it. So if your baby doesn't enjoy it at first, try again."

WALKERS

Like exercisers, walkers have a suspended seat in the center of a supporting frame that has legs and wheels. The baby moves the walker around using a scuttling action with her feet and toes. Walkers vary in shape—some are simple, others are molded to look like cars or trucks. Some have trays, toys, and/or sounds and lights.

In spite of numerous safety warnings, lots of parents are eager to find and buy walkers for their babies during the pre-walking stage, in the belief that it will help their babies walk sooner, entertain them, or somehow be educational.

The truth is there is absolutely no scientific evidence that putting a baby in a walker will help her walk sooner or improve her development in any way. In fact, some studies appear to show that walkers actually interfere with a baby's acquisition of walking skills.

Exerciser and walker safety tips

Here are important ways to protect your baby from exerciser and walker hazards.

✔ **Buy certified models only.** Consider a model that has a "JPMA Certified" sticker on the frame or seat.

✔ **Use them on a floor with no descending stairs.** They're safest in a single-story dwelling.

✔ **Use walkers sparingly.** Limit your baby's time in the walker to only 30 minutes per day.

✔ **Babyproof for your baby's height.** Make sure there are no dangling cords, hot spots, drawers, or cabinets that might be hazardous to your baby.

✔ **Stay close.** Never let your baby out of your sight while she's wheeling around.

✔ **Use walkers only indoors.** Don't be tempted to use one on the deck, patio, or near a pool.

WARNING

Certified walkers don't always put on the brakes!
Even though most certified walkers have skid-resistant tabs or presser feet underneath their frames to stop a walker from going over the edge of a step, the mechanisms can give parents a false sense of security. Such safety stops may not work if the baby approaches the step sideways or backs into it, and slip-resistant stoppers may fail to hold if they're dirty or covered with lint. The tops of staircases should always be protected by a screwed-in safety gate.

✔ **Don't let it be used as a plaything.** Don't allow your baby to push the walker around from the outside or let other children use it as a plaything. Children can get hurt falling into the frame.

✔ **Don't attempt to lift the walker with your baby inside.** You might trip, your baby could fall out from the side, or the frame could break from the pressure.

Highs & lows of walkers

Highs. Babies seem to enjoy being given a taste of what it's like to move around on their own.

Lows. They have a limited span of usefulness. Serious safety problems have figured in severe baby injuries to thousands of babies and over 100 deaths, especially from head trauma, drowning, and burns. Overuse of a walker may slow down a baby's walking independently or enforce abnormal foot and leg actions.

SAFETY CONSIDERATIONS

Although stationary exercisers are considered relatively safe for baby play, walkers have serious safety problems. The U.S. Consumer Product Safety Commission reports that an estimated 197,200 babies were treated in emergency rooms in the U.S. for walker-related injuries over a period of 11 years, with the most serious injuries caused when walkers tipped over on a hard surface or down stairs. Tots have also drowned after rolling into water and been seriously injured when their walkers rolled into hot ovens, cups of coffee, and heavy objects. Surveys show that in 78 to 80 percent of walker-related accidents, the babies were being supervised—the walkers simply scooted too fast.

Fortunately, the introduction of stationary activity centers in the mid-'90s as a substitute for walkers on wheels, along with the creation of a voluntary walker certification standard by the Juvenile Products Manufacturers Association (JPMA) and the American Society of Testing and Materials (ASTM), have helped to drastically reduce walker-related baby injuries nationwide.

The biggest safety concern regarding exercisers is their ability to "walk" from baby's motions when there's a saucer-shaped rocking disk for a base. For walkers, it's that the wheels fastened to the frame may allow the baby to move faster than parents can keep up with them.

With either product, the baby can propel himself toward hot stoves and fireplaces, menacing stairwells, suspended appliance and lamp cords, and outdoor swimming pools and open bodies of water that pose a drowning threat. Moving over rough or uneven surfaces could cause the device to fall over, hurting the baby inside.

Babies are also hurt when they try to stand up and fall out of the units, since the products have no seat belts. Components, such as seats, sometimes give way, allowing the baby to fall or get wedged between the tray and the seat. And toys fastened onto the trays may work loose, exposing the baby to the bolts, sharp tips, or small parts that could choke her.

Manufacturers who wish to have their activity centers or walkers certified by the JPMA and ASTM agree to have their products tested by an impartial testing facility to ensure they meet exacting safety and durability standards. (Note: The standard is voluntary, and manufacturers can elect not to have their products tested. On the other hand, being certified does not make a product immune to having flaws or undergoing recalls.)

The certification program for activity centers addresses the stability of the exerciser if a baby leans over; the structural integrity of the exerciser by giving it weight tests; checks how well the leg holes of the seat hold the baby inside; component strength and other issues; and the wording and placement of warning labels.

The walker standard requires that they help to prevent falls down stairs, by requiring either a base wide enough that it can't roll through standard doorways or special stoppers on the base of the walker that bring it to a halt when it comes to the edge of a step. Walkers are also tested for structural integrity by how they hold up to weights and being pulled with specified pounds of force, and how well they hold babies inside.

You can find exerciser and walker recalls by going to www.recalls.gov and searching the Consumer Product Safety Commission's site (www.cpsc.gov) and entering "exercisers" or "walkers" or the specific brand name of the product you want to check. Our recommendation is to buy an exerciser instead of a walker.

13

GATES & ENCLOSURES

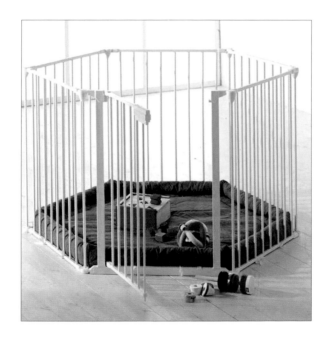

Safety gates will help protect your baby from stairways, pets, and unsafe situations at home. Enclosures can provide a fenced-in place for play. This chapter offers suggestions on choosing the best gates and enclosures for your space needs. You'll find detailed shopping hints and a discussion of critical safety issues.

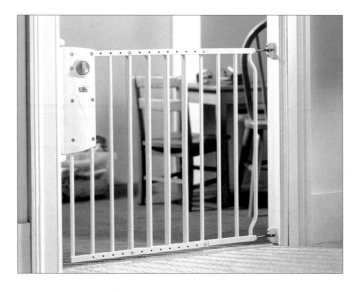

INSIDE THE GUARDING GATE

Gates are just what they sound like—small locking barriers to keep your toddler out of mischief while still allowing him a certain amount of freedom to move around.

The prime time that parents purchase gates is as soon as their babies start to crawl and become mobile—between 6 and 9 months of age—and they're one of the top 10 biggest baby-product sellers.

One word of caution from the start: No gate can completely stop a determined toddler from getting a leg up over the top of the gate and flinging himself over the other side; nor are there any guarantees that he won't figure out how to open it. As with any other accident-prevention product, a gate simply buys you time.

When to Buy

Purchase gates soon as your baby starts to become mobile, at around 6 to 8 months, and use them to guard unsafe spaces, such as stairways, until your baby is a sturdy walker and climber, between 24 and 36 months.

How gates work

Gates are constructed from wood, metal, plastic, or a combination of these materials. While wooden gates are more compatible with most interiors, those made from metal with welded parts and those made of dense molded plastic tend to be sturdier.

Gates are categorized by how they fasten to the wall: (1) those that attach to walls using screws, which are called hardware mounted, and (2) those that cling by using rubber gaskets pressed into the wall, called pressure-mounted gates.

While pressure-mounted gates are reasonably safe for less risky door openings, such as the bathroom, the kitchen, or another child's room, the gate guarding the top of a staircase should always be screw-mounted directly onto the wall.

That's because a pressure-mounted gate, especially a flimsy one, can readily be dislodged by a child (or a dog), especially if he falls into the gates tries to climb over it, or when an object, such as a walker, is rolled into it. And if the gate gives way, both baby and gate could tumble down the stairs, potentially causing far more serious head and body injuries than if the baby had simply tumbled down on his own.

Most gates are made of panels fastened to a stationary frame that fastens to a hinge on one side, with a latch on the opposite side that locks the gate shut with an audible click.

Locking devices are usually spring-action and made of metal, and they're designed to be tricky, requiring feats that thwart intrepid toddlers. How easily a gate locks or opens varies with brands and models; some are more ergonomically friendly and easier to use than others. Some gates swing closed on their own power, others don't. And some models, especially those designed for guarding stairs, allow the gate to be locked into a single swinging direction so that it won't open out over the stairway.

WARNING

Destroy killer accordion gates!
Old-fashioned, folding accordion gates with wooden slats are still around, but they're dangerous and shouldn't be used. The gates' wide diamond-shape gaps and the V shape at the top create a choking hazard. The gates also have a history of crushing fingers when the gates' slats squeeze together during opening. If you come across such a gate, don't buy it, and destroy any you have around the house.

Areas of Possible Head Entrapment

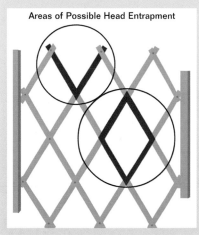

WARNING

Gates hurt parents!

Gates are supposed to protect babies, but they don't protect parents and other family members. Tens of thousands of adults and children have required emergency room treatment because they've tripped trying to step over gates. Typical gate-related injuries include painful back and knee injuries, broken wrists and elbows. Enforce this household rule: "Stop, open the gate, walk through, and close the gate behind you." (And select a gate that's easy for everyone to unlock.)

Gates for unusual openings

The architecture of some homes requires more than just a standard wall-to-wall doorway gate. As a result, manufacturers have responded by creating odd-sized gates and those with special adaptive hardware for installing across openings that don't fit traditional dimensions.

Some models come with end posts that rotate and fasten to angled surfaces. If you want to attach safety gates to banisters, wrought iron, brick, or any other nonstandard doorway material you will probably have to order separate parts. Most gate manufacturers also sell adapters that make their gates wider.

Six strategies for selecting a gate

Lots of parents end up taking gates back to the store because they don't fit doorways and other openings that they want to block off at home. Here's a list of what to do in advance to save you extra trips back to the store.

1. First, measure the openings. Doorways and openings vary widely from home to home. Some openings are 30 inches wide; others are even wider. If the doorway opening has a baseboard, measure from that part. The packaging and instructions for the gate will specify exactly how narrow or wide the gate can be. Trying to stretch the gate beyond the maximum width recommended by the manufacturer substantially weakens its ability to hold and could cause it to break.

2. Decide on the type of wall fastener. Gates with sides that screw into the wall have more staying power than models that use nonslip rubber gaskets to hold the gate on the wall. Screw-mounted versions should always be used at the tops of stairs.

3. Deal with the screw problem. If you live in a rental property with rules about not nailing anything into the wall, ask your landlord's permission and explain the safety (and liability) problems. Promise to repair the screw holes when you move out. Or, if you have no other option, choose a high-quality pressure-mounted gate and install it with sufficient pressure so that it won't budge.

4. Note special problems. If the area you're planning to fasten the gate to has banisters on one or both sides, or if the wall is angled or there are other unusual configurations, you'll need a gate that comes with special adapters. (Or purchase them separately.)

5. Choose the right material. If you're concerned about decorative appearances, then you may want to choose a wooden gate in a neutral or darker wood finish, but metal or plastic gates tend to be sturdier.

6. Compare prices. Browse around first to find the gate models that will work for your openings and then plan to compare prices on the Internet. Make sure to write down the exact model number, since more than one gate may have the same brand and model name. Also check out the retailer's return policy and factor in shipping and handling costs, including what it would cost you to return the gate if it doesn't fit or if you decide you don't like it. (An excellent Internet source for gates for hard-to-find openings is www.onestepahead.com.)

Checklist

Gate shopping

✔ **JPMA/ASTM certified.** A certification sticker offers extra assurance that the gate has been tested for safety and durability. (See certification discussion on page 191.)

✔ **The tallest version.** The taller the gate, the more protection from a climbing toddler or nosy pet (or the temptation to step over).

✔ **One-hand operation.** Locking mechanisms should be easy for you to use, but hard for a tot to manipulate.

✔ **Vertical slats.** Gates with vertical slats resembling crib bars are easier to see through and discourage tots from climbing over.

✔ **Sturdy.** Look for strong hardware and materials.

✔ **Smooth finish.** All gate surfaces should be smooth—no sharp edges, roughly welded seams, or protruding staples or nails that could hurt small mouths and fingers.

Avoid:

✗ **Crossbars on the floor.** Avoid gates that have a bar across the floor of the opening to support their frames, which could trip family members.

✗ **Gaps that could be used for toe-holds.** Avoid gates with center panels made of plastic mesh or with gaps, which your tot could use as a foothold for climbing over.

✗ **Sharp or hostile parts.** There should be no sharp corners or parts that could hurt a baby if he falls into them. Be sure hinges and closures can't pinch or injure small fingers.

✗ **Ineffective pressure gaskets.** Avoid pressure-mounted gates with gaskets that readily compress, making the gate likely to fall.

> **❝We saved money by purchasing the gate at a discount pet outlet. The gate was almost identical to the one in the baby store, but taller, which we felt was an advantage.❞**

Learning Curve's The First Years Simple and Secure Stair Gate

($60)

This is a hardware-mounted gate designed for the tops of stairs or any other household use.

It closes securely with a clicking sound when it locks. The two-stage push-and-turn knob action for unlocking the gate is manageable for adults, but too difficult for a child under 2. Vertical metal bars discourage toddler climbing while allowing a view to the next room. Adjustment slots allow you to customize the gate's expansion width between 29½ inches and 44 inches. For babies 6 to 24 months.

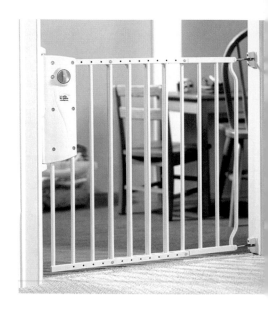

Evenflo's Secure Step Top of Stair Wooden Gate

($50)

The Secure Step is an expanding wooden gate that fits spaces 28 inches to 42 inches wide. It has steel hardware and opens using a simple one-handed lever. The gate's wood finish is nontoxic and can be wiped clean. Even though the gate comes preassembled, it requires a 5-step installation process using a Phillips screwdriver and electric drill with a ⅛-inch drill bit. A special hinge allows the gate to be locked so that it can't swing out over stairs.

ENCLOSURES

Corrals for young cowpokes

While safety gates are designed to protect babies from falling down stairs or getting into unsafe areas, enclosures are made from hinged gatelike panels that provide a corral for keeping tots in one place so they can't roam around the house.

Most come with one hinged panel that operates as a gate for putting children inside and getting them out. Generally, the enclosure package comes with a starter set of panels to form a compact circular corral, with extra panels available for separate purchase to make a larger circle. And most come with hardware that allows you to fasten both ends of the enclosure to the wall to form a shield to protect your baby from the fireplace, a wood stove, your computer, or other spaces that you want to make off-limits to him.

Just as with safety gates, enclosures aren't a substitute for constant parental supervision, and you should never let babies and toddlers out of sight while they're playing inside an enclosure (or outside one keeping them from danger areas).

When to Buy

After your baby can safely sit up on his own (6 to 8 months). Constantly supervise and discontinue use when your child attempts to climb over or can open the gate (24 to 36 months).

Highs & lows of enclosures

Highs. Like the large square playpens of years past, an enclosure can restrain your baby and keep him (and other siblings) in one place while you focus on cleaning or doing other chores nearby. It can help to cordon off unsafe areas, like the fireplace and its sharp brick ledge.

Lows. A baby knows when he's being locked off and may protest at being kept away from your side. Enclosures can be heavy and cumbersome to move around and store, and they eat up a lot of space. They're costly for the short period of time that toddlers will use them. They shouldn't be used on uneven surfaces, such as outdoors, where a gap underneath could entrap an arm or body should the baby try to escape.

✔ Checklist

Enclosure shopping

✔ **Easy-to-open gate.** The entry gate should be easy for you to operate but hard for a tot to open.

✔ **Compact fold.** Sections should fold together compactly enough to fit in the closet.

✔ **Portability.** Light enough that you can easily carry it from one place to another.

✔ **Available panel additions.** You should be able to buy or order extra panels to expand the size of the enclosure if you wish.

Kidco's PlayDen
($180)

This large tubular-steel enclosure lets babies and toddlers roam free and play in a large section of a room while still protecting them from dangerous or unsupervised areas. The set comes with three interlocking sections, each one measuring 29 inches high and 24 inches long. Sections lock together in a moveable configuration that fits an area of your home, and additional 2-foot extensions are available. The gate requires wall mounting on both sides and comes with a gate for entering and exiting.

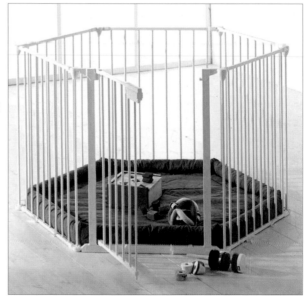

SAFETY CONSIDERATIONS

Safety gates and enclosures are not fail-safe! Typical injuries include fingers cut or pinched by sharp parts, hinges, and locking mechanisms. Unsafe gaps in the panel entrap toddlers' necks or allow small children to get a toehold to climb over.

Pressure-mounted gates can detach from the wall, allowing them to fall (especially dangerous at the tops of stairs), which can cause more injury to the baby than if he fell without the gate. Thousands of children and adults have been injured when they tripped on a crossbar at the base of the frame or attempted to step over the gate rather than opening it and walking through.

Sometimes adults forget to close the gate after going through, allowing their tots access to stairs and other unsafe places. If enclosures are used on uneven surfaces, such as outdoors, a gap underneath could entrap an arm or body should the baby try to escape.

Gates are recalled when components fail or when babies are injured by them, such as when babies become entrapped in a gate's components or have their fingers or toes hurt by them. To find gate and enclosure recalls, use www.recalls.gov to search the Consumer Product Safety Commission's site (www.cpsc.gov). And be sure to return the registration card that comes with your gates or enclosures or to register them online at the manufacturer's site so that you will notified if there is a safety recall.

Gates and enclosures both come under the voluntary certification program for the Juvenile Products Manufacturers Association (JPMA) in cooperation with the American Society of Testing and Materials (ASTM) If the manufacturer complies with the standard and has its gates tested by an independent laboratory, the gate will have a sticker stating "JPMA Certified."

14

HIGH CHAIRS, BOOSTER SEATS & HOOK-ON HIGH CHAIRS

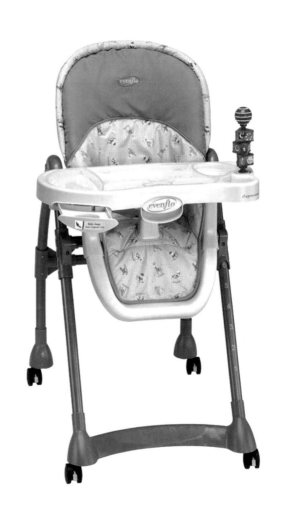

Here's all you need to know about the many seating options for feeding your baby. High chairs, the most popular option, are discussed first, followed by other seating alternatives such as booster seats that fasten onto adult-size chairs and hook-on chairs that are secured to the edge of a table. You'll find in-depth product discussions, detailed shopping hints, and information on product safety.

HIGH CHAIRS

The lowdown on high chairs

High chairs are designed to bring babies to parent level, making baby feeding easier. By necessity, these baby-seats-on-stilts have widely spaced legs to keep them from toppling over if an active tot tries to climb them.

> **"Even when we weren't using our baby's high chair to feed her, we liked having it in the kitchen to keep her out from under foot when we were cooking, cleaning,or loading the dishwasher. "**

With the exception of restaurant-style boosters designed to be pulled up to the table, most high chairs have removable trays that glide on and off using squeeze clips that lock onto the arms of the chair in one of several positions, but getting the tray on and off can be a hassle. The trays aren't made to hold a baby in place and shouldn't be used as a restraint.

For safety's sake, all newer-model high chairs come with adjustable seatbelts that are secured to the back or sides of the chair's frame to keep small diners from standing up and falling out. Almost all also come with between-the-legs posts in the front of the seat to protect babies from getting captured by sliding underneath the tray ("submarining").

Some chairs recline, which can make the chair substitute as an infant seat (with the tray removed) before the baby is ready to sit up and try solids. A word of caution, though: Always use the seat's safety belts, and keep an eye on your baby, since no chair can be trusted to fully protect her by itself.

Wooden high chairs tend to be bulky and awkward and don't come with wheels, while most tubular-framed models are more streamlined and mobile. Being able to roll a high chair, however, can be both a blessing and a curse. The good news: You can wheel the baby around from room to room while you do chores. The bad news: Unlocked wheels compromise the chair's stability and may cause it to fall over on a climbing tot, and there's a good chance the chair will become a large push toy for an active toddler.

You really won't need to purchase a high chair until your baby has gained enough neck and back strength to sit up on her own—between 6 and 8 months. And if you postpone acquiring one until then, you can take the baby shopping with you to test features such as the fit of the safety belt, the comfort of the seat cushions, and how well the seat dimensions and tray height work for you both.

What you get for the money

Models at the bottom of the high-chair price range usually have frames constructed of lightweight metal tubing, thin vinyl seat covers that are heat-sealed around the edges, vinyl or thin mesh waist belts and buckles, and small trays. Even though an inexpensive model may come in handy at Grandma's, it can't be relied on to hold up to the everyday wear and tear that a toddler can dish out.

You can expect to pay between $40 and $50 for the lowest-priced high-chair models. Examples in this category include Cosco's Simple Start High Chair with a molded unibody seat that includes a snack tray and a full-size tray and a tray topper. J. Mason's Compact High Chair, about $47, has a larger tray, vinyl-padded seat cushions, and folds compactly on its X-shape tubular frame. Just a little higher in price, Evenflo's Expressions High Chair models start around $50. The most basic model in this product line has locking wheels, multiple seat and recline options, and a removable cushioned and washable seat cover to top vinyl seat cushions.

Moderately priced chair lines, such as those from Evenflo's mid-price Expressions versions, Baby Trend's Trend Chair ($89), and Graco's Contempo ($100+), feature roomier seats with deeper cushioning and can adjust to various heights when a latch is squeezed on each side of the seat's frame.

Some of these models offer an additional thickly padded fabric seat cover that can be removed for washing. The seatbelt will be made of sturdy nylon webbing with a 5-point positive-lock belting system to hold a baby at the shoulders, around the waist, and between the legs. The trays are larger than less expensive models, and many newer models offer removable dishwasher-safe plastic tray inserts. Most have seats with several recline positions, which makes them able to support babies too young to sit up on their own. Graco's top-of-the-line chairs come with detachable toys,

When to Buy

Six months to 3 years and/or 40 pounds, younger for reclining chairs. (Always follow the manufacturer's age and weight guidelines for your chair.)

WARNING

Prevent baby falls

Each year, nearly 8,000 babies are rushed to emergency rooms as the result of high-chair-related injuries. Most often, the baby tries to stand up in the chair and topples overboard, sometimes sustaining serious head injury from the fall. Don't depend upon the tray to hold your baby inside. Always use high-chair seat-belts to secure your baby, and stay in the same room whenever your baby is in the chair, even if she's dozing.

and others offer adjustable footrests for increased baby comfort.

The costliest chairs are usually sleek imports, such as Italian-made Peg Pérego's Prima Pappa Diner ($170 and up) that uses trendy color schemes on the seats and trim. However, pricier imports won't perform any better when it comes to functionality and ease of use than less expensive and often lighter-weight U.S. versions. Some very expensive high chair/youth chair combinations with wood frames actually lack both the comfort and convenience of standard chairs, in spite of costing hundreds of dollars.

Mid-price chairs are the best investments on a feature-by-feature basis.

10 shopping strategies for buying high chairs

1. Test products yourself. Test the tray to see if it goes on and releases smoothly with one hand while you're holding a baby in the other. Try raising and lowering the seat, reclining the seatback, and folding the chair if these features are offered. If you wait to buy the chair until your baby's almost ready to start solids, test the height of the tray to make sure it's not so high your baby disappears behind it.

2. Take notes. You may discover an acceptably priced chair at a local store. Once you settle on the best model, take detailed notes, including the manufacturer's name, the model name, the model number, and the price, and then comparison shop several other sources for the same chair before you buy.

3. Have the facts. If you buy sight unseen, make sure you're getting the exact name and model number of the product you want, since high-chair lines that carry the same company and model name can range from a bare bones unit to a posh has-everything version, depending upon the model number. You may believe you're getting a great deal but instead receive fewer features.

4. Watch for sales. Just as with cars, baby products have seasons. New products typically are released around the end of the year, and you may be able to get last year's version on sale if you time it right. Also keep your eyes out for special discount coupons or other end-of-season baby sales that are periodically offered by Toys "Я" Us, Babies "Я" Us, and other big discounters.

5. Factor in hidden costs. Not all online discounts for high chairs turn out to be bargains after all. If you decide to order a high chair online or from a catalog, don't forget to factor in shipping and handling when you compare costs.

6. Don't back-order. Unless you're assured the product will be delivered within a reasonable amount of time—say, three weeks—don't have the product back-ordered or delayed. You may end up with long delays and not get the chair by the time your baby needs it.

7. Read the fine print. The seller should give you full return privileges if the product doesn't work for you. Ask about

Q/A

Q I'm 7 months pregnant. My mother-in-law wants to lend us the antique high chair that my husband used as a baby. The top tray is on hinges and swings down over the baby. Is it okay to use it?

Although antique high chairs can be charming, they don't have the safety features of newer chairs, including seat belts to keep the baby from standing up and falling out and a center post to keep babies from sliding out from under the tray. Older models are also harder to keep clean. If you still want to use the chair, we recommend purchasing an adjustable front-zippered harness that you securely fasten to the chair and use with your baby to make sure she doesn't get hurt by falling overboard. Damp mop and dry the high chair after each use to keep the sticky stuff from drying on the chair and ruining the finish.

Q Our baby is almost 8 months old, but we have the hardest time getting her to sit up in her high chair. She always seems to slouch, especially if the tray's not pushed up against her chest. Any suggestions?

If the chair's footrest is adjustable, try raising it so your baby's legs can stretch out. Also, placing a rolled bath towel under your baby's thighs may help press her into the back of the chair so

that she sits up better. Just make sure that nothing you put into the chair interferes with the seatbelts that help to hold her safely inside.

Q My baby had a scary accident when the plastic seat on her chair broke and fell to the floor when I reclined it. I called the manufacturer's customer service number, but the person on the other end of the line made me feel like I was to blame for the accident. What should I do?

By law, manufacturers are required to report to the Consumer Product Safety Commission (CPSC) any accidents involving their products reported by parents. But some unscrupulous manufacturers may try to avoid reporting the problem by attempting to diminish the importance of what you are describing. In addition to reporting the accident on the company's toll-free number, we suggest filing a detailed report of the accident by fax or in writing to the president of the company, and that you also file an accident report on CPSC's toll-free consumer hotline (800-638-CPSC). If you report an accident, make sure to include the model name and number of the chair and where you bought it. You could be protecting other babies from harm, since sometimes the CPSC issues recalls for "near misses" as well as for products that actually cause injuries.

return policies before you buy, otherwise you may be stuck with an awkward, uncomfortable, or malfunctioning (and therefore unsafe) chair and not be able to return it.

8. Be cautious about buying used items online. It's hard to assess a product's flaws and problems from a photo on an auction site such as eBay. Ask questions, and make sure the seller will allow you to return the

product if something isn't right.

9. Keep your receipts and register the product. Once you've bought the high chair, be sure to keep the receipts in a safe place. If there's a registration card, fill it out and send it in immediately. That tells the manufacturer how to contact you if there's a recall for a serious safety issue.

10. Set aside assembly time. Putting a high chair together out of a carton can

Checklist

What to look for when high chair shopping:

✔**JPMA approved.** "JPMA Certified" sticker on the chair.

✔**Seat belt.** 5-point seat belt with toddler-resistant buckle.

✔**Tray.** Easy to slide on and off with one hand. Deep rim for spills.

✔**Crotch post.** To prevent baby from sliding under the tray (submarining) and from deadly entrapment.

✔**Seat height.** Multiple seat heights so that the chair can fit under the table or lower to the floor so your tot can use it as a seat.

✔**Stability.** Hard to tilt or pull over. Casters lock.

✔**Cleaning ease.** Smooth surfaces that won't capture crumbs and baby food.

✔**Folding.** Folds easily and compactly for storing.

sometimes be exasperating, and sharp tubes can even draw blood! Allow at least 30 minutes (preferably without your baby anywhere nearby) to attach the legs and wheels, unwrap and wash the tray and components, wipe down the vinyl seat, launder the fabric insert, and test out the seat positions—you get the picture!

Avoid:

✗ **Unsafe components.** Sharp edges and pinch points under the tray. Protruding legs at the base of the chair could cause tripping and stubbed toes.

✗ **Too big.** Small eating areas call for a small footprint (or a strap-on booster.) If the tray's too high, it may dwarf your baby.

✗ **Hard to clean.** Upholstery with nooks and crannies that harbor crusted food (and germs).

✗ **Safety problems.** Flimsy seat belts and lack of a center post (to prevent sliding under the tray) compromise the chair's safety.

✗ **No wheel locks.** Locking wheels are important for stabilizing the chair and keeping it from being pushed around by a tot.

✗ **Awkward features.** Hard-to-operate height adjustments and overly large trays that are cumbersome to put on and take off.

> **"Don't buy a high chair until you meet and get to know your child. We invested in a trendy Scandinavian wooden chair before our baby was born. It was the wrong choice! We ended up trading it in for a standard chair with multiple seat positions, a vinyl seat, a washable seat cover, and wheels that let us roll the baby around."**

Highs & lows of high chairs

Highs. High chairs raise your baby up to your level for feeding, and they give her a bird's-eye view of the kitchen while you're preparing meals. Reclining models can be used like baby seats on wheels until your baby's old enough to sit up on her own. Seat heights adjust on most models so you can lower the chair and remove the tray when you want to pull your baby up to the table during family meals. Trays with deep rims can help to catch spills and slosh. One-handed tray removal on some models makes putting baby inside easier.

Lows. Assembling the high chair out of the carton can be time-consuming and challenging. Babies stand up and fall out, or they can slip out under the seat when they're not safely belted in. High chairs aren't reliable babysitters, and parents always need to stay close. Trays can sometimes jam, and folding the chair may pinch parents' fingers. High chairs eat up a lot of kitchen space—a problem in small kitchens.

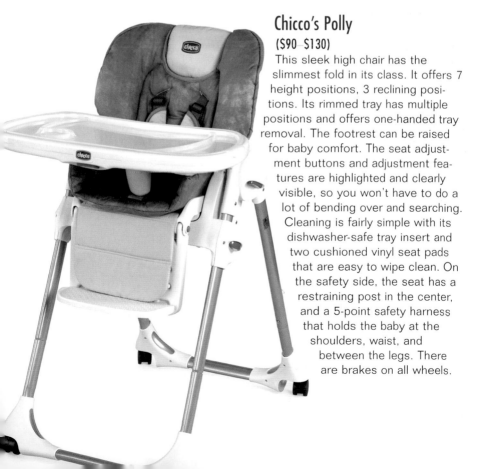

Chicco's Polly
($90–$130)

This sleek high chair has the slimmest fold in its class. It offers 7 height positions, 3 reclining positions. Its rimmed tray has multiple positions and offers one-handed tray removal. The footrest can be raised for baby comfort. The seat adjustment buttons and adjustment features are highlighted and clearly visible, so you won't have to do a lot of bending over and searching. Cleaning is fairly simple with its dishwasher-safe tray insert and two cushioned vinyl seat pads that are easy to wipe clean. On the safety side, the seat has a restraining post in the center, and a 5-point safety harness that holds the baby at the shoulders, waist, and between the legs. There are brakes on all wheels.

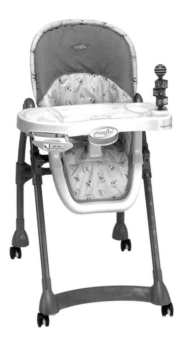

Evenflo's Expressions High Chair
($60)

The slender profile of the seats in this line helps it fit into smaller kitchens. It offers 7 seat heights and 3 reclining positions. The tray has multiple positions and can be removed with one hand. It comes with a dishwasher-safe tray insert. There's a slide-away organizer in the front to hold baby food jars and utensils. Three-point harness system.

> **"I really like the fact that my baby's high chair has a post that goes between the legs so she doesn't go sliding down. No matter how snugly I strapped her into other high chairs, she kept sliding down, and the post made it easier for her to sit up."**

BOOSTER SEATS

The baby booster club

Booster seats—not to be confused with booster car restraints for kids—are small square seats that take the place of the phone book used on top of the dining room chair in Granny's day.

They're designed to sit on top of an adult-size chair to raise a child to dining-table height. Some seats come with removable trays. The seats are generally much less expensive than a standard high chair, and some parents prefer them as a lightweight, portable substitute for a full-size (and floor-hogging) high chair.

The adult chair that holds the seat is important. It should be stable and have a wide, flat seat part that's wider than the booster to ensure that it won't wobble or slip off sideways.

Boosters usually come with two sets of safety straps, one that fastens around the base of the adult chair and the other that fastens around the chair's back to keep the booster frozen in place even when there's a wiggly child inside. (They're not safe when used on stools, folding chairs, or other unstable seats.)

When to Buy

Approximate age and weight for use: 6 months to 49 pounds, younger for reclining chairs. (Always follow the manufacturer's age and weight guidelines for your booster.)

Some booster models have seat backs that recline for use with infants, or adjustable seat levels to grow with the child. As with full-size high chairs, if the booster has a tray, it should not be pressed into the baby's chest or belly as a way of restraining and keeping her in the seat. Instead, always rely on a sturdy adjustable seat belt and buckle, and fasten your baby in every time you put her in the seat.

Avoid:

✗ **Inadequate restraints.** Lack of seat belt, or flimsy seat belt and buckle. No crotch belt.

✗ **Poor finishing.** Sharp edges that could cut a child.

✗ **No chair fastener.** Lacking straps to secure the seat to the chair.

✗ **Hard to clean.** Nooks and crannies that make cleaning a chore.

✗ **Tray problems.** Hard-to-adjust tray or one that reclines with the seat.

✗ **Not very portable.** Clumsy for carrying and storage.

Highs & lows of booster seats

Highs. Boosters take up less space than traditional high chairs and cost substantially less, while serving essentially the same function. Most come with removable, washable trays, and nearly all have safety belts. Most models also fold compactly for use not only at home but also for carrying to restaurants and for travel. Some models adjust to different heights as the child grows, and some come with a washable padded seat cover.

Lows. Not as convenient to use as a rolling high chair, and may not fit young babies well. Safety issues: A toddler may pull the seat on top of herself when trying to mount it on her own. An improper fit between the host chair and the booster can compromise the safety of the seat, possibly leading to the fall of both baby and seat. Seat belts tend to be flimsier, and the buckle's plastic components may break. The seat's back or base may separate from the frame, which could lead to an injury. Not for use in vehicles.

 # Checklist

Booster seat shopping

There are not a lot of booster models from which to choose, but there are noticeable differences in the features that boosters offer. Here's what to look for:

✔ **Wide base.** Will sit solidly on a chair.

✔ **Skid resistance.** Nonskid surfacing on base to keep the seat from sliding.

✔ **Seat belt.** Seat belt for crotch and waist, with toddler-resistant buckle.

✔ **Safety belts.** Two sets: one to fasten to the chair back, the other to go underneath the chair.

✔ **Cleaning ease.** Smooth surfaces that won't capture crumbs and baby food.

✔ **Tray** (optional). Easy to slide it on and off.

✔ **Recline** (optional). Easy to operate, allowing tray to stay upright when reclined.

✔ **Storage** (optional). Comes with a storage pouch or straps for carrying.

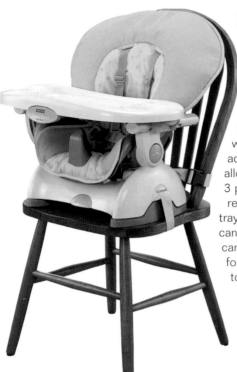

Fisher-Price's Spacesaver High Chair
($50)

With many of the features of a full-size chair, the Spacesaver straps down on a kitchen or dining-room chair from underneath and behind. It comes with a 5-point harness to hold baby inside and features a roomy, deeply cushioned seat with a wipe-clean pad. There are 3 height adjustments and a 3-position recline that allows the deep-rimmed tray (which also has 3 positions and is dishwasher safe) to remain level when the seat is reclined. The tray can be removed with one hand. The seat can be used like a high chair, or the seat back can be detached to make a toddler booster for the table. The base has nonslip surfacing to help keep the seat in place.

❝I'm loving our baby's booster seat! It straps onto a regular dining chair, the seat lowers as my baby grows, and it offers a 3-position recline. The pad's easy to remove for cleaning, and the tray doesn't have any awkward crevices to clean❞

Learning Curve's First Years On the Go Booster Seat
($25)

This handy, pack-and-go booster is about the size of a lunch box when deflated and zippered closed, but then it self-inflates with an air valve to expand into a full-sized chair booster. The T-strap waist restraint goes between the baby's legs and there are 2 anchor straps for fastening the inflatable underneath the seat portion of most dining chairs. A carry handle as well as an outside mesh pocket make the closed, 1-pound seat great for travel. For 9 months up to 40 pounds, or about 4 years.

HOOK-ON HIGH CHAIRS

Table toppers for tots

Hook-on high chairs fasten onto tables to enable children to use the surface for eating. Although the concept of fastening a chair directly onto a table sounds like a great concept, these have serious flaws. The original chairs could be hooked onto tables using long arms on top and bars underneath that pressed into the table when the weight of the baby was added to the seats, but most tables aren't designed to hold a 15- to 30-pound weight on one edge without tipping over.

There have been numerous accidents, some involving head or body injuries, when the seats have fallen over with the table or slipped off from babies' motions. The chairs can't be used on glass table tops, card tables, the foldout wings of tables, or on tables that don't have sufficient surface area to support the chair's hardware. And they shouldn't be used with a chair underneath, which could enable a child to lift himself and loosen the seat's hold on the table ledge.

When to Buy

Approximate age and weight for use: 6 months to 3 years and/or 36 pounds, younger for reclining chairs. (Always follow the manufacturer's age and weight guidelines for your chair.)

Avoid:

✗ **Poor safety features.** Chairs that have a flimsy seat belt or buckle and/or lack a crotch belt.

✗ **Flimsy construction.** Weak hardware that could bend, or thin upholstery and inadequate stitching that could fray or tear.

✗ **No locking mechanism.** Hook-ons that rely on pressure, rather than positive locks that hold it on to the table.

✗ **Hard to clean.** Nooks and crannies that trap food and make cleaning a chore.

Highs & lows of hook-on high chairs

Highs. Hook-on chairs are lightweight and fold easily and compactly, and may come in handy for travel.

Lows. The types of tables they can be safely attached to are limited. Most models pose a serious falling hazard for your baby, especially if they're used incorrectly.

Chicco's Caddy Hook-on High Chair
($40)

This model is our only product choice. Seats from other manufacturers in the category simply don't measure up. The Caddy's strong rubber feet cling to the top of the table. Underneath, it relies on ratcheting feet that press into the table's base and release with a simple squeeze-and-release latch. The seat comes with a 3-point harness. It folds compactly for travel and storage in its own case, and the seat's fabric can be removed for machine washing. Make sure to follow all of the manufacturer's safety precautions.

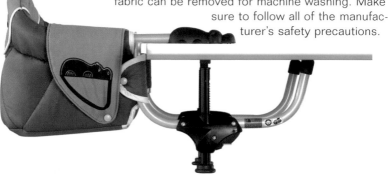

 # Checklist

Hook-on high chair shopping

Here's what to look for when you're shopping for hook-on high chairs:

✔ **Comfortable seat.** Seat offers adequate support for the baby.

✔ **Skid resistance.** Nonskid surfacing on all contact points with the table.

✔ **Seat belt.** Seat belt for crotch and waist with toddler-resistant buckle.

✔ **Compact folding.** Folds or disassembles easily for carrying and storage.

SAFETY CONSIDERATIONS

High-chair accidents include head and face injuries when unrestrained babies fall out of chairs as they try to stand up or when the tray fails, allowing baby and tray to fall forward out of the seat. Babies are also hurt when they attempt to climb into the chair on their own, pulling the chair over on top of themselves. Fingers can sometimes get pinched or cut from sharp hardware components on the underside of the tray. Some babies have strangled when their heads have become entrapped as their bodies slipped out from under the tray. And parents and other family members are injured when they stub their toes on the legs or wheels of the chair.

Boosters cause accidents when they slip off chairs or allow the baby to fall out. Hook-on chairs injure babies when they slip off the table, or when the table or tabletop tips over or breaks from the added weight of the baby.

High chairs, booster seats, and hook-on chairs have undergone a series of recalls over the years for component failures and safety problems, such as when high-chair seats have accidentally detached from their frames or when hook-ons have allowed babies to detach their chairs from the table by bouncing and pushing on table edges or chair bottoms.

All three product categories have voluntary certification standards. Those products that are certified will display a "JPMA Certified" sticker on the unit or packing carton. The sticker indicates that the product's manufacturer complies with rigorous safety standards, including periodic testing of product lines set up by the Juvenile Products Manufacturers Association in compliance with the American Society of Testing and Materials (ASTM.)

Being certified does not mean the particular product your baby is using has been individually tested for flaws, or that the design or unit is fail-safe. Numerous products that have been certified have also faced recalls when they were shown to have major baby-harming flaws.

Note that some manufacturers of quality products have elected not to be involved in the certification process, but their product may be safe even though it doesn't sport a certification sticker. (Search the CPSC recalls list from www. recalls.gov.)

15

MONITORS

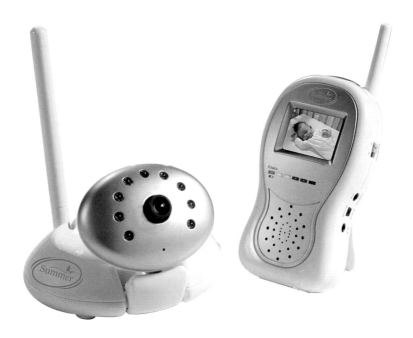

Nursery (or baby) monitors use electronic transmitters and receivers to allow you to hear your baby's every whimper from another room or even when you're on the way to the mailbox. This chapter walks you through all of their techy details to help you choose the sharpest one for hearing and even seeing your little snoozer.

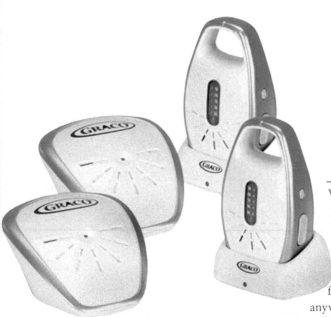

STOP, LOOK, AND LISTEN!

Whether you take the plunge the first night you bring your baby home from the hospital or months later, you're likely to feel uneasy the first time your baby sleeps anywhere but in the same room with you. A baby monitor can help you feel more connected when your baby's sleeping down the hall or you're in the kitchen, by supplying you with a second set of ears (and possibly extra eyes, too) to stay in contact.

Monitors have two basic parts: a transmitter that sends a baby's sound—or sound plus image—and a receiver that you carry around to pick up on your baby's signals. There are four basic types of monitors: audio versions that transmit only a baby's sounds to a small receiver that parents carry or clip on; intercom monitors, similar to walkie-talkies that allow parents to both hear and talk to their babies; video monitors that allow parents to both hear and see their babies via small video cameras and portable picture screens; and motion sensors that register the lack of baby's breathing and sound an alarm when the baby stays still for too long. These are used mainly for special-needs babies.

The transmitter part of monitors and cameras that is kept near your baby usually comes with adapters that plug into an electrical outlet and are designed to sit on a chest or shelf within a few feet of the baby's crib. The part that parents use to receive the baby's audio signal is usually a small handheld battery-operated device with a flexible antenna for picking up the sound signals broadcast by the baby's unit. Motion and breathing alarms rely on sensors placed directly on the baby's body or on the crib's mattress and sound an alarm if the baby stays motionless after a matter of seconds.

AUDIO MONITORS

Baby monitors send out signals, just as radios do, and the Federal Communications Commission (FCC) governs which wavelengths the monitor manufacturers can use. How well a monitor will perform depends primarily on how crowded the monitor's selected wavelength is, how its particular frequency handles obstructions such as concrete walls, and the strength of the monitor's signal.

Most monitors rely on batteries or on a combination of batteries and charging stations with plug-in electrical adapters to run, and many parents complain that they eat up lots of batteries. As with cell phones, a receiver takes a lot of juice. If it runs out of batteries, if it's not rechargeable, or if you forget to rest it in its docking station, the unit will fade and then go dead. (Some units have low-battery indicators.)

Many of the features on today's baby monitors have migrated from other high-tech devices. Most offer on/off switches, volume controls, rows of small lights that let you see as well as hear the intensity of baby sounds, a selection of broadcast channels (such as channel A or B) for getting the clearest and most static-free reception on your receiver, electrical outlet adapters, and low-battery indicator lights. Some receivers come with a battery pack and a small docking station for recharging when batteries run out of juice.

A few of the more sophisticated models offer a vibration mode, as cell phones often do. And other packages include an extra receiver so both you and your partner can listen in on your baby at the same time—or you can leave one receiver permanently stationed in your bedroom and carry the other one around.

Standard baby monitors compete for limited bandwidths, and lots of parents complain that their receivers experience interference from cell phones or CB radio signals, or that their monitors pick up snippets of cordless-phone conversations. And if you're able to overhear neighbors talking near their babies' monitors or someone else's baby crying on yours, the chances are pretty good that you and

When to Buy

From late pregnancy through the first 6 months if you feel you need to keep tabs on your baby's sleeping and waking.

your baby are being overheard, too.

Static noise on receivers is another problem. You may experience buzzing from household electrical devices, such as when your receiver nears the base of your cordless phone, when the refrigerator chunks on, when you turn on the television, or when you use the microwave. And that same interference can affect both the sound and the image of an audio/video monitoring system.

A monitor's packaging will say whether the set uses the 49 MHz, 900 MHz, or 2.4 GHz bands. The 2.4GHz band is the likeliest to have interference, since microwave ovens, wireless networks, and most wireless home phones use this same frequency; and the monitor may also interfere with your wireless reception when you're using your computer. Some older-model cordless phones operate on 49 MHz and 900 MHz bands that could also interfere with reception.

The distance that a monitor claims you can move from your baby and still pick up his signals ranges from as little as 200 feet up to 2,000 feet. But even though a monitor may boast that it has a transmission distance over 900 feet, that doesn't mean you'll get good transmission if you have electrical devices that are transmitting on the same wavelength. In fact, lower-range wavelengths are better at bouncing around obstacles if your baby's nearby. And no matter what monitor manufacturers guarantee, most monitors will lose their signal if concrete walls or other dense obstacles come between your baby's unit and yours.

While regular analog baby monitors operate on a frequency much like a radio, more recent designs use Digital Spread Spectrum (DSS) technology to modulate the baby's signal and scramble it as it travels between the monitor and the receiver, making eavesdropping almost impossible and reducing interference and static.

As with any product, not all brands perform equally well, and a higher price tag

> **❝ It took a few months for us to realize that the baby monitor wasn't helping us, especially at night. One of us (usually me) would jump up every time there was a sound. Finally we decided just to turn it off, trusting that if our baby really needed us, he'd let us know. ❞**

doesn't always guarantee superior performance. It makes sense to try out the monitor at home, and if it doesn't transmit clearly because of interference in your environment, then to consider returning it for another brand. Make sure to check out the retailer's return policy before you buy, keep the receipt for your purchase, and carefully repack the monitor in its original packaging when you take it back.

What you get for the money

At the bottom end of the monitor price scale are simple analog (radio-style) monitors that are available for about $20. These models have several channels that access commonly used monitor wavebands, a power switch and "on" light, a light display to show the intensity of the baby's noise, a volume control, and an electrical adapter for the transmitter.

Technology improves as prices rise. In the $35–$45 range, you can get multiple channels to choose from to minimize interference from other monitors using the same frequency, or you may have the choice of the less-populated 900 MHz range and a longer transmission range of, say, 1,500 feet. Some offer a voice-activated sound-and-light show on the baby's unit, with soft music and nature sounds—even a flashing and dimming ceiling show to soothe him back into dreamland (as found on the Fisher-Price Sound and Lights Baby Monitor).

Digital monitors—the wave of the future—kick in at $50 and up. These scramble and modulate signals using computer technology. Some monitors in this price range, such as Evenflo's Whisper Connect Two-Way analog monitor, offer features that allow your voice to be transmitted to your baby's room.

For $150 to $250 you can purchase a video monitor with a small camera that mounts on the wall or sits on a shelf near your baby. Most have night sensors that enable you to watch your baby on a small handheld color monitor even when the lights are dim. Some monitors may have an add-on that allows you to pick up a visual signal of your baby on your own television. It's important to remember that sleeping babies aren't all that interesting to watch; and once they're awake, they demand to be picked up and tended to, not watched from afar.

Future electronics can be expected to improve the sound quality, signal strength, and distance signals can travel, as well as becoming more sophisticated as features migrate from cell phone and other technologies. You may be able to receive a call when baby cries or check in on him using your phone's screen with a dialing code. But no matter how well monitors perform or how sophisticated they become, they can't take the place of parents' own ears and eyes for keeping constant watch over babies.

Quick tips

Monitors don't protect your baby from SIDS

When it comes to Sudden Infant Death Syndrome (SIDS), it's not the baby who's making noise that's of concern, but the one who isn't. According to the American Academy of Pediatrics, regular baby monitors are not effective in protecting babies from SIDS. Having your baby in the same room with you during the first 6 months of life is. The simplest and least-expensive option is to allow your baby to sleep in your room in a small-sized crib, bassinet, or cradle (discussed on pages 52–67.)

Highs & lows of audio monitors

Highs. A monitor can give you peace of mind that your baby isn't crying when you're out of earshot. Walkie-talkie versions may let you whisper sweet nothings to your baby or talk with your spouse in the nursery.

Lows. A monitor can't tell you if your baby has stopped breathing—a deeper concern for most parents of newborns. Monitor sounds could make you more jumpy about normal baby sounds and momentary fussiness, since they're usually amplified by the receiver. Static and interference are often problems unless the monitor uses digital technology. If the receiver's not rechargeable, it can eat up a lot of batteries.

Checklist

Audio monitor shopping

Here's what to look for when you're monitor shopping.

✔ **Clear reception.** A monitor with a different channel mix, such as channels A plus D instead of only A and B, and one that uses 900 MHz, which is less crowded and picks up clearer signals. Digital models allow less interference and static than analog versions.

✔ **Rechargeable batteries.** Monitors gobble up batteries. Rechargeable receivers can save up to $50 a year in battery costs. Also make sure both the transmitter (baby's unit) and the receiver (yours) have plug-in electric outlet adapters and a low-battery indicator.

✔ **Portability.** An easy-to-use belt clip and flexible antenna improve portability. Some models offer a pager feature to help parents find a lost unit.

✔ **Sound lights.** Indicators that light up to signal the intensity of baby's sound are useful for judging when it's time to head for the nursery, even when you're vacuuming.

✔ **Optional extras.** A warning light or alarm that signals when you're out of range, a night light feature for the baby's room, a 2-way walkie-talkie feature that lets you talk to your baby or others in the nursery, vibration to alert you to baby's crying when there's other noise going on.

Avoid:

✗ **Buying too early.** Most babies are pretty loud, and unless your house is very large and soundproofed, you may find a monitor more of an irritant than a help.

✗ **Battery eaters.** Monitors that use standard batteries, instead of being rechargeable.

✗ **Too-small receiver.** Can disappear between couch pillows and underneath papers.

✗ **Your neighbor's monitor.** With the same brand and model as the apartment next door, you may end up listening to the wrong baby! (Unless the monitor uses digital technology to keep the signal private.)

✗ **Video monitor.** If you're on a tight budget, a video monitor could be considered overkill.

Sony NTM-910 900 MHz BabyCall Nursery Monitor
($40)

Sony's monitor bandwidth allows you to carry the receiver farther than conventional (43–49 MHz) monitors yet still hear activities in the nursery. It offers 27 chan-

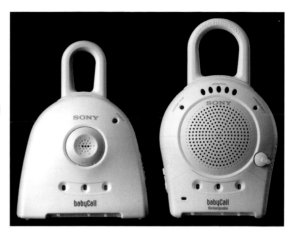

nels, to select the clearest one. The receiver is water resistant for use in the bathroom or kitchen. The voice-activated receiver eliminates most extraneous background noise for clearer transmission. It has a belt clip for wearing around the house. The transmitter can be operated either by rechargeable batteries or using a standard outlet with its AC/DC adapter. Activity lights indicate baby sound levels. An out-of-range indicator beeps and lights up when you exceed the transmitter's range. The units operate on standard household current or rechargeable batteries (furnished).

Graco iMonitor Digital Monitor with 2 Units
($85)

Since this monitor is totally digital, it helps to ensure privacy and to prevent eavesdropping. The manufacturer claims that the units work up to 2,000 feet. The monitor comes with 2 rechargeable parent units and 2 docking stations for them. There is also a parent-unit finder feature for locating misplaced units. The child unit uses an electrical outlet, but also has battery backup in case of electrical failure. Lights offer a visual signal that shows the strength of baby's crying. Newer models will have an adjustable vibration to feel the baby's call.

AUDIO/VIDEO MONITORS

Today's video monitors for the nursery use a small camera, similar to one you would perch on top of your computer screen. Most transmit both sound and color-image signals to a small handheld receiver with a screen not much larger than a cell phone's.

Video monitors simply don't have the same transmission power that audio monitors do. This means that you may only be able to get a clear video picture from about 200 to 300 feet, and walls or other obstacles may impede the transmission or cause the image to become blurry.

Most units come equipped with infrared technology that allows the small camera to pick up images in your baby's darkened room. The camera on some newer units gives you the power to pan the camera around the room upon command so that you can see your baby (or another child, pet, or caregiver).

With models priced between $100 and $250 (or more), a video moniter isn't an inexpensive investment. And in this case, quality and price often go hand in hand. The same interference issues that plague audio-only monitors also afflict combination audio/video ones.

Most units offer both battery operation and electrical outlet adapters. Expect that batteries will run out quickly—so rechargeable batteries and a charger are a good investment, especially if the parent part of the unit doesn't come with a charging dock.

Safe use tips

As with all electronic devices, safe use of your monitor is important. Here are some guidelines to follow.

■ **Beware a false sense of security.** Babies require continuous surveillance. Check on your newborn frequently, and pick up your baby as soon as you're sure he's awake, rather than relying on the monitor to oversee him.

■ **Keep away from water.** As with radios and hair dryers, a monitor is an electrical device that could shock you. Don't get any components near the bathtub, the kitchen sink, buckets of water, and don't put them in a wet basement.

■ **Watch out for cords.** Keep the transmitter well away from your baby's crib and the adapter cord out of reach so your baby can't become entangled in it, pull it down, or play with it at the electrical outlet.

■ **Keep away from heat.** Monitors are vulnerable to heat, so keep the units away from direct sunlight and don't set them near a register or radiator.

SAFETY CONSIDERATIONS

Monitors don't come under the certification program for the Juvenile Products Safety Commission (JPMA). They have infrequently been involved in recalls by the U.S. Consumer Product Safety Commission (CPSC), usually due to electronic flaws that could lead to shocks or their overheating. Monitor recalls can be searched by going to www.recalls.gov, the government's recall site, and entering the word "monitors," or the specific name of a monitor on the CPSC site (www.cpsc.gov).

Mobi Technologies MobiCam Ultra Wireless Monitoring System
($190)

The MobiCam system includes a 2.4 GHz handheld, wireless audio and video receiver with a small, 1.8-inch, color screen. It promises a reception range of about 300 feet. The camera has an infrared mode for night viewing up to 25 feet in total darkness. The unit also has a voice-activation function that automatically turns the camera on. The camera unit is designed to sit in one place, with limited angle control. Both the camera and the receiver require batteries and use them quickly, but the system comes with plug-in adapters to extend battery life. It has a belt clip, viewing stand, and hanging loop. An optional wireless camera and software products allow computer or PDA viewing.(Note: The unit's 2.4 GHz band may interfere with wireless computer connections.)

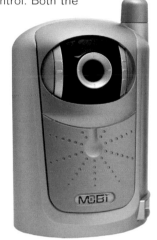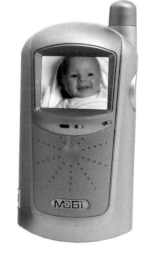

Summer Infant's Day & Night Handheld Color Video Monitor
($200)

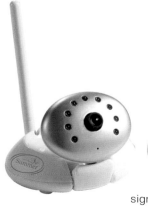

One of a series of audio/video monitors with similar names from Summer Infant, the parent unit of this version has a small, lightweight, 2.5-inch color LCD screen and a 900 MHz audio monitor with 2 channels and approximately a 350-foot audio range. An on/off button allows for audio-only signals. It can be hand-carried, clipped onto a belt, or propped on a flat surface using its flip stand, and lights indicate the strength of the audio signal. The camera has night vision and is designed to sit on a flat surface. Both units come with A/C adapters and use rechargeable batteries that last up to 10 hours. A power-saver feature times out after 3 minutes when battery power is running low.

16

PLAY YARDS & PLAYPENS

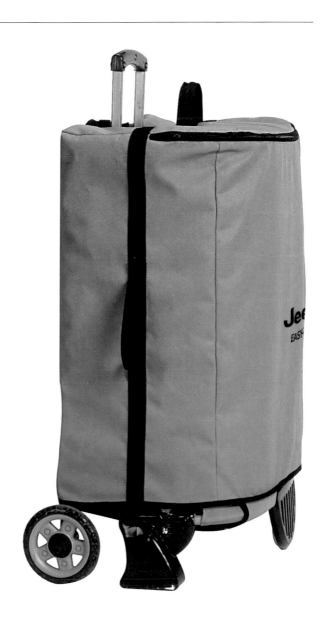

This chapter is all about playpens and play yards—foldable baby enclosures sometimes called port-a-cribs or pack-and-plays after name-brand models. Here's what you need to know to make a wise choice, along with shopping tips and serious safety warnings.

PENS FOR PETITE PLAYERS

Portable play yards are rectangular enclosures, usually with mesh sides. Since play yards are compact, foldable, and weigh much less than cribs, parents like to use them as convenient baby holders for indoors, on decks outdoors, or when traveling. But their disadvantage, especially with young babies, is that they sit close to the ground, which makes lifting and lowering a baby more of a strain for parents' backs.

> **"Our baby sleeps more soundly in her play yard than she does in the crib upstairs. The mobile and vibrations have been fun, too."**

Today's play yards are distant relatives of the old-fashioned square playpens of yester-year that were heavy and bulky and ate up a lot of living room (or closet) space. Instead of being constructed from wood, modern versions have frames of lightweight tubular metal components and mesh sides. Most of today's designs use sturdy moisture-resistant ripstop nylon, similar to tent material. And like tents, these man-made frame-and-fabric contraptions can be a challenge to put up and take down!

Most frames have wheels on at least two legs, for rolling around. And most also come with generous elasticized pockets on one or two of the end panels, for holding baby stuff. All yards come with a thin fabric-covered pad for the floor. It's worth noting that the fabric covering the pen and its padded floor are not removable and washable, as pads on other products are—such as bouncers, car seats, high chairs, and strollers—although some manufacturers sell removable washable sheets to cover the padded floorboards of their models.

What you get for the money

Lower-priced play yards start around $40 to $50. For that investment, you'll get a simple rectangular model with mesh sides but no extras. Example: Cosco's Passport ($40–$50).

Add $10 to $20 to that and other options are added, such as elasticized storage pockets on the outside of the yard, as well as a full-size or three-quarter-size bassinet that clips onto the railings to form a raised bed for young babies weighing under 15 pounds. Examples include basic models in Evenflo's BabyGo or Graco's Pack 'n Play lines, with Graco also offering extra fitted sheets for purchase. Larger, square models, similar in shape to old-fashioned playpens with padded railings and floorboards, also fall into this price range.

Models in the $80 to $100 range add a padded, indented diaper-changing unit that hooks over the top rails (safety belt included), such as Evenflo's Madison line or Graco's Baby Einstein's Discover yard. Over the long haul, most parents find that they have to bend over too low to use the changer, and they quickly resort to a standard diaper-changing table since it's more comfortable to use.

Other accessories as prices rise: roll-down flaps that act as sunshades, and bat-tery-operated features such as a rotating mobile, a vibrator that buzzes, a night-light, and other light and sound extras.

At the top of the price chain—$150 and up—are the sophisticated models that carry everything less-expensive models do, but with added fashion touches, such as trendy coordinated fabric patterns and rounded C shaped legs. They have thicker padding all around and a pull-down canopy. And they offer more battery-operated features, such as multiple music and sound choices, rotating mobiles with toys, and lights and vibrations that switch on and off with the touch of a button, and even consoles to hold diaper wipes.

Graco's Pack 'n Play Suite Solutions, sold at Babies " Я " Us, boasts an oval bassinet in the season's hottest shades and patterns. These also have a baby organizer that includes a diaper stacker, a wipes container and storage pockets, a 2-speed electronic mobile, switch-operated vibration, 5 nature sounds and songs, a full-length canopy, a night-light, and easy-to-operate squeeze latches that reduce the "fumble factor."

To induce parents and gift givers to buy more products, some manufacturers have created entire suites of coordinated baby

When to Buy

Wait until after the birth to be sure you really need one. Most manufacturers suggest that play yards can be used from birth until your baby reaches 30 pounds or 34 inches, or about 3 years of age, but most toddlers protest to being caged in such narrow confines long before that.

products, called collections, that use identical colors and fabric themes on multiple products. The baby's play yard will be designed to match his infant seat, his stroller, and possibly his high chair. There's only one problem with acquiring a matching, multiple-product suite: Individual products need to be evaluated on their own merits on critical points such as safety, ease of use, and comfort for the baby.

It's worth noting that the extras on the highest-priced play-yard models not only raise the price, they also add to the play yard's weight. While the loaded Graco Suite Solutions weighs 33 pounds, a simple J. Mason unit weighs only 13. Heavily accessorized units also require more storage space and increase the time and attention required to set up and break down the unit, and units loaded with electronics eat up batteries.

Do you really need a play yard?

Granted, play yards are very popular with most parents, but before you purchase a play yard, weigh these other options:

Better sleeping alternatives.
Newborns sleep a lot, and a portable crib, bassinet, bedside sleeper, or cradle will give your newborn a compact, secure, and moveable sleeping place for the same price or less than a mid- or upper-priced play yard, while eating up less space. Plus, you won't have to bend down so far, and you'll be able to remove the sheets to wash them (See "Bassinets & Crib Alternatives," starting on page 52.)

Baby comfort issues. Play yards force babies under 5 months of age to remain in a completely reclined position on their backs, and they have only semitransparent sides. A high chair with a reclining seat and wheels or a bouncer seat with

rocking, vibrating, and sound features will perform the same functions as a top-of-the-line play yard, yet cost considerably less while giving your baby a better view of you and her world. (See bouncer discussion starting on page 76.)

Toddlers don't like them. When it comes to restraining toddlers and keeping them out of trouble, babyproofing an area and then cordoning it off using safety gates or an enclosure will probably be more appealing (and appeasing) to your tot than confining her in the tiny cramped space afforded by a play yard. Enclosing your baby like that can thwart her natural drive to crawl and actively explore her environment, which is essential to strengthening her muscles and refining her motor skills and eye–hand coordination. And most babies protest when their parents move out of their sight. (Gates and enclosures are reviewed starting on page 182.)

WARNING

Read the directions!
Although play yards look simple when they're set up, it's important to read the directions before you open and fold down the first few times. They'll tell you exactly how to do that and how to use the play yard, and warn you of potential safety hazards. The instructions will also tell you how to contact the manufacturer if there's a problem or you have questions regarding assembly and setup. Store the directions for your play yard with all the instructions for other baby products, so you can easily access them.

✔ Checklist

Play yard & playpen shopping

If you decide to purchase a play yard after all these considerations, here are some basic features to look for (or avoid) when you shop.

✔ **No frills.** Considering the limited use that the product offers, it's probably best to err on the basic (read, less expensive) side.

✔ **Certified.** A "JPMA Certified" sticker on the frame or carton indicates that the play yard's manufacturer complies with the rigorous safety and durability tests of the Juvenile Products Manufacturers Association.

✔ **Firm cushioning.** Firm, not mushy, padding on the floor; less than 1 inch thick, so that a "suffocation pocket" can't be formed around the baby's face should she inadvertently turn face down or get captured in the side.

✔ **Lightweight.** You can lift it and fold it without straining your back.

✔ **Tight mesh.** The mesh is dense enough so it can't capture small fingers or toes, but you can easily see through it to keep an eye on your baby inside.

✔ **Hinges.** No exposed sharp edges or pinch points on the folding hinges in the center of the yard and at its four corners that could injure or capture your baby's fingers.

✔ **Padded railings.** The yard's railings are well cushioned to protect the baby during falls.

✔ **Easy folding.** Most play yards are very challenging to open and fold until you get the hang of it. Try it once or twice with the model you're thinking of buying.

✔ **Wheels.** Having at least 2 wheels on one end will make moving easier.

✔ **Carry case.** A zippered fabric carrier or a floor pad with Velcro straps designed to wrap around the folded frame makes toting and storing more convenient.

Avoid:

✗ **Recalled used models.** More than 10 million play yards have been recalled over the years when the sides didn't lock securely and made a fatal V configuration that strangled babies. Before using a hand-me-down play yard, make sure it's not on the recall list.

✗ **Capturing gaps.** Floor padding must fit flush against the edges of the yard, with no gaps or edges that could compress your baby's neck and airway.

✗ **Exposed or protruding hardware.** Sharp hardware anywhere on the unit or protruding bolts under the floor padding could injure your baby.

✗ **Hostile exterior.** Sharp edges on the outside of the yard could hurt a baby or child who falls on them.

✗ **Flimsy construction.** Avoid models with flimsy, too-soft floor pads or rickety frames.

✗ **Electronic overkill.** Too many lights, moving toys, and other frivolous add-ons will increase the unit's price and weight but not the soothing.

Q I'm pregnant, but I'm not sure whether to put a play yard on my gift registry's wish list. My friends with children all love theirs, but I'm wondering if I'd be better off asking for something more practical.

Whether a play yard works for you depends a lot upon your baby and how she responds to being inside one. A small baby bed, such as a portable crib or bassinet, might be a better place for your young baby sleep until you're ready for her to move into a full-size crib. Some toddlers adapt to sitting in play yards, but most won't. We'd suggest postponing buying a yard until later, then borrowing one from a friend or neighbor (as long as it hasn't faced a recall) to see how one works with your baby before you take the plunge. You may discover that the yard wasn't as much of a necessity as you thought.

Q My baby had a "near miss" when her play yard bar didn't lock open completely and she hurt her finger under the hinge's padding. It made her cry, but she was okay after we picked her up. It was definitely my fault for not making sure the sides were locked into place, as they should have been. Should I report what happened to the CPSC, even though I was the one at fault?

Absolutely! Consider it your duty to help protect other babies and not just your own. Many recalls happen not just because babies have been seriously injured, but also because enough parents have reported incidents that *could* have been serious or life threatening. File a report not only with the Consumer Product Safety Commission but also with the manufacturer, and stop using the yard. Hold onto the unit for a while in case an investigation ensues. (You can find the full contact information for the CPSC on page 360.)

Q When I put the baby in the play yard, her older sister wants to get in, too. I like that she wants to play with her, but I wonder if it's safe to have two children inside.

Read the manufacturer's instructions. Most warn parents that the yard should be used with only one child. Children can bump into one another, use one another to climb out, which can lead to falls, and their combined weight may stress the yard's fabric and frame.

❝A portable play yard is great when you're going somewhere that isn't childproofed (like the park or your mother's house) or when you know you'll be visiting somewhere during baby's naptime. ❞

Highs & lows of play yards

Highs. Most portable play yards are lightweight, come with wheels, and fold compactly for storing or for travel. Their dimensions allow them to be rolled through doorways—something a full-size crib can't do. The mesh sides allow babies to peer out. The clip-on bassinet feature provides a place for small babies to nap, which is especially handy if your house has two stories and baby's crib is on another floor. Some come with a carry case to make transporting easier.

Lows. Opening and folding a play yard can be a hassle. If the side bars don't click solidly into place, as with some older models, the bars' V-shaped indentation could be life threatening. Mattress pads tend to be soft and cushy, and their moisture resistance makes them less porous and breathable, which could affect your baby's air supply should she entangle, or even strangle your baby. (Read the manufacturer's instructions about coverings for the play yard floor.)

WARNING

Play yards aren't babysitters!
Most of the serious, life-threatening play-yard accidents happen to babies when their parents mistakenly rely on play yards to serve as babysitters. The typical scenario is that a parent leaves her baby alone in a separate room, only to discover that something happened while she was away. Manufacturers and safety experts alike recommend that parents never leave a baby unattended, whether asleep or awake, inside a play yard.

Graco's Pack 'n Play Playard (Model 9241SBA)
($60)

This basic model (15 pounds) in the Graco Pack 'n Play Playard line offers see-through mesh on all sides and wheels on one end. It comes with a removable U-shaped toy bar with 3 dangling toys. The play yard's bottom pad can hook onto the sides of the yard to make a suspended bassinet. The unit opens by pressing down on the center floorboard, then locking the side rails, followed by installing and fastening down the mattress pad. It folds into a compact M shape by removing the pad, pulling up on a handle in the center of the floorboard, and lifting and releasing side locks by pushing buttons so that the sidebars can fold while the center floor rises. The pad then wraps around the unit, and the whole thing fits into a zippered carry bag. (Carefully follow the manufacturer's directions!) Optional sheets are available that fit the floor pad. For babies weighing up to 30 pounds.

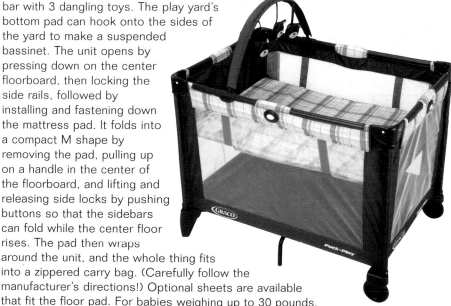

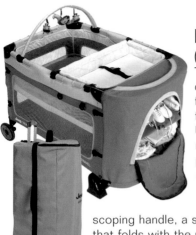

Kolcraft's Easy-Travel Playard

(S110)

This new and innovative play yard style is designed for portability and is much simpler to fold than typical portables. It has an aluminum frame, a full-length, removable bassinet, and a U shaped removable toy bar. There is vented mesh on all sides, and a folding shelf with a zippered cover on one end. The unit has a luggage-style telescoping handle for rolling, and goes into its own zippered case for a good fit in the closet or trunk of the car. Its features include a telescoping handle, a set of large wheels, a side storage shelf for toys that folds with the unit while still holding its stuff, and a changing table unit with belts. For babies weighing up to 30 pounds.

Safe use tips

Safety precautions for play yards

■ Double-check the yard each time. Check all the bars and components every time you set up the yard, to ensure that everything is locked and fastened into place before you place your baby inside. The floorboard should be completely flattened and secured to the sides of the yard.

■ Follow manufacturer's precautions. Don't exceed the recommended age and weight guidelines that come with the yard; don't put more than one child inside.

■ Protect baby from falling out. Once your baby can stand up, remove toys or bumpers that she could use to get over the railing; and don't allow her or other children to play near the yard if there is a danger they could fall into it.

■ Remove add-on components. Don't put a baby or child in the yard while hook-on features such as the bassinet or diaper-changing unit are attached to it.

■ Keep baby out of the sun. Babies are very vulnerable to sunburn and sunstroke. The yard shouldn't be used in direct sun; and even in the shade, limit your baby's time outdoors and protect her with sunscreen lotion.

■ Don't use a dome. Some older-model play yards came with a ribbed dome that completely covered the top, to shield the baby from direct sunlight. The dome came with sewn-on warning patches not to use it in direct sunlight because of the danger of serious heat buildup inside, and most manufacturers discontinued the domes because of the danger of babies getting heatstroke.

■ Destroy it if it's broken. Don't use a broken or malfunctioning play yard with your baby, and destroy it so that other parents won't pick it up from the curb or dump and try to use it. One way to do that is to cut the mesh and pads with scissors. Duct tape a sign on the floorboard that warns "UNSAFE!"

WARNING

Playing it safe with play yards

While other products, like toys and baby clothing, make great buys at yard sales, thrift stores, or even on eBay, buying a used play yard can be risky. A bent frame or weakened component could elude the federal recall list and not be visible on an Internet photo. Don't take the risk on a used yard unless you can inspect the unit in person and you're certain it hasn't appeared on a recall list from years past.

Don't add extras!

Unfortunately, some parents mistakenly attempt to add extra padding to the play-yard floor to make it more bedlike, or they add a pillowcase, a crib sheet, or even a plastic garbage or dry-cleaning bag over the floor pad for protection. A baby can suffocate if her face or neck becomes entangled in the extra padding, is pressed against the plastic, or gets between the add-ons and the sides of the yard. Don't add anything to the bottom or sides of the yard that didn't come with it.

SAFETY CONSIDERATIONS

Typical play-yard injuries include babies falling into the play yard's frame from outside, climbing over the bars and hitting their heads when they fall out, and falling inside the yard and striking the frame or hard objects inside. More seriously, baby deaths have been caused by serious flaws in play-yard designs in the past.

Over a period of a decade, more than 200 babies have died in play-yard related accidents, making this product category second only to cribs for serious risks. More than 10 million portable play yards units manufactured in the past decade have undergone federal recalls or corrective actions.

The biggest recalls were for units with protruding bolts that presented the potential of capturing babies' pacifier strings or garments, resulting in hangings, or for play yards with defective side locks that allowed a V shape to form at the center hinges, causing babies to strangle when their necks became captured there.

Most manufacturers involved in play-yard recalls have agreed to provide parents with repair kits or other remedies for recalled models. In some cases, manufacturers are now offering repair kits, monetary rewards for turning in defective play yards, or the opportunity to trade in unsafe yards for new models. If you're not sure about the safety status of an older model, we recommend contacting the manufacturer before using it. Or visit www.recall.gov on the Internet and search "play yards" on the link to CPSC. But note: In some cases, very old recalled models may not appear on the Internet list.

Play yards have a voluntary safety standard overseen by the Juvenile Products Manufacturers Association (JPMA) and the American Society of Testing and Materials (ASTM). Manufacturers that want their play yards certified must have them tested for compliance, to help minimize the potential of baby injuries. If the play yard is certified, a "JPMA Certified" sticker will appear on the play yard as well as on its packaging.

17

POTTIES & STEP STOOLS

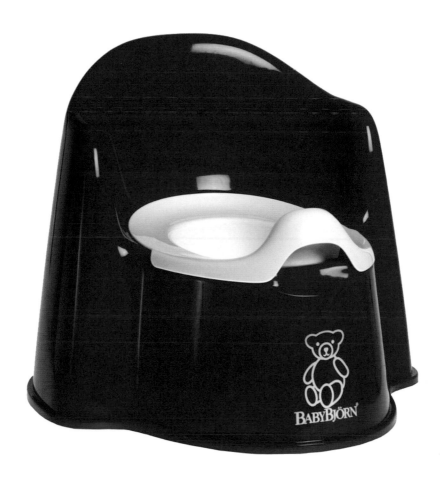

Consider this chapter advance potty planning. Most parents start thinking about potty training around the time their babies turn one, but there's no need. The average age these days for potty mastery is 34 months for girls and 37.5 months for boys, since it takes a long time for children to master such a complex set of skills. In anticipation of when that glorious phase arrives, here's the poop on potties, plus step stools, which also belong in the hygiene department.

GETTING TO THE BOTTOM LINE

Showing interest in the toilet, enjoying praise from grownups, and disliking the dirty-diaper sensation are all good signs that your child is ready to begin the learning process of self-toileting. Mastering all of the steps is a big deal for kids, and learning is a months-long process involving plenty of accidents and misses between hits.

Most children simply aren't developmentally ready to master the muscular control it takes to make more hits than misses on the toilet until about three to four years of age. Although some playgroup moms may brag that they had junior potty trained by 18 months or within the space of a day, most likely these moms aren't including a lot of dirty underwear in their definitions of success.

Signs it's potty-training time

Here are some signs that your child's probably ready to start the potty-training process.

✔ Can pull pants and underpants up and down without help
✔ Can back into a potty and sit down
✔ Is able to sit still for 5 minutes at a time
✔ Can follow one or two simple directions
✔ Can answer simple yes and no questions
✔ Is aware of bodily functions
✔ Can take naps without having an accident
✔ Likes imitating others

Once you get the signs that your child is physically ready, then what?

We suggest reading about potty training in one of the many toilet-training instruction books available in bookstores and libraries. Or you can access some of the many how-to articles on the subject that can be found on the Internet. Your pediatrician can also be a great source of helpful information.

When you feel the time is right, start talking about using potties and toilets and all of the fabulous advantages that come with having these skills. Ask your child to tell you when he needs to "go," and heap on praise when he does.

As you've probably noticed, bathrooms aren't built for the convenience of persons who are three feet tall. You're going to need to make some modifications so that your child's transition out of diapers is safe, hygienic, and convenient for both of you—and the rest of the family. Plus, you'll need potty emergency plans while you and your child are away from home.

Buying a potty

The range of potties available goes from simple one-piece chamber pots or child-size adapters that fit over the adult seat to multiple-component floor pots—with battery-operated features, such as liquid sensors that reward the child for hitting the mark and those that even make mock toilet-flushing sounds.

Accessories can help make the learning process more fun. There are picture books for children about using the potty, and dolls that drink water and use miniature toilets so your child can practice through play. Some great DVDs are also available, with catchy songs and eye-catching characters who can help inspire kids and show them what to do.

Adult-toilet ring adapters are an inexpensive toilet-training option, and are certainly a more pleasant option for the adult on duty, since they take advantage of normal toilet flushing. Their prices range between $10 and $20. At the lowest price are simple folding plastic inserts designed to sit on top of the adult seat, such as the Cushie Traveler that is cushioned and folds compactly (between $10 and $15). Zeets Disposable cardboard toilet-seat adapters for travel come five to a box ($10–$12). Contoured seat adapters with handles are priced between $15 and $20 with higher prices for more ergonomic handles and seat shapes and adjusters to fit the seat to both round and oval toilet-seat shapes.

Simple one-piece floor potties resemble old-fashioned chamber pots and have a price range similar to toilet-seat adapters. They're a good option for children who are intimidated by the large toilet and scared of being flushed away. And having one's own private (and comfortable) seat may be motivating. At the low end of the spectrum is the BABYBJÖRN Little Potty ($10–$12), and further up the price chain are heftier, anatomically shaped pots with high backs, some with removable pots, such as BABYBJÖRN's Potty Chair ($20–$25).

Complete potty packages are bigger investments. Some come with wetting dolls and children's toilet-training manuals to boot. Fisher-Price's Potty Elmo ($25–$30) asks for a drink when his hand is squeezed. Afterward, he announces he needs to use the potty, and once he's seated he'll sing a fun song. Elmo's clothes, a small book, and a sippy cup come along with a simple pot to complete the set.

Floor pots with removable toilet-seat adapters are in the same price range option. Basic models include Graco's Soft Seat Potty Trainer, which sells for about $20, has a lift-out toilet-seat adapter with side handles, and a removable collection pot. Learning Curve's 3-in-1 Toilet Training System, at about $18, offers a removable collection pot and a seat top that fits adult toilets.

Note: Sometimes too many bells and whistles can be counterproductive. Fisher-Price's Laugh and Learn Potty, around $35, makes so many sounds that children are tempted to use it as a toy, rather than a serious place to take care of business.

Five potty-shopping strategies

Here are some tips when buying adapter rings or potties.

1. Invite your child to shop with you, and let him have a say in picking the potty or seat style, as well as helping to choose at least 6 to 12 pairs of "big kid" underpants. (You'll also still need disposable pull-ups or diapers for overnight protection.) The best underpants are those that have action or princess figures imprinted on them or some other novelty or color that makes the pants seem like a huge step up from diapers.

2. Advanced reconnaissance. Take a look at the adapters and potties available at local stores before you invite your child along for the final selection, so you'll know what to show him and what to avoid.

3. Measure for fit. If you're getting a toilet-seat ring or a floor potty that includes an adapter, write down the measurements for the dimensions of the inside of your toilet's seat to make sure that the ring will fit well on all sides. This is especially important if your home toilet seat is elongated or not a standard shape. At the same time, measure from the floor to the top of the adult seat to help in choosing the right-height step stool.

4. Buy separate units. Adults and other children are going to need easy access to the toilet, too, and items such as a seat with attached steps are awkward to dismantle or remove. A separate easy-to-remove ring or a flip-up seat adapter will work best.

5. Safety concerns. Make sure that all components of rings and potty seats are smooth and rounded, with no sharp edges or unfinished seams that could scratch or cut a child.

✔ ══ Checklist ════

Potty shopping:

Here's what to look for when potty shopping:

✔ **Easy to clean.** Parts should be easy to separate for cleaning, but not so easy that your tot disassembles them for fun.

✔ **Ring won't come loose.** To help prevent falls, an adapter ring should attach firmly to the adult seat, using either a locking mechanism or a deep rim underneath.

✔ **Carry handle for ring.** So you or your child can easily move it from one bathroom to another, and you can throw it in the car for trips.

✔ **Comfortable backrest.** Your child will be leaning back on the lid of a floor potty.

✔ **Slip resistant.** You don't want a potty turning over or scooting around the floor! Look for a wide base with slip-resistant pads underneath.

✔ **Easy-to-remove collection pot.** The best models have cups that lift up from the top of the ring, without getting caught on the frame.

✔ **A safe, smooth splash guard in front.** Little boys have terrible aim; a well-designed front shield or removable soft guard will help contain accidents.

Avoid:

✗ **Too many bells and whistles.** Not only do electronic features eat up batteries, they may keep children from concentrating on doing their jobs.

✗ **Hostile underside.** Make sure that if the seat accidentally tips over as your tot backs into it, he won't be injured by the potty's feet or a sharp underside.

✗ **Too many components.** Simpler is better. The fewer the components, the easier the pot is to use and clean.

✗ **Sharp edges or seams.** No plastic tags and sharp edges that could scratch your child.

When to Buy

When your child shows sure signs of being able to follow a chain of commands and manage the physical skills needed to master self-toileting, usually between 24 and 36 months.

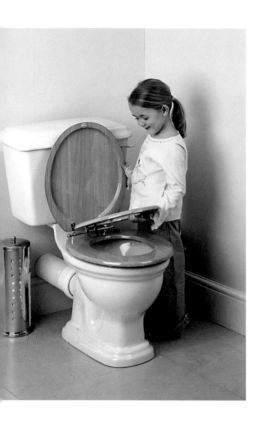

ADAPTER RINGS

TrendyKid's Family Seat
($40 wood, $30 plastic)

A round toilet seat for tots, kids, and adults, the Family Seat screws onto a standard toilet just as a regular ring and lid would. The only difference is that it has a smaller tot ring that fits up into the lid but can be pulled down when your child needs to use it. Available in wood or white plastic, with magnets to make the ring stay up until it's ready for use. No fastening or removing a seat adapter every time someone else wants to use the john. How convenient is that? (Available in specialty stores and baby-product catalogs.)

Munchkin's Deluxe Potty Seat
($20)

A soft seat for small bottoms, this easily removable toilet-seat adapter ring has a cushiony center and adjustable handles on the sides for different-sized kids. The padded vinyl-covered seat has a gentle rise in the front for a splash guard, and an extended ring inside holds it inside standard toilet seats. The back has two feet, so it can stand on the floor in the upright position. Nicely portable from one bathroom to another.

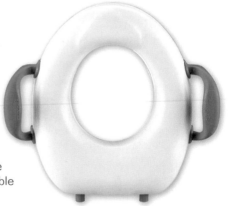

FLOOR POTTIES

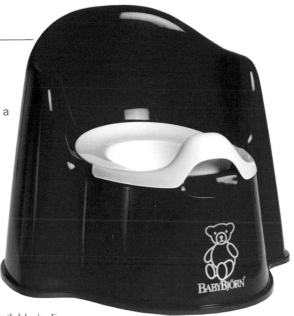

BABYBJÖRN's Potty Chair

($25)

This Swedish import is made
from thick molded plastic with a
smooth, easy-to-wipe finish.
The pot easily removes from
the front. The chair's
ergonomic design gives your
child plenty of legroom,
allowing him to get closer to
the potty inside. It has a
rubber skid-proof base and
gently sloped spray shield.
According to the manufac-
turer, all plastics used in the
potty are PVC-free and recy-
clable. In addition to the red
version shown at right, it is available in 5
other color selections, including pink for girls
and blue for boys.

Visionaire Products'
Peter Potty Flushable Toddler Urinal

($40)

Parents with boys rave about the Peter Potty, a
freestanding height-adjustable urinal for boys
that does not require plumbing. It flushes with a
push-button, using water from a removable top
reservoir, and empties into a waste catcher
below. A target in the base of the potty helps
boys to aim better. The potty part can be wall-
mounted to save space.

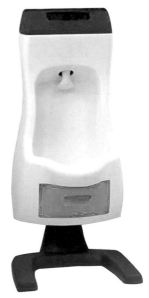

STEPPING HIGH WITH STEP STOOLS

Step stools are useful for helping a child get up to a standard toilet seat and for reaching the sink for hand washing and tooth brushing. Most step stools are simple one-piece units. They can be wood and have a single or double step, or molded plastic with wood costing a little more. Some multiple-component children's potties have flip-down lids and claim they can also be used as step stools, but they're generally not as stable or safe as dedicated stools are.

The best step stools are high enough to support a child's feet at the toilet. Prices range from $15 to $50, with most in the $30 range.

Levels of Discovery's Toad Stool ($45)

This clever green step stool has a chip in its base that makes a "ribbit" sound when stepped on. It's constructed of wood and is hand-painted green with frog-y features including large, googly eyes. It's made for toddlers with good body control and balance (2 to 5 years). Can support 250–300 pounds. Dimensions: 5 inches by 10 inches by 5½ inches tall. Includes lithium batteries.

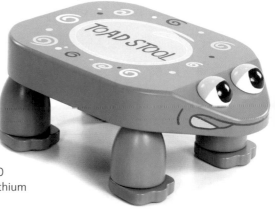

✔ Checklist

Step-stool shopping:

Here's what to look for when shopping for a step-stool:

✔ **Wide, stable base.** The stool won't tip over if your child trips on the edge.

✔ **Nonslip base and top.** Grippers on the bottom help it stay in place. Grids on the top help prevent slipping.

✔ **The right height.** Tall enough to support your child's feet when he's sitting on the john, and to reach the faucets at the back of the sink.

✔ **Easy to carry.** Lightweight enough for a child to move from one place to another. Handles help.

✔ **Easy to climb and descend without falling.** Large enough that your child can climb up and move around on the top without falling off.

✔ **Water resistant.** Able to hold up to lots of splashes.

Avoid:

✗ **Sharp edges.** The overall finishing should be smooth and rounded.

✗ **Too-small dimensions.** Needs to be tall enough and wide enough for tots to use.

✗ **Combination stools.** A folding stool back or other add-ons defeat the purpose of the stool and only eat up more bathroom space.

Dorel Juvenile Group's Eddie Bauer 2-Step Stool

($30)

This quality wooden step stool has a foldaway bottom step to save room. The stool's edges are rounded, and its top surfaces are grooved to prevent slipping. Its weight and bulk make it less easy to move around than lighter plastic models. On the plus side, it offers an easier climb, a taller top step, and its weight and stability make it less likely to slide out from under your child.

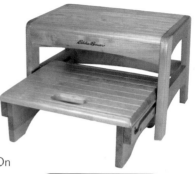

When to Buy

Your child needs to be a good walker and have good balance to safely use a step stool (2 to 5 years).

SAFETY CONSIDERATIONS

With potties and toilet seat adapters, typical injuries include children hurt by sharp components on the seats and adapter or falling off the toilet and hitting the floor when adapters fail to hold onto the adult seat. Typical injuries with step stools occur when children misstep and fall off or when they trip and fall into an edge of the product. The most common injuries that occur in these accidents are a split lip, a bad bruise, or, more rarely, a broken arm. Recalls for potties and stepstools are rare.

Potties and step stools do not come under voluntary certification standards from the Juvenile Products Manufacturers Association (JPMA) and the American Society of Testing and Materials (ASTM), and recalls are rare. However, several thousand children a year are sent to emergency rooms from potty- or step-stool-related injuries.

Here are some tips for keeping your child safe when it's toilet-training time.

✔ **Supervise.** To protect your child from injuries, supervise him in the bathroom.

✔ **Cushion for falls.** Keep a soft, cushiony bathroom rug around the toilet seat and under the step stool to cushion falls.

✔ **Demonstrate.** Teach your child how to get up and down safely from the toilet and the step stool. Have him run his hand around the surface of the step stool and to feel the edges of the stool with his feet while standing on it with your support, so that he becomes more aware of its boundaries.

18

SAFETY PRODUCTS

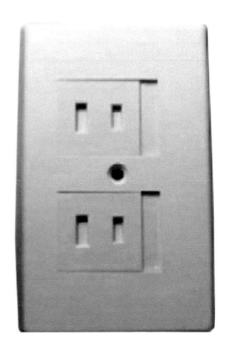

This chapter is all about accidentproofing your home to help keep your exploring baby safe from household hazards, including poisons, electrical outlets, and kitchen dangers. Here you'll learn about common baby perils, plus you'll find suggested products to help guard your baby (or at least slow her down).

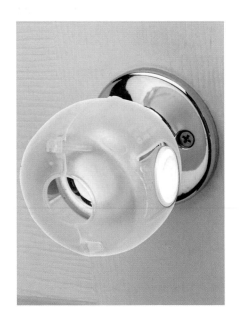

HOME SAFE HOME

Hundreds of thousands of babies are raced to emergency rooms every year with serious injuries sustained from accidents in and around their homes, and even at playgrounds that are supposedly designed for children. Most often, accidents aren't caused by specific products.

Babies are simply curious, lack judgment, and will put about anything in their mouths—even dish detergent, wires, and houseplants. And some babies just seem to have the urge to climb and will scale any height, even if it's an unstable shelf, television stand, or dresser. The best ways to prevent accidents are vigilance, removing likely hazards from baby's way, and keeping a constant eye on your little explorer.

Safety checklist

Here's a quick list of products that need to be well out of babies' and children's reach:

✔ **Aspirin and Tylenol** (acetaminophen) and other over-the-counter remedies for fevers, coughs and colds, and other ailments.

✔ **Cold and cough medicines** that carry the word 'infant' on the label have been withdrawn by the FDA and pharmaceutical manufacturers to help protect babies and toddlers under 2 years of age from accidental overdose. All nonprescription medications for infants should be used only on the advice of your baby's physician.

✔ **Vitamins and iron tablets.**

✔ **Prescription medications** (medications for heart conditions, antidepressants, and blood pressure can be harmful and possibly fatal to a child).

✔ **Toothpaste** (a swallowed pea-size amount of one containing fluoride can be toxic to a child).

✔ **Mouthwash.**

✔ **Talcum powder.**

✔ **Cosmetics and body lotions.**

✔ **Shampoo and conditioner.**

✔ **Salt** (more than $1\frac{1}{2}$ swallowed tablespoons can be lethal to a toddler).

✔ **Cleaning products and bleach.**

✔ **Dry-cleaning bags and other plastic bags.**

✔ **Tobacco products and ashtrays.**

✔ **Matches.**

✔ **Electrical cords and cables.**

✔ **Alcoholic beverages.**

✔ **Tools,** especially with cutting edges or sharp points.

✔ **Paint and paint thinners.**

✔ **Propane, kerosene, lighter fluid, and other fuels.**

Be prepared!

Be sure to sign up for a first aid course at your local Red Cross, Y, or rescue squad and learn CPR and the baby Heimlich maneuver. It could save your baby's life.

GETTING STARTED ON BABYPROOFING

The best way to start protecting your baby from home accidents is to get down on your hands and knees in every room of your house, so that you can spot dangers from your baby's eye level. Look for unprotected electric sockets, dangling electrical cords, and low-level window-shade cords. Also secure any and all potential poisons: powdered dish detergent, medications, vermin poison, vitamin supplements, antifreeze, plant fertilizer, and so on.

Shelves, chests, and TV sets are dangerous if they're not secured to the wall. Tots can and do pull these heavy objects on top of themselves when they try to climb them.

Look for sharp-edged furniture, which can injure sleep-deprived adults, too. Surprisingly, the most dangerous object in the house can be a coffee table. A whopping 70,000 tots are rushed to emergency rooms every year from falling into

When to Buy

Purchase and begin installing babyproofing products as soon as your baby starts to roll over, pull up, and show signs of becoming mobile, at around 6 to 8 months. Use indefinitely to protect your toddler or preschooler from household dangers.

Quick tip

Is a professional babyproofer for you? If you have an active crawler, you may want to hire a professional babyproofer (also known as a child safety consultant) to assess your home for potential hazards and make safety recommendations. To locate a professional in your area, contact the International Association for Child Safety, www.iafcs.com.

sharp edges and corners of furniture.

Water sources also require extra vigilance. Babies have drowned in toilets, bathtubs, and even buckets of mop water.

Safety products are designed to help protect your baby from all these household hazards. Covers make it harder for your baby to fiddle with outlets. Cord shorteners help put electric and blind cords out of reach. Corner guards soften table and fireplace edges when there's a fall. Cabinet and drawer latches allow you access but make it hard for your tot to open them. Doorknob covers keep the knob from being turned by anyone but an adult. Doorstops protect small fingers from getting smashed when doors slam. Lid locks are designed to hold toilet seat covers down. Faucet covers will help keep your tot from touching hot bathtub plumbing. Appliance latches help keep refrigerator doors and medicine-cabinet doors shut.

It's important to point out, though, that no safety product is fail-safe. It may help slow your tot down, but *nothing* can protect your baby as well as your own watchfulness. Take time to instruct babysitters before you leave the house about how to handle an emergency. Have emergency telephone numbers and directions to your house posted in bright letters next to the kitchen phone, and make sure your house numbers are easy for rescue workers to find.

Help for poisoning

If you suspect your baby has swallowed a toxic substance, the American Association of Poison Control Centers offers a toll-free, 24-hour-a-day Poison Help Line: 1-800-222-1222.

The baby safety dozen

Here are the greatest baby dangers and how you can plan ahead to prevent them.

1. Car accidents. Install and use an approved car seat. (Find more information about car seats starting on page 84.)

2. Falls. Never leave your baby on a raised, unguarded surface, even in a bouncer or car seat.

3. Heatstroke. Never leave your baby in the sun, or in a parked car.

4. Drowning. Never leave your baby alone near *any* open water, large or small.

5. Burns. Set the water heater to 120° F or less, and always check the temperature of bathwater carefully. Reduce the heat before turning off the faucet, to cool down the metal surface, and use faucet covers.

6. Fires. Install smoke detectors, and test them periodically.

7. SIDS. Always put your baby on her back for sleeping.

8. Suffocation. Don't let your baby sleep on couch cushions, beanbag chairs, waterbeds, or other soft surfaces. (See Chapter 9, *Cribs, Mattresses & Bedding*, for more information on suffocation.)

9. Poisoning. Keep caustic chemicals such as kerosene and drain cleaner out of the house. Keep medications and chemicals in their original containers that have child-resistant caps (don't change containers!). Throw away all medications. Protect your child from lead poisoning caused by ingesting lead found in old paint chips and paint dust, lead in drinking water, and gnawing on brass keys and key rings.

10. Choking. Don't let your baby play with toys or small objects that could be swallowed. Don't feed your baby hot dogs, nuts, grapes, or other foods that could get caught in her throat. Don't let your baby play with deflated balloons, plastic bags, or plastic wrap.

11. Strangulation. Don't tie a pacifier around your baby's neck. Secure cords of curtains, wall hangings, and blinds out of your baby's reach. Never tie cords or ribbons across cribs or playpens, and remove mobiles by the time your baby is old enough to roll over or pull up.

12. Electrocution. Cover electrical outlets, and use only newer extension cords with prong-hole covers. Don't use hair dryers or other electrical devices near sinks or tubs. Keep baby away from appliance wires, extension cords, and power strips.

Safe use tips

Here's a list of common hazards around the home and where they can be found.

✔ **Chests with drawers.** Simple bureaus and dressers don't look dangerous, but they can fall on tots who try to use the pulled-out drawers as steps for getting to the top. Toddlers also like to pull out drawers, and if they come out easily, they can fall on your baby and injure her. Fasten the chest in your child's room to the wall using a special safety strap or an L shaped bracket found in hardware stores, and install stops at the back of all drawers so they can't be pulled out and fall.

✔ **Cribs.** More babies die from crib-related accidents than from any other baby product. Old heirloom cradles and hand-me-down cribs are the most dangerous, because they're not up to modern safety standards and can have broken hardware or crib bars, gaps between crib bars or between the mattress and the sides of the crib, and corner posts that can hook neck holes in babies' clothing or strings on pacifiers, causing strangulation. It's worth it to buy a new crib. See Chapter 9 for specific crib hazards.

4 Dangerous chemicals. Babies aren't discerning about what's safe to put in their mouths and what's not. *All* medicines and over-the-counter remedies are hazardous to children. Childproof caps on medicines aren't childproof, they just slow down inquisitive children. Bleach, cleaners, and detergents are dangerous! Dishwashing detergent, both gels and powders, can cause severe mouth and throat burns, although they smell delicious. Deadly poisons such as paint thinners, weed killers, and antifreeze should be stored on a high shelf, preferably in a locked shed or far from living areas.

✔ **Dogs.** Dogs bite millions of people in the United States annually and send more than 800,000 a year to emergency rooms. Most victims are children, attacked by known dogs. Be especially wary of animals, such as guard dogs, that are kept in kennels or behind fences, since they could attack your child or bite through the fence. Teach your child proper animal manners, and warn her not to approach unfamiliar animals, even dogs and cats, or any animal that has been injured or is eating. Do not keep a dog (no matter the breed or size) that you can't control, and don't bring a new dog into your home until your child is mature enough to be taught how to relate to it.

✔ **Garage door openers.** Make sure your automatic garage door will stop and reverse when it encounters any resistance. Test it with a brick or some other object.

✔ **Gas water heaters.** The pilot lights on water heaters can present a fire hazard, especially in a garage where fuel is stored. Don't pour gas in an enclosed space or near a pilot light of any kind.

✔ **Electric appliances.** Especially if you have an older home without a circuit breaker, keep radios, hair dryers, and other electrical appliances far away from sinks and bathtubs. Cover your electrical outlets, especially those at child's-eye level. The sockets may look like appealing places to stick metal objects, which can have fatal results. Make sure that your bathroom has GFI (Ground Fault Interrupter) electrical receptacles, to instantly shut off electric current if a hair dryer or other electrical appliance should fall into water.

✔ **Ladders and shelves.** Toddlers love to climb and don't understand that shelves and ladders will fall over if they pull on them. Hang ladders on hooks in a safe place, and be sure shelves are held by strong supports bolted securely to the wall.

✔ **Lawnmowers.** Parents and grandparents alike are guilty of believing that giving a tot a joy ride on a ride-on mower is a fun idea, but babies and small children have been horribly injured from falls, being run over by mowers, or being injured when the mowers threw up sticks and rocks. Don't teach your tot that lawnmowers are safe and friendly. They're not. Keep your baby safely inside while mowing is going on.

✔ **Plants.** Many household plants and blossoming flowers can be toxic. Though most are not fatal if swallowed, they can cause burning to the mouth as well as stomach pain. For a more extensive list of poisonous plants, the Canadian site "Safe Baby" (www.safebaby.net) offers a list of common plant dangers.

✔ **Ride-on toys.** Often parents make the mistake of buying a ride-on toy, tricycle, or beginner's bicycle that's too large, hoping their child will grow into it. The danger is that ride-on toys don't have brakes, and they can fall over when the front wheel is turned too far to one side, making them more difficult to control. Children have been killed when a ride-on rolls into the street or a vehicle backs into them. Don't let your tot use a ride-on toy outdoors until she is at least three years old and has the body skills and judgment to protect herself from harm. Before she rides, teach her how to steer and stop. Make sure she wears a well-fitted helmet on any ride-on, especially on tricycles, which turn over easily. Ride in parks or other areas where there is no vehicle traffic nearby.

✔ **Suctioned baby bathtub seats.** Avoid these seats at all costs. More than 40 babies have died in accidents associated with them. The problem is these seats give parents a false sense of security about their baby's safety. Drowning occurs when a parent leaves the baby happily playing in the water to answer the doorbell or the telephone; suction cups on the seat release, and the baby falls face-forward into the water and drowns.

✔ **Tools.** Tots like to imitate what their moms and dads do. They will pull down and handle drills, saws, and other dangerous tools, and may even succeed in turning them on. Put a safety gate on the door to your work area. Shorten cords so they are out of reach, and unplug tools and store them safely out of reach when not in use. Keep tots away or restrained while you're working.

✔ **Toys and chests.** Dangerous toys send thousands of kids to emergency rooms every year. Make sure your baby's toys are age appropriate, and inspect them for sturdiness; make sure there are no sharp corners and edges that could hurt a child who fell on them. Also don't store your toys in a chest with a heavy lid that can cause injuries. (See our baby toy suggestions on page 318).

✔ **Walkers.** New or old, baby walkers are extremely dangerous and send about 3,000 babies to emergency rooms every year, mostly for serious head injuries when a walker has tumbled down a staircase or into a pool. If your baby has the urge to stretch her legs, try a stationary exerciser instead.

✔ **Water.** Drowning is a major killer of small children, who can drown in as little as an inch of water within a few minutes. Babies drown in bathtubs, wading pools, diaper pails, and mop buckets. Protect an outdoor pool with a fence and a gate that locks automatically. Drain all buckets and wading pools and store them upside down. If there's an unprotected pool or body of water nearby (even something as small as a goldfish pond), teach your tot about the dangers of water and don't leave her unattended around it.

✔ **Playgrounds.** Although they appear to be great for meeting children's play needs, most playgrounds have serious hazards, too. For example, children have sustained severe head injuries and broken bones by falling from playground equipment such as monkey bars and climbers onto uncushioned hard surfaces like asphalt and compacted earth. Even a headfirst fall from just two feet can cause a serious head injury. Sliding boards strangle children when their hood strings become entangled in hardware. Toddlers are routinely struck by swings. Sandboxes are breeding grounds for parasites. Always supervise your kids at play and make sure they follow safety rules. Be wary of public sandboxes—don't let baby eat the sand, wash her hands thoroughly after play, and keep home sandboxes covered when not in use.

Lurking kitchen hazards

Kitchens and babies don't mix. Try getting down to baby-eye level so you can see the tempting objects and dangers that might appeal to your toddler. You'll find drawers with sharp knives, cabinets with breakable glass items, dangerous chemicals under the sink, scalding-hot cooking surfaces, and electrical appliance cords that a baby could pull, causing spills and other injuries.

For maximum safety, keep your baby out of the kitchen when you cook. One way to achieve this is to install a gate at the kitchen door; another is to place your baby in a play yard, a baby seat, or a high chair out of harm's way. Here are some danger zones to watch out for.

✔ **Dishwasher.** Dishwasher detergent can cause severe, disfiguring chemical burns to a child's mouth. Store it out of baby's reach, don't leave the dishwasher door open, wash dishes immediately after loading, and wipe up any detergent residues with paper towels that you can dispose of safely.

✔ **Storage.** Remove all detergents and chemicals from under the sink and place them in a locked closet or up high enough that they can't be reached by a curious tot. Keep plastic bags and kitchen wraps out of reach—they pose a suffocation hazard, and some cartons have sharp serrated edges.

✔ **Small appliances.** In the kitchen, babies can injure themselves by tugging on cords to pull over coffeemakers, food processors, toaster ovens, and other appliances. Use twist ties or rubber bands to wrap up and fasten cords so they can't be reached, or tape loose cords to the wall with duct tape. Unplug appliances when they're not in use, since some appliances, such as coffeemakers, have caused fires even when they appear to be turned off.

✔ **Refrigerators.** Keep small refrigerator magnets out of your baby's reach. Your baby can choke on them and they can be deadly if ingested.

✔ **Stoves/ovens.** If your range has front knobs, pull them off and store them out of reach until you need to cook. (Stove knob safety covers are available, but they are easily defeated and may make your little one even more fascinated with the stove and the challenge of getting the covers off!) Turn all pot handles toward the back of the stove when you're cooking, so that they can't get pulled on by children. When possible, cook on the back burners. Does the front door of your oven become hot enough to cause burns? Remember, a baby's skin burns a lot easier than yours does. If the oven is within reach of your baby and has a front window that gets really hot, or if you have an older model with poor insulation, consider replacing it with a newer, better-insulated model.

✔ **Microwave ovens.** They're handy for heating foods, but they shouldn't be used for heating baby-food jars or milk bottles because they create hard-to-detect hot spots of food or milk that could burn a baby's mouth and throat, and sometimes the heat can cause baby food jars, glass bottles, or vinyl bottle liners to melt or even explode.

✔ **Cabinets and drawers.** Keep knives, scissors, and other sharp objects in drawers with child-resistant safety latches installed from the inside. Lock beer, wine, and liquor away. Put protective pads on the sharp corners of countertops if they're low enough for baby to knock into them. Keep stools and chairs out of reach so your baby won't be tempted to use them for climbing.

✔ **Telephone cord.** A long cord on your telephone may make it easier for you to walk around in the kitchen, but it is tempting for a baby to chew on the cord, and a tot may get it caught around her neck. Shift to a shorter cord or a cordless portable.

Fire precautions

Make sure smoke detectors and a carbon monoxide detector are installed and in working order. Check their operation every few months and replace dead batteries. Also have a viable fire plan, including marking the window of your baby's room with a safety sticker, having a folding ladder in case you have to exit the second story from a window, and installing large, highly visible address numbers to help rescue personnel to find you in an emergency. These easy-to-do precautions could make the difference between life and death for your baby and other members of your family.

SAFETY PRODUCTS

Railing Guard

Dorel Juvenile Group's Safety 1st Railnet

($20)

If you have a multilevel home or an outdoor deck with railings that are placed far apart, or a tot who likes to push toys through the railing onto the level below, a mesh or plastic guard that ties around banisters and railings can give you peace of mind. This one comes in 10-foot lengths. Look for a guard that's easy to install and won't damage railings.

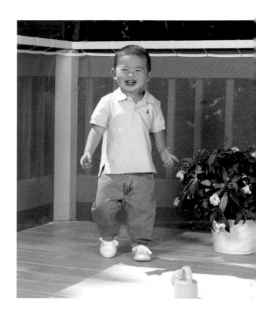

Gates

See our selections starting on page 188 in Chapter 13, *Gates & Enclosures.*

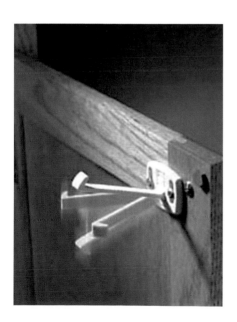

Cabinet Lock

KidCo's Swivel Cabinet & Drawer Lock

(4 for $4)

Some toddlers love opening doors and cabinets and pulling out everything inside, which can be both annoying and dangerous. Cabinet latches and locks can prevent this, at least until the toddler figures out how to open them. The best cabinet latches make access easy for an adult but prevent a child from opening the cabinet, and from pinching her little fingers when the door swings shut. The KidCo cabinet and drawer latch features a press-down hook that allows the cabinet door or drawer to be opened about an inch so an adult finger can press down firmly on the swiveling hook to release it. The hook automatically engages again when the gap is shut. The package comes with catches, mounting plates, hooks, and wood screws. Available in different amounts per package.

Cord and Outlet Shield

Double-Touch Plug'N Outlet Cover
(2/$2.00)

Some babies are fascinated with electrical cords and try to unplug them from the wall. This 2-piece, plastic electrical cord-and-outlet shield fits over the outlet plate, allowing electrical wires to exit underneath. It requires an adult hand to open.

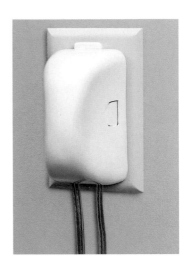

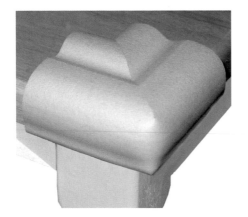

Cushioned Corner Covers

KidKusion's Corner Kushions
(4 for $8)

For babies who are just starting to pull up on furniture (and for sleep-deprived adults stumbling through living rooms in the dark), corner protectors for tables, window ledges, and other hard corners can help prevent bruises. The KidKusion Corner Kushions attach with foam tape and promise not to mar furniture.

Doorknob Cover

Dorel Juvenile Group's Safety 1st Clear Grip Door Knob Covers

(3 for $3.50)

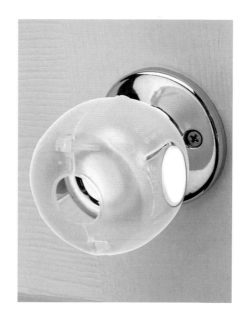

Doorknob covers are designed to keep curious kids out of rooms where they don't belong, and from locking themselves in rooms accidentally. They allow the door to be opened by an adult but not by a child. But this type of product is sometimes more aggravating than useful. It's much simpler to lock off-limits doors (like the door to the basement steps, for instance) with a simple up-high hook-and-loop latch on the outside.

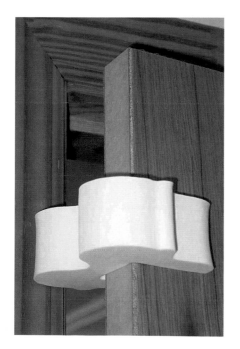

Door Positioner

KidKusion's Door Mouse Finger Guard

($6)

A nonmarring foam guard that creates a gap between the doorframe and the door, so that the door will not close and crush small fingers. Patented design keeps "Door Mouse" securely in place on the door. It slides onto the side of the door above a child's reach.

Electrical Outlet Cover

KidCo's Decora Outlet Cover
($4)

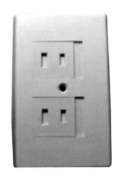

Plastic electrical outlet plugs are cheap and easy to come by. The problem is that determined tots can pull them off and may even chew on them and choke. A better, more lasting solution is a safety plate with a sliding cover that snaps shut as soon as a plug is pulled out.

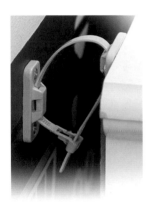

Furniture Safety Brackets

Mommy's Helper's Tip-Resistant Furniture Safety Brackets
(8 for $6)

Even the most stable-looking furniture can come crashing down if a toddler tries to climb it. Furniture brackets strap armoires, bookshelves, file cabinets, and chests of drawers solidly to the wall. They're a must-have if you've got a climber.

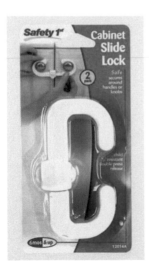

Cabinet Lock

Dorel Juvenile Group's Safety 1st Cabinet Slide Lock
(2 for $4)

This is a lock for the knobs or handles of adjoining cabinets with doors that open side by side. It can be used to help secure cabinets where poisonous chemicals or sharp objects are stored. Push buttons make it easy for adults to stretch and crimp the lock, but it's hard for kids.

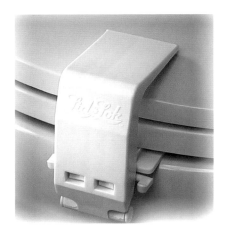

Toilet Seat Lock

Mommy's Helper's Lid-Lok
($10)

The toilet can be a fascinating whirlpool of delight to tots, who are top-heavy enough to fall headfirst into them and drown. Plus, kids like playing in it and throwing toys, hairbrushes, and other objects in and flushing them down to see what happens. Lid-Lok is a durable plastic lock with a special two-point latching system that requires adults and older children to push in on both side buttons at the same time to lock and release. It easily mounts to standard or padded toilet seats.

Window Guard

Angel Guard Guardian Angel's Window Guard

($50)

Open windows and window screens can pose a real hazard, especially to toddlers. Window screens, designed only to keep bugs out, just aren't strong enough to keep toddlers in. Be sure to move furniture away from windows, and use window guards on any window above the first floor. The Guardian Angel, made of steel tubing, is a good value, with a button-release for emergencies.

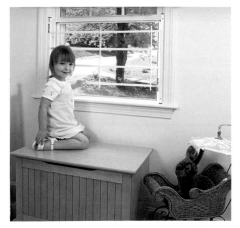

19

SOFT CARRIERS

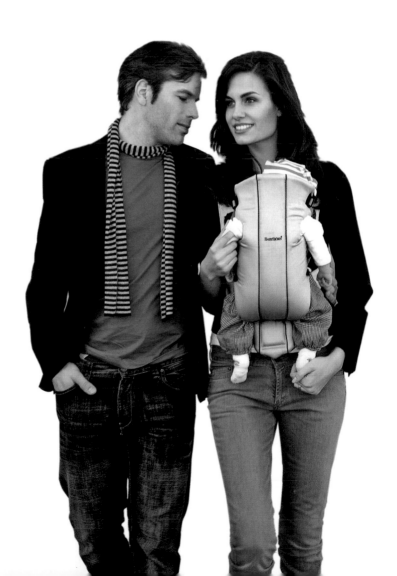

Soft carriers are fabric baby holders that let you tote baby on your body, hands-free. This category includes slings, wraparounds, and soft carriers with straps. This chapter describes all your soft-carrier options and offers lots of shopping and safety tips.

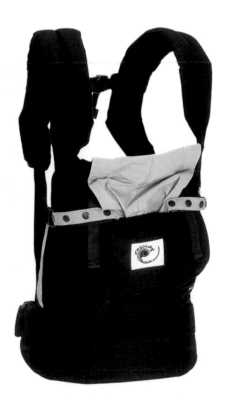

SOFT CARRIERS: WOMB WITH A VIEW

Parents have been figuring out hands-free ways to carry infants for much of human history. In comparison to the cost and bulk of a stroller, soft carriers offer an economical and compact solution. They work especially well if you use stairs, escalators, and public transportation a lot, or need to negotiate crowded places.

There are basically four types of carriers: pleated slings that wrap around one shoulder and enfold the baby in a small hammock in front; tie-on carriers in a variety of configurations from a single piece of cloth to those that use sashes; carriers for front (or back) that suspend a soft baby seat with leg holes and are secured by shoulder straps; and hip carriers that go over one shoulder and are specifically designed to help support a toddler while he straddles a parent's hip. (Framed backpacks for babies who can sit up independently are discussed starting on page 42.)

Carriers are available in a variety of

colors and materials. Fabrics include corduroys, soft canvases, stretchy knits, ripstop nylon, micromesh, and upholstery fabric. And there are even leather front carriers lined in lamb's wool if you're willing to fork over nearly $800 to sport the designer image. Some carriers are suitable for warm weather, while others work better in cooler climates.

Extras include padded head supports for small babies, snap-on burp bibs, back supports for parents, thick padding for the baby's seat or on the rim or base of slings, elasticized outer pockets, and special privacy features to allow discreet nursing.

Prices begin around $25 for a no-frills simple pouch, but slings and carriers average between $45 and $75. Organic cotton slings and soft front carriers with thick padding and air-vent mesh can edge up to nearly $100, while leather and designer slings that cost hundreds of dollars may not deliver as much comfort as softer, less expensive, and more flexible models.

> **"I couldn't live without my BABYBJÖRN. It's been through two babies and hundreds of washings, and it's still almost like new. I carry my baby around while I do laundry, vacuuming, and other chores. I'd put it in my 'favorite baby product' category."**

Important baby comfort issues

Your baby's posture and ability to breathe are important issues with a soft carrier. A baby's head is huge and heavy compared to the rest of his body, so it's important that a carrier keeps his spine straight in a natural sitting position that doesn't stress his spine and hips or allow his head to wobble. Also, if the carrier fits too loosely around the baby's body and doesn't offer adequate support, it could allow baby to slump forward, which might suppress breathing, especially in vulnerable babies such as those suffering from apnea. This is why most manufacturers of soft front carriers don't recommend their products for newborns.

If you use a front carrier for your baby, make sure your baby's face is never buried in the carrier's fabric. Inspect the leg holes to make sure the seat isn't lower than the openings, and if your baby's legs start to turn blue or show pressure marks on the backs of his thighs after he's been carried around for a while, stop using the carrier.

When to Buy

Have one on hand for use with your newborn. Usually used until your baby can sit up independently, around 6 to 8 months, when a framed carrier may be more comfortable.

Q I tried using a baby carrier that I got for my shower, but it made my back hurt, so I had to give it up. I'd still like to use one, but it seems like too much of a pain. What do you recommend?

How you position your baby in a carrier makes a big difference in your comfort. He should ride high—basically in the same position he would be in if you were carrying him in your arms. Any lower or having the carrier too loose can cause back strain. The straps of the carrier should be centered in the middle of each shoulder, and a pelvic belt that buckles around your waist can help distribute your baby's weight more evenly.

Q I thought my baby would love being in a carrier, but he hated it and protested every time I put him in it until I took him out. Is he just unusual, or is there something I missed?

Some babies seem to hate being confined, especially around their heads; others like keeping their legs curled up instead of being forced into a straight position by a carrier. If your baby seems soothed by certain positions, then a carrier that allows him to ride in that same position may work best. If

he hates being cradled in your arms or seems unnerved by being touched, then it's likely he'll also dislike the same position inside a carrier. Some babies fuss just at the beginning of getting in the sling, but start relaxing once their parents begin walking, which provides a soothing rhythm.

Q At what point should we stop using a soft carrier and move the baby into a framed backpack?

A framed backpack will cost a lot more than a soft carrier, but if you're serious about hiking or camping with your baby or just plan to do more than a few hours of toting your baby throughout the week, then you should consider moving up to a serious pack. Backpacks should be used only once your baby has strong sitting skills, certainly no younger than 6 months of age. The pack's frames, thickly padded pelvic belts, and well-padded shoulder straps will offer more body comfort for you, and the frame will help to distribute your baby's weight more evenly on your body than a saggy fabric carrier. But no matter how much you pay, the pack won't make your baby any lighter. (See our discussion of backpacks starting on page 42.)

Avoid:

✗ **Poor construction.** Don't use carriers made with flimsy fabric and unreinforced seams.

✗ **Weak buckles.** Flimsy buckles, snaps, or rings might accidentally release from the weight or motion of the baby.

✗ **Confusing straps.** Too many straps, snaps, and fasteners make it difficult to use.

✗ **Leg holes too large or uncomfortable.** Big leg holes could let the baby could slip through. If the seat is lower than the leg holes, that could constrict the circulation in his legs.

✗ **Uncomfortable sides.** Your baby's arms and underarms may become chafed if the sides of the carrier are too high, aren't padded, or have straps that rub against them.

✔ Checklist

Soft carrier shopping

✔ **Comfortable fit.** Be sure it fits your particular body and baby. The sling should adjust to the right length for your body and offer adequate room for your baby without enveloping him or squeezing him too tightly.

✔ **Sturdy and washable.** Quality fabric can withstand lots of machine washings without fraying or shrinking. It should be double-stitched and reinforced where straps join the carrier's body.

✔ **Safe buckles and latches.** Strong fasteners that won't release unexpectedly and cause the baby to fall. They should not have small parts that can come loose and be swallowed by the baby nor sharp edges that could cut or pinch him.

✔ **Simple to use.** Putting the carrier on and taking it off should be simple and self-evident, without too many entangling straps and latches.

✔ **Comfortable shoulder straps.** Parents' shoulder straps should be adjustable, densely padded, and spaced so they don't rub the neck or slip off the shoulders.

✔ **Head support.** Your baby will need a cushioned head support for the first few months. After that, you can fold the support down or snap it off.

✔ **Adjustable seat.** The baby's seat should adjust to different heights and have sturdy snaps that won't rub his belly. (Extra safety loops or a backup pouch will help prevent accidental falls.)

✔ **Front or rear facing.** Some models allow baby to face either out or toward mom or dad's chest, and some are designed to be carried on the back—a handy option for toting toddlers.

✔ **Extras.** Options may include snap-on flannel burp bibs, elasticized pockets for small items, panels for discreet nursing, reflector strips for evening strolls, breathable mesh, or special porous fabric for air circulation.

✔ **Adaptable.** Choose a carrier that can be adjusted to other carriers' body sizes.

> **❝** I'm only 5 feet tall, and the sling never worked for me and my baby. I could never adjust it to fit right, and my baby hung down. I finally gave in and bought a stretchy one-piece carrier in the small size. It fit around my baby like a tee shirt and worked much better. **❞**

Getting the right fit

Not only does your baby need to feel comfortable with a carrier, but so do you. If you and your partner are different sizes and both of you plan to use the carrier, get one that accommodates both of you (or buy two different sizes). Some slings come in plus and petite sizes as well as standard sizes.

Tube-style carriers are sized according to chest size and height. BABYBJÖRN's carrier, the most popular U.S. one, offers an extra-large version for taller people and custom-made carriers, too. Try on different carriers, just as though you were selecting a piece of clothing, and don't settle for one that isn't comfortable or that swallows your baby.

Most parents feel awkward the first time they try to figure out how to use a sling or soft carrier. It helps to read the directions first, or to watch the DVD if one comes with the carrier. And before you put your baby in the carrier for the first time, practice all positions with a pillow or teddy bear first until you can perform all of the adjustments smoothly. Fatigue and muscle aches, particularly a backache, are signs that you haven't adjusted the carrier correctly, the carrier is the wrong size for you, or that it's poorly designed and probably should be returned to the store.

> **❝I guess I thought the carrier would make the baby feel lighter. It didn't. It's not something you can do all day. After a while, your shoulders or back (or both) will start aching and you'll be glad to take it off.❞**

SLINGS AND WRAPS

Slings resemble small, pleated fabric hammocks that have a single large strap. The sling loops over one of the parent's shoulders and forms a circle under the parent's opposite arm. It can carry a baby in front, or it can be moved to one side and serve as a seat to help support an upright tot straddling his parent's hip.

Most slings use a fastener at the shoulder, such as two O-rings placed next to each other so the sling's tail can be folded over on itself to cinch and tighten the sling. Rings can be made of metal, molded plastic, or nylon. Some parents don't like the O-ring configuration because it could allow the fabric to gradually work loose. The rings can sometimes strike the baby's head, and they make a lot of bumping sounds in the dryer.

Other models, called wraps, use no fasteners at all but are long lengths of soft fabric that loop around parent and baby in a series of X's to hold the baby in place while his legs hang down. Another type is a presewn stretchy tube that comes in a selection of sizes and is folded and looped to form the baby's seat. The advantage of the tubes is that they are lightweight and easy to fold into a pocket or purse, and they fit the baby more closely than hammock-style slings that could allow the baby to fall out when the parent bends over.

While most slings are "one size fits all," other models offer small, medium, and large options—a distinct advantage for petite moms who may find they can't cinch a regular-sized sling tight enough to bring the baby high enough for comfortable carrying.

Slings come in a wide choice of fabric

colors and patterns as well as different fabric thicknesses. Fabric that is too thin may not support the baby well enough, while very thick fabric may make it too hot for use in warm weather. Models are made of a single length of fabric or a series of fabric pieces sewn together, to form the hammock and the straps. The width of slings varies, but it should be wide enough so the baby won't be cramped inside.

Padding is sometimes sewn inside of slings to form a cushioned surface for the baby's back, and some models offer a cushioned pad for the parent's shoulder. If you plan to tuck your baby and sling under your coat in cold weather, you may prefer a fairly compact model without the extra shoulder padding. And a wider hammock may be needed if you plan to use it to the side to help support a hip-straddling toddler.

Over the Shoulder Baby Holder
($45)

Clearly the most popular sling with parents, the Over the Shoulder Baby Holder (OTSBH), for babies up to 35 pounds, has thick padding on the shoulder and sides ("rails"). It's essentially a large piece of fabric sewn with a front-pleated hammock to form a pouch for carrying the baby. The tail is threaded through two nylon rings that are sewn into a pocket at the end of the carrier and allow the sling to be adjusted to different lengths and configurations. The bottom of the tail has a third nylon ring as an extra safety precaution. The sling can be used in a variety of positions—for a reclining newborn, to a semi-upright 1- or 2-month-old, to a side (or even back) carrier for an older baby. Adjusting the sling can feel awkward at first and require practice, and it's more bulky and hot than lighter weight (and less padded) models; but once mastered, positioning the baby (or putting him down) takes only seconds. Sizes include small (parents 70–120 lbs.), medium (110–180 lbs.), large (140–250 lbs.) with XL, XXL, and XXXL available by special order for a $10 charge. Available in a wide variety of all-cotton fabric choices in florals, solids, and prints.

Highs & lows of slings and wraps

Highs. Provides a semireclining position suitable for young babies, but also can be used to support a toddler on your hip. Slings can be positioned for discreet nursing, are usually completely washable, and are more comfortable than carrying an infant car seat.

Lows. Getting the right adjustment and tightness takes know-how (follow the directions and the instructional DVD if one comes with the product). There are no safety straps to hold the baby in, which could be a problem if you lean over to pick up something and the baby is pitched forward. The pressure of the baby's weight is carried on one shoulder and across the back, which could cause aches and body-alignment problems. Not recommended for strenuous activities, such as hiking.

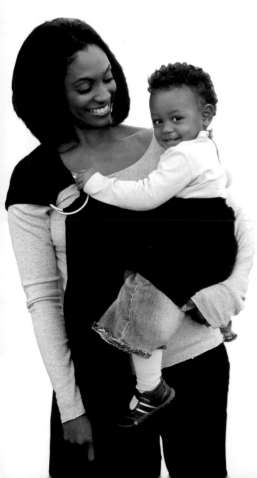

Maya's Wrap Baby Sling
($36)

More compact and less bulky than the Over the Shoulder sling, the Maya wrap is a single length of fabric with no padding that fastens using double rings to allow you to adjust the fit. It can be used from birth to 35 pounds, and it adjusts easily by loosening or tightening different sections of the fabric. (Previous ring problems that caused a recall have been repaired.)

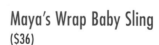

SOFT FRONT CARRIERS

Soft carriers usually consist of an inner seat pocket for the baby, an outer fabric covering that also offers a fold-down firm headrest for newborns, padded shoulder straps for the parent, and waist straps to help support the baby's weight. Because they force the baby into an upright position, they're not recommended for babies younger than two months old.

Some soft carriers have seats that adjust to different depths as the baby grows, and some are also designed to allow a child to face forward during infancy and then to face outward toward the world when the child reaches 3 or 4 months of age.

For maximum comfort, the shoulder straps should be wide and padded to dis-tribute the baby's weight evenly across the shoulders and back. And the carrier should be designed to allow the baby to ride high on the chest—the rule of thumb being that you should be able to kiss your baby's forehead when you look down.

Getting the baby inside the carrier and mounting the carrier on your body can be a hassle, and it takes practice to master the skill. Some have a confusing jumble of straps—for the shoulders, for the baby, for around the back, for adjusting the baby's headrest—so ease of use is impor-tant. An easy-release feature that allows you to remove a sleeping baby without waking him up can be a godsend.

BABYBJÖRN's Baby Carrier Original
($75–$80)

The most popular soft carrier in the U.S., this Swedish import for babies 8 to 22 pounds is simple, easy to put on, well cushioned, and comfortable for both par-ents and baby. It is completely machine washable, has excellent back support, is easy to get the baby in and out, and adjusts as your baby grows with snaps to modify the seat's height. It's pricey, too, but many owners say it's worth the extra cost. Like any other carrier, it can be hot in the summer; but in winter, you can wear it comfortably with a roomy jacket or coat buttoned over the carrier. Available in a variety of colors. An extra large version is available for about $15 more.

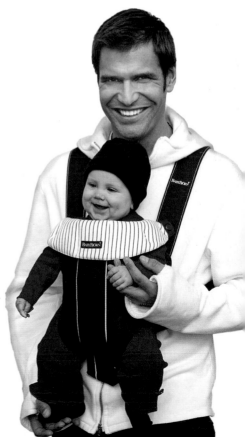

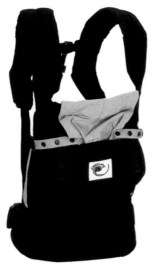

ERGObaby's Carrier
($90)

Compact, comfortable, and sturdy, the ERGObaby carrier is for babies from 15 to 40 pounds (although that may be too much weight for some parents to bear). It's made of machine-washable cotton. And parents rave about its comfort and how their babies enjoy riding in it. It can be worn in front, in back, or on the hip. The wide, sturdy waist belt fastens securely to place most of the weight of the baby on the parent's hips instead of the waist. It accommodates parents' waists from 27 to 45 inches, and an optional waist expander is available for waists up to 54 inches. A wide, rectangular fabric section sits above the waistband for the baby to rest on, which allows the baby to sit on his rump rather than being suspended by the crotch as with some carriers. It comes with an attached sleeping hood to support baby's head during sleep and a zippered storage pouch in the rear. You'll need to purchase a soft cushioned infant insert separately if you plan to use it with a young baby ($25).

Highs & lows of soft front carriers

Highs. They're made of comfortable fabric, which is easy to wear. They put your baby's head at your chin, and you can provide natural warmth and comfort with your hand on baby's back. They're a convenient and comfortable alternative to using a car seat as a carrier.

Lows. Some models have complex straps that make putting them on a challenge. They can be hot in the summer. Poor hardware or overly large leg holes have led to baby injuries in the past.

Safe use tips

Here are some practical tips for helping to keep your baby safe while you're wearing a soft carrier.

✔ **Watch your step!** A baby can sustain head injury if a parent trips and falls forward, causing the baby's head to hit the floor. The most severe injuries happen when the baby's head strikes a hard surface, such as a concrete or tile floor. Wear sturdy, stable shoes, and proceed with caution when your baby is onboard.

✔ **Remember: your dimensions change.** It's easy to forget that you're wider with a carrier on or that your baby's head is behind you and could strike the top of the car or the trunk lid when you lean over to reach inside.

✔ **Avoid hot beverages and foods.** Your baby could be burned if he hits your hand and causes you to spill hot liquids or food on his head or arms.

✔ **Don't cook with your baby in front.** Your baby could be burned by hot grease or steam. Place your baby in a baby seat or high chair away from the cooking.

✔ **Don't roll with the baby in a carrier.** Don't use the carrier on a bicycle, in a vehicle, or on skates or a skateboard.

SAFETY CONSIDERATIONS

Typical injuries involving soft carriers include fastener and seam failures that allow the carrier to open and the baby to fall out, overly wide leg openings that allow the baby to fall through, and injuries to the baby when a parent falls or knocks into something while wearing the carrier.

The Consumer Product Safety Commission (CPSC) has recalled carriers because of product failures that allowed babies to be injured in falls. To research soft carrier recalls, go to www.recalls.gov to search the CPSC's site.

The Juvenile Products Manufacturers Association (JPMA), along with the American Society of Testing and Materials (ASTM), has created a voluntary certification standard for soft infant carriers. That standard requires that manufacturers use an independent testing laboratory to validate that their carriers comply with specific safety and durability standards. If a soft carrier is certified, a certification sticker can be found somewhere on the product. Note: Being certified does not mean that a soft carrier is immune to recalls, and not being certified does not necessarily indicate that it is unsafe.

20

STROLLERS & OTHER BABY WHEELS

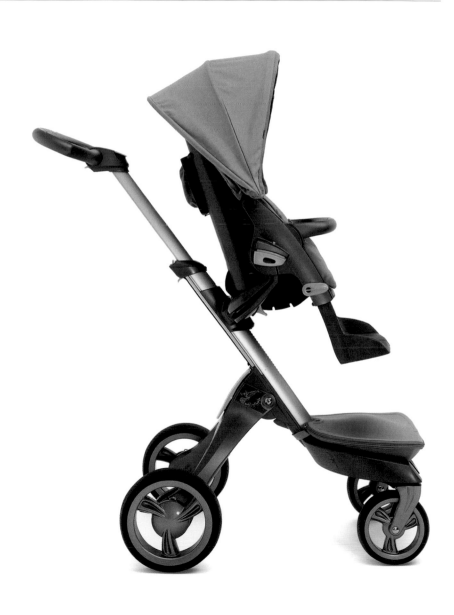

Strollers, called pushchairs in the U.K., are foldable kid-size wheeled chairs made especially for rolling around the young and the restless. There are hundreds of strollers from which to choose—from inexpensive umbrella styles, to mid-weights, sophisticated imports, and specialty strollers for joggers or for transporting more than one child. This chapter will help you weigh all of your stroller options and guide you in choosing the best and safest models.

ON YOUR MARK, GET SET, ROLL!

When your baby weighs less than 15 pounds or so, a soft carrier or sling is fine, even best, for a trip to the store, speeding through an airport, or for a walk around town. But as your baby gets heavier, carrying her can get tiresome. That's when it's time to buy a stroller. But what kind?

Strollers are probably the most challenging baby item to shop for, because there are hundreds of models and designs from which to choose. As with cars and other consumer products these days, strollers often serve as personal statements about the lifestyle and aesthetic of their owners.

The price range for this baby-product category is widespread—from simple fabric-and-frame "umbrella" models that you can acquire for about $20 to sophisticated state-of-the-art contraptions with frames made from aircraft-quality aluminum and equipped with options like cup holders, MP3 speakers, mosquito- and UV-blocking canopies, shock absorbers, winter buntings, and snap-on rain shields.

For parents with tons of money to spend on baby products and who seek to be the envy of their babies' playgroups, there are over-the-top models, including the $729 (plus accessories) patented Bugaboo Frog, or Silver Cross's $3,000 Balmoral pram suitable for the heir to the British throne.

Up until recent years, parents were offered only two color choices for strollers: navy and navy with one other color, usually yellow or beige. Now, strollers come in a huge palette of colors and patterns, including plaids, animal prints, princess pink, and G.I. camouflage. They're also customizable to parents' lifestyles, whether they're joggers, city dwellers, or suburban SUV drivers.

As with any other product, the price of your baby's wheels depends upon a series of factors: the quality of materials and manufacturing, the brand name, and the options.

Don't fall into the trap that so many parents do of believing that if a stroller costs more, it will automatically be better. As you will see, quality and cost don't necessarily go hand in hand, and there's always the risk of being seduced by the image that a stroller conveys, when a more economical model or one with fewer options might meet your (and your baby's) needs just as efficiently—and be lighter and easier to fold.

When to Buy

Purchase a stroller that reclines during the last months of pregnancy for use during your baby's first year. Later, consider other models that mesh well with your lifestyle and transportation needs. Most children stop using strollers by 3 or 4 years of age.

Features to consider

The stroller features your baby needs change over time. Newborns need to be able to fully recline (or nearly so), and most parents of new babies prefer that their babies face them, which is why specially equipped strollers that allow infant-only car seats to be snapped onto their frames facing parents are so popular.

Once your baby has more postural control and is able to sit up for periods of time, a stroller with several upright positions will work best. At that stage, babies are much more interested in looking out on the world than facing their parents. To be comfortable, toddlers and young children need strollers with wider and deeper seats—dimensions that would swallow a young baby.

When it comes to selecting the best stroller for your baby, the other important consideration is how you plan to use it. If you live in a city and you'll be using the stroller in tight places—rolling between narrow store aisles; repeatedly folding and lifting the stroller in and out of cars, cabs, or buses; or racing through airport terminals—you'll get the best service from a lightweight, nimble model with one-handed steering and folding.

If you're a suburban dweller who drives a minivan or has ample trunk space in your car, and if you only take outings to the mall, the zoo, or other easy-to-navigate places, you'll be best served by a heftier mid-weight model with larger wheels and lots of storage space.

If you're buying a stroller with the intent of taking long walks or running on uneven terrain, a model with big wheels and spring-action shock absorbers and lots of space between the rear handlebar and the stroller's axle will work best for you.

TYPES OF STROLLERS

Here's a chart showing the general categories that strollers fall into by size, price, and function.

TYPE	DESCRIPTION	USE	PRICE RANGE
Lightweight, inexpensive strollers	Small frame, often flimsy. Small wheels, hammock-like or lightly padded seats. Few or no recline options. Skimpy storage and small or no sun canopy.	For brief jaunts and travel. Suitable for children who can sit up on their own.	$15–$60
Mid-weight strollers	4- or 3-wheel ("sports") configu-rations on a medium-sized frame. Front trays, multiple recline positions, deep storage bins.	For long walks and negotiating curbs and uneven terrain. Suitable for young babies and toddlers.	$125–$350
Lightweight portables	Light and nimble with compact, complex frame. Loaded with all the bells and whistles, including easy steering, thickly padded seats, multiple recline positions, a front tray, and an ample storage bin.	For urban use, mall shopping, and travel. Suitable for young babies through toddlers.	$120–$500
Multi-component stroller systems	Interchangeable seat and bassinet units click in and out of the stroller's frame. Seats can be placed in a variety of positions (reclining or upright; rear facing or forward facing).	For city, suburban, and neighborhood use. Suitable for newborns through toddlers.	$600–$900+

TYPE	DESCRIPTION	USE	PRICE RANGE
Full-size carriage/ strollers	Heavy, large frames, and big wheels. Thick upholstery. Fully reclined, forms a baby bed. Adjustable footrest, deep storage bin, numerous extra accessories.	For suburban and rural use. Adaptable for newborns through 4-year-olds.	$200–$600
Travel systems	Mid-weight or full-size strollers with frame components that come with a matching infant-only car seat to be transferred from car to stroller.	City and neighborhood use. Stroller can be used 6 months (or longer) with the car seat installed, and it then converts to a standard stroller.	$100–$300
Jogging strollers	Heavy, bulky frames that may partially fold. 3-wheel configuration with a single wheel in front. Large pneumatic wheels removable for storage. Locking hand brakes, limited seat positions, and often limited storage capacity.	Useful for running on both even and rough terrain or in the snow, but extremely awkward in tight quarters.	$150–$250
Multiseat strollers	Heavy-duty frames to support 2 or more seats installed side by side or one behind the other (called tandem strollers).	For siblings, twins, or multiples.	$200–$660

TYPES OF STROLLERS (Continued)

TYPE	DESCRIPTION	USE	PRICE RANGE
Wheeled car seat frames	A lightweight folding frame designed only for supporting rear-facing infant-only car seats, but with no seat of its own.	For babies under one year seated in their infant-size car seats.	$50–$90

Smart shopping tips

■ **Don't buy on impulse.** Simply because you've fallen in love with a leopard-print stroller that goes with your favorite purse doesn't mean that it will be the most comfortable for you and your baby, or that it will be the most serviceable over the next 4 years. Compare feature-by-feature for weight, seat recline, folding ease, brakes, storage, seat belts, sun shield, and other essentials.

■ **Shop around.** Once you've pinpointed the stroller you want, write down the manufacturer, the stroller name, and the specific model number. Then browse big discount chains, such as Wal-Mart, Babies "Я" Us, and Toys "Я" Us, as well as such Internet sites as www.amazon.com, www.Target.com, and other reputable e-tailers to search out bargains. But beware of hefty shipping and handling charges.

■ **Track the model.** Remember that stroller manufacturers change model names, numbers, features, and fabrics virtually every year, and not all models carrying a given manufacturer's logo perform equally well. There can be variations on models carrying identical names. So what might seem like a real bargain could simply be a stripped down no-frills model.

■ **Know return policies.** Before you finalize the stroller sale, find out what the return policy is, in case the stroller turns out to be a lemon or you (or your baby) simply don't like it. Some retailers only allow 14 or 30 days to return the product for a refund; or you could be forced into exchanging an undesirable model for an identical version. Especially if you're buying from the Internet or a catalog, also check the seller's shipping and handling costs for returns; and think twice about back-ordering the stroller, since months could pass before it finally arrives.

■ **Be cautious about used strollers.** Buying used strollers on the Internet, such as at an eBay auction or thrift store, could backfire. Frames are easily knocked out of whack, and misaligned wheels are common, causing the stroller to wobble or veer. The seat's upholstery or safety belt may be soiled or frayed. Even what appears to be a new stroller could be outdated or have undergone a recall.

■ **Read what reviewers say.** It helps to know what the experts are saying about particular stroller models, such as www.Consumersearch.com, www.BabyBargains.com, and www.epinions.com. *Consumer Reports* also occasionally rates strollers. Their ratings can be accessed online at www.ConsumerReports.org when you pay an annual subscription fee. Avoid stroller reviews on sites that also sell them; and keep in mind that some parent-reviewers, having invested hundreds of dollars on a costly stroller model, may feel the need to justify their purchase.

■ **Buy preassembled.** If possible, buy the stroller already assembled and ready to roll out of the store. Otherwise you may be in for an exasperating time trying to assemble all the various parts. Plus, if it's already assembled, you can troubleshoot for problems before you leave the store.

■ **Search for seasonal sales and discount coupons.** New stroller models typically ship in early September through late December. Toward the end of the year, you may be able to get a great discount on outdated or discontinued stroller models. Some major stores host seasonal "baby weeks" when they offer discount coupons on major baby-product lines (but watch out for bare-bones loss leaders—priced to draw you into the store in hopes you'll buy a more expensive, feature-loaded one instead). Baby fairs, held in major metropolitan areas, are great places to haggle for a stroller, too, since manufacturers' reps don't want to have to pay to ship their display models back to the warehouse.

■ **Nix unnecessary extras (or purchase them separately).** You and your baby can probably do without a lot of add-ons, or you can purchase them separately for much less than what they add to the stroller's final price. Examples: clear vinyl all-weather shields, snap-on leg bags, small speakers for broadcasting iPod tunes to your baby, a removable case for toting your belongings. Extras bump up a stroller's price (and weight).

Avoid:

✗ **Pinch points and protrusions.** Babies can be hurt when strollers accidentally collapse, capturing their fingers in sharp X joints; and tots outside the stroller could fall into sharp components.

✗ **Wobbly wheels.** Wheel-alignment problems are the number one complaint of parents. Many strollers now have snap-off wheel assemblies to simplify replacing them.

✗ **Flimsy seat belts.** Your baby could be hurt if the seat belts don't hold, or they fray and pull off.

✗ **Awkward folding.** You'll open and fold the unit hundreds of times. Make sure that isn't awkward or difficult to do.

✗ **Oversize models.** Large strollers may be difficult to store in your home or car.

✗ **Unneeded extras.** Don't pay for extras that aren't important and only make the stroller heavier and harder to fold.

Checklist

Stroller shopping

Here's what to look for when you shop for a stroller for your baby.

✔ **Manageable weight and size.** A huge, bulky model eats up trunk space in your car and may squeeze out suitcases or groceries. But if you live in an urban area, you'll need one with large enough wheels to tackle uneven sidewalks and deep curbs.

✔ **Durable frame.** Stroller frames bend and get out of whack. An aluminum frame, although usually more expensive than a steel one, is lighter and sturdier. Give the stroller a "jiggle" test by rattling the frame with the handlebar. A well-constructed frame will feel sturdy and tightly put together.

✔ **Certification.** A "JPMA Certified" sticker on the stroller's frame indicates that the manufacturer has agreed to have its stroller models undergo rigorous voluntary safety and durability tests.

✔ **Safety harnesses.** Superior 5-point harness systems have shoulder straps, in addition to waist and crotch straps, to keep the child from standing up or sliding out.

✔ **Brakes.** Engage the brakes and try pushing the stroller forward to ensure they are easy to use and won't accidentally release.

✔ **Folding ease.** Test how readily the stroller folds and reopens. When the stroller frame is fully opened, it should lock into place and not fold unexpectedly. (Most stroller folding requires a series of actions, and you may need a sales clerk to demonstrate how to do it the first time.)

✔ **Seat recline options.** Your baby will need sturdy back support at a comfortable angle so she doesn't slump forward. Check how easily the back reclines. The more positions offered, the better, although a semi-recline is adequate. (Generally, only large multi-component stroller systems and combination carriage/stroller models recline fully to create a bed.) When the seat back is in its deepest recline, the baby's head and arms should be protected from being captured in gaps in the frame.

✔ **Maneuverability.** Give the stroller a test drive before buying (preferably with your baby inside). The stroller should corner well, allow one-handed steering, and roll straight ahead without veering.

✔ **Wheels and shocks.** Most strollers offer wheels that can swivel for easy cornering but that can also be locked in the forward position for rough terrain. Rubber or cushioned foam tires are better at absorbing jolts than hard, rigid tires made from molded plastic. Look for shock absorbers just above the wheel assemblies in the front, or on both front and rear wheels.

✔ **Handlebar comfort.** The stroller's handles or handlebars should be either adjustable or at a comfortable height for you and others without anyone's having to lean over or push from an awkward position. Your hand position should be natural, with no strain on your wrists. Cushioning for the handles or bar makes steering more comfortable.

✔ **Canopy or sunshade.** A deep, folding sunshade will help to protect your baby from wind, rain, and glare. Some models place a vinyl or mesh window on the top of the canopy so parents can keep an eye on their babies.

✔ **Storage.** A roomy storage bin underneath the stroller seat will come in handy for toting your purse, a diaper bag, or other items. If the bin sags too much when you press down on it, it may drag and scrape when it's loaded, especially when the stroller goes over curbs.

✔ **Possible extras.** Although they're not necessities, you may want a removable cushioned head support for small babies; shoulder-belt padding to protect the baby's neck area from shoulder straps; a removable front tray with a bottle/snack holder for baby; a cup or key holder for you; a zippered clear weather guard, or a snap-on cover for the baby's legs during cold or inclement weather.

Quick tips

The 3-stroller family. With so many stroller options out there, you may end up investing in not just one stroller but two, or even three, before your child becomes a true biped.

Problems with 3-wheelers. Strollers with only one wheel in the front are more tippy and unstable, especially when being lowered down a curb. They may also abruptly come to a stop if the single front wheel swivels into a sideways position.

Buy the bag separately. Diaper bags designed to match a stroller and to hook onto the stroller's arms are likely to be overpriced and bulky, and most parents don't find them as comfortable or convenient to use as softer purse-style bags.

Protect your stroller in flight. Most airlines don't allow strollers to be carried on board. Keep your stroller's delicate frame from getting bent and small accessories broken or lost when you check it as baggage. Plan ahead to pack the stroller in a box designed for golf bags, or wrap it in a blanket or clothing and stuff it in a zippered duffel bag.

Sun protection. Babies are much more vulnerable to sunburn than children or adults. Make sure to use the proper sunscreen on your baby's skin when she's out in the stroller. If the stroller's sunshade is too high to protect your baby's skin and eyes, use a protective brimmed hat. And consider purchasing a snap-on umbrella that fastens to the stroller frame—available as a stroller accessory in most baby stores.

A cheap twin solution. One temporary and inexpensive solution for rolling two children around together is to purchase two lightweight strollers and use screw-on metal connectors to fasten them together. You'll find them for sale in baby specialty stores. That way, you can separate the strollers as needed.

Q I'm pregnant, and I'd like to put a high-quality stroller that we can use for the first few years on my baby registry list. Should I select a large, fully reclining model with lots of padding that I know will make my baby (and later my child) the most comfortable? Or should I list something that's smaller and easier to wheel around?

Strollers can be heavy and awkward. Even though you could purchase a huge stroller with a seat back that folds to form a miniature baby bed, you may want to consider a unit that offers a partial but adequate recline for a young baby but will be serviceable for the next three years. Our suggestion would be to ask for a mid-weight and mid-price stroller (with an adapter that fits most brands of infant-only car seats if you decide to use one of those). The model you choose should be easy to steer and fold, preferably with an aluminum frame.

Q We're hoping to take a long airplane trip with several layovers, and we'll need a stroller for moving the baby around while we're passing through airports. My understanding is that strollers have to be checked at the gate, and that means we'll be without a stroller when we get off to change planes. What do you suggest we do?

Strollers aren't usually allowed onboard most commercial airlines (check with your carrier to be sure). If you're using an infant car seat, consider purchasing a lightweight folding stroller frame (without a seat) made just for infant car seats, which will make navigating the airport easier. Your carrier will probably allow you to check the frame just before you enter the plane and will have it ready for you when you deboard. Also consider carrying a small strap-on soft baby carrier for lugging your other stuff on and off the plane.

WARNING

Strollers hurt tots! Make sure your baby isn't close to the stroller when you fold it, since the joints and sharp components could crush or cut small fingers. Keep your toddler safely secured when in the stroller so she can't wriggle out, and never let her push it like a plaything, since she could get hurt falling into the sharp edges of the frame.

Cars hit strollers! Cross only at intersections, and be very cautious when pushing your baby's stroller out into the street. The front of your baby's stroller precedes you by several feet, and motorists are not likely to see your stroller, emerging between parked cars.

LIGHTWEIGHT, INEXPENSIVE STROLLERS

Sometimes called "umbrella strollers," these are the most basic of strollers. They're usually priced between $19 and around $75. Parents sometimes call them disposables, as in "So what if the wheels get wobbly? Just throw the thing away and buy another one!"

The umbrella designation comes from the curved umbrella-like handles of early models. This line of very basic strollers is not to be confused with fancier light-weights that may also be described as umbrellas but are much more costly and are chock full of special features.

Usually these bantamweights are quite easy to open and fold with one hand, and they're especially handy when scrambling into cabs or racing to airport gates. But when it comes to withstanding the wear and tear of heavy use, especially negotiating lots of uneven sidewalks and steep curbs, they don't hold up very well.

At the lowest price, wheels may be fixed permanently in the forward-facing position rather than being able to swivel. Wheels are usually quite small, and there may be no shocks in the wheel assembly to dampen the jarring. On the most basic level, the seat could be a simple fabric sling made of coarse cloth or vinyl mesh, with little if any padding or back support for the baby and no recline options. Seat belts could also be flimsy and thin, with a poor quality buckle and no shoulder straps to hold in a toddler.

But these cost-cutting flaws aren't always the case. Some mainstream manufacturers are now producing inexpensive models while still maintaining a service-able product. If you hunt around, you may be able to find a real bargain, with features that mimic models that are much pricier. (See our featured models on page 282.)

Highs & lows of umbrella strollers

Highs. The biggest advantage of choosing a low-priced umbrella stroller, of course, is the money you save. And without all the extras piled on, an inexpensive stroller can be amazingly light-weight. Just flip open and go. Some companies have managed to mass-produce very economical strollers that hold up pretty well and that carry some of the most important features, such as several seat reclines, a sunshade, and a storage bin. Should your child demand to be carried, you can probably roll the folded stroller behind you or stick it under your arm.

Lows. Predictably, a lower price tag for a stroller could translate into a flimsy product. Thin tubing and poorly mounted wheels may cause the stroller frame to bend or break or the wheels to veer or fall off. The sling seats found on some bottom-line models aren't comfortable for babies and children of any size. The sharp angle of the bottom edge of the seat could cut off the baby's circulation from under the knees. Many have either no sunshade or one that is too high and flat to protect the baby from glare (and sunburn). Storage bins and pockets may also be limited or missing altogether.

Dorel Juvenile Group's Safety 1st Altura Stroller
($55)

Inexpensive but not rickety, the Altura delivers lots of features for its low-end price. It has large dual front wheels that swivel and can lock into the forward-facing position. Its well-padded seat has a 3-position recline and comes with a removable cushioned headrest. Its 3-section canopy is deeper than most in its category and offers a fold-down tinted visor with a peek-in window on top for peering in on the baby. There's a removable front tray for the baby with 3 deep cupholders, as well as a parent console with cupholders just below the padded handlebar. Underneath is a generous mesh storage bin with an easy-access spring-down lip at the rear. The unit folds with one hand, using a simple maneuver from the handlebar to stand upright on its own. One drawback: As with other strollers in this price class, the unit offers only a 3-point harness (waist and crotch belts). If you're concerned about your restless toddler standing up or wriggling out, we suggest buying an attachable harness to get needed shoulder straps.

MID-WEIGHT STROLLERS

Mid-weight strollers are the standard workhorses of the stroller kingdom. They aren't thin and frail like their lightweight, inexpensive umbrella cousins; nor do they have wobbly frames like some compact, costlier lightweights. And they are not behemoths with cumbersome frames and oversize wheels that eat up trunk space and give parents backaches from lifting them. Instead, they convey a feeling of compactness, sturdiness, and stability.

There is an enormous array of models from which to choose in this mainstream category. The first choice you'll have to make is whether to get a model with a 3-wheeled triangular frame or the more standard square 4-wheeled frame.

We find the 4-wheelers to be more stable and less likely to tip over sideways, particularly when you are heading the stroller down steep curbs. Plus, 3-wheelers have the annoying problem of having the front wheel get stuck in the sideways position, bringing the stroller to an abrupt halt; and they offer less open space for toddlers wanting to climb in the stroller on their own.

Front wheels on standard 4-wheelers

Kolcraft's Jeep Wrangler XT All-Weather Umbrella Stroller

($40)

This 14-pound steel-framed stroller for babies from 6 months of age to 35 pounds offers a lot of bang for the buck. It has dual wheels on all sides and folds easily and quickly. The mesh-back seat has a roll-up panel for use as a headrest and to help ventilation in hot weather. The seat back also reclines for naps, and the manufacturer recommends using it in the reclined position for pre-sitting babies. The stroller has an adjustable canopy, foam-padded grip-style handles, a removable parent cupholder and 2 removable cargo bags. The unit offers only a 3-point harness (waist and crotch), so we suggest an attachable harness with shoulder straps if you're concerned about your restless toddler. Available in a series of colors, including pink and purple for girls and dark blue for boys.

usually swivel but can be locked into a forward-facing position by pressing down pedals above each wheel or applying a rapid pull-back and push-forward maneuver. The swiveling is useful for tight spaces and everyday strolling, while the forward-facing wheel position is desirable for fast walking or navigating rough terrain.

Most of the seats of these models are fixed to face the front, but rarely you may find a model with a reversible seat or a reversible handlebar, to give you the option of facing the baby either toward you or toward the direction of travel. The hardware for reversing handlebars usually adds substantially to the stroller's weight, and most parents ultimately settle for the baby-facing-forward position.

There may be dual tires in the front on each side, which help to give the stroller more stability. Although tire treads are mostly a cosmetic feature, some type of cushioning or shock absorbers should be supplied to soften your baby's ride.

Cushy tires can help, as can suspension springs mounted above the wheels. You can test for springiness by pressing down on the front of the stroller's seat or also on the handlebar in the back.

Good seat belts are essential. With an estimated 12,000 babies rushed to emergency rooms in stroller-related accidents, mostly from falling out, you'll want an easy-to-adjust 5-point harness (providing shoulder harnesses as well as straps for the waist and crotch) to keep your tot from trying to stand up or wriggle out of the stroller.

There may be several reclining positions for the seat. That's useful, especially if you plan to use the stroller while your baby is small. Adjustment may be via a simple lift-to-release mechanism on both sides of the back, or you may have to fiddle with straps or zippers.

Note: If the seat doesn't fully recline, it's most likely because federal regulations won't allow a stroller's seat back to assume a totally flat, bedlike position unless it also offers some type of cover for the stroller's leg holes, to prevent the baby from submarining—slipping out of the hole—when the seat is used as a baby bed. The rationale is that babies have died when they managed to wriggle out one of the stroller's leg holes feet first, strangling themselves in the process.

The seat should be comfortably cushioned, and the seat covers removable and washable. Metal components on the sides of the seating area should be shielded with fabric and/or padding so your baby's arms don't contact metal, and there should be no open gaps between frame components that could conceivably capture your baby's head or limbs.

Options may differ according to the model. A deep pull-down canopy will help shield your youngster from glare and rain (and from nosy onlookers). Being removable is a plus, especially if you've got a small or cluttered trunk. So is having a vinyl window on the roof that lets you peer in to see if your baby is asleep or awake.

A zippered vinyl weather shield, a mesh insect shield, or a snap-on cover to keep your baby's legs warm and dry are all extras that add more to the cost of the stroller. (Consider using a blanket for a foot covering and purchasing the other items separately when you're sure you need them.)

It should be simple to locate the latches on either side of the stroller—levers in the back, or a release on the handlebar to start the folding process. The stroller should readily snap back into a locked, upright position, too. Latches to compress the stroller in the folded position and stand upright on its own in the folded position are useful, especially in grocery or airport lines.

The stroller should steer nimbly with one hand, and wheels shouldn't come to an abrupt halt if they turn sideways. Handlebars for pushing the stroller should not force your hands or wrists into an awkward position. And they should be exactly the right height for your pushing comfort so that you don't have to lean over or reach too far upward. Adjustable handles or handlebars may be the best solution, especially if the person pushing the stroller is unusually short or tall.

Figuring out what to do with your purse and with shopping bags when you're pushing your baby around is a perennial problem. Look for an ample storage bin underneath the stroller that can hold weighty packages without dragging on the ground. The bin should be easy to access from the outside without forcing you to squat or crane to move things in and out.

Highs & lows of mid-weight strollers

Highs. Comfortable and stable (when there are 4 wheels on a square frame), generally reliable. Possibly strong enough to last the whole 4 years. Five-point harnesses with shoulder straps offer good protection from falls or sliding out. A reclining seat is great for napping. Your tot may appreciate a front tray or bars to hold on to, as long as they can be removed when she's old enough to scramble into the stroller on her own.

Lows. Heavier than umbrella strollers and more sophisticated (and costlier) than lightweight models. Wheel problems are a constant complaint from parents. Sometimes components fail, and the frame can get bent out of shape. May be too large to store in the trunks of compact and subcompact cars. Three-wheel models are less stable, can screech to a halt when the front wheel gets stuck sideways, and sometimes make it harder for children to scramble inside.

Graco's Quattro Tour Deluxe Stroller

($130)

Large but sturdy, the Quattro Tour weighs in at 25 pounds. It offers an easy one-hand fold and is for babies from 6 to 36 months and weighing up to 39 pounds. There is a 4-position reclining seat, including full recline, with a removable infant head support and a 5-point harness for both waist and shoulders. The front tray with cup holders can pivot and hang to the side but is not removable. The folding canopy has a tinted foldaway sun visor along the front edge and a see-in window on top. The padded handlebar has an attached organizer tray with 2 cup/juice box holders. There are 10-inch wheels on the rear and 8-inch dual wheels with spring-action shocks in front that swivel or lock into the forward-facing position. There is a roomy storage bin below plus a time and temperature tracker. The stroller adapts to hold Graco and most other mainstream infant-only car seats in the rear-facing position, or it is available as a travel system accompanied by a coordinating Graco SnugRide rear-facing infant-only car seat.

Chicco's Cortina
($150)

This roomy 25-pound aluminum-framed stroller is designed for use from birth to 50 pounds. It comes with a deeply-padded seat that reclines to multiple positions, including a full recline for infants, using a squeeze-release handle in the rear of the back seat. Straps under the adjustable leg rest allow the legholes to be safely sealed off in the full recline position. Padding is removable and can be machine washed and drip dried. The stroller folds using a pull handle in the center of the parent console and stands by itself in the folded position. Dual swiveling wheels in the front lock into the forward position for rough terrain. All wheels have shock absorbers. The removable child's tray in the front opens using buttons on either side and comes with a lift-out, washable tray insert with 2 cup holders. The adult's console also has dual cup holders. The angled padded handlebar adjusts to different heights. The spacious storage bin underneath the unit is easily accessed from the rear. The stroller is designed to support the Chicco KeyFit 30 Infant Car Seat (sold separately), or you can purchase a Cortina travel system with the KeyFit included for about $290.

"Surprisingly, the cheap little umbrella stroller I bought at the grocery store for $20 has turned out to be a gem. It's so simple to fold, is lightweight enough to be dragged around by the handle when my baby wants to be carried on my hip, and I don't have to worry about tossing it into the trunk. "

LIGHTWEIGHT PORTABLES

Lightweight portables (usually imports) are the BMWs of the stroller world. They're highly sophisticated, with an incredible number of comfort and convenience features. But unlike the midweights, their skillful engineering enables them to carry a lot of extras while remaining light and nimble.

Usually, these models handle beautifully, but with a wobblier feel than the ride from bigger and more rigidly assembled models, and their seats may be smaller and more compact.

You'll find extraordinarily plush interiors, excellent recline features, fully adjustable 5-point harness systems, deep fold-down canopies, adjustable footrests, and rapid-fire folding and opening capabilities. Some models come with carry handles on the side or shoulder straps, to make toting them easier. All these amenities packed into a small frame come with a hefty price tag, too, especially the trendiest European and Japanese brands. (Think: Aprica, Combi, Chicco, Peg Perego, and Maclaren.)

Most models in this category have smaller-than-standard wheels, which is great if you're seeking compactness and have limited storage space. But as we've mentioned, miniwheels become a disadvantage if the stroller has to constantly negotiate potholes, roll through grass, make it over tree roots and tilted sidewalk slabs, or head down steep curbs.

You could pay hundreds of dollars less for models with many comparable features from mainstream U.S. stroller manufacturers. In truth, a large proportion of stroller models sold in the U.S., whether with American or European brand names, are actually rolling off identical conveyor belts in Asian factories that are mass-producing models to the specifications of any particular brand.

In some cases, all the bells and whistles can be a bother. Call it the fumble factor. Expect to feel awkward bent over the stroller trying to figure out how to make the frame fold, to clasp its components together once that's accomplished, and to make the stroller snap to attention again when your baby's installed, strapped down, front bar is fastened, seat is reclined, and you're ready to roll again.

Maclaren models, for example, require the edge of a shoe to push down a tab on one side to engage the brakes, and then a similar metal tab on the opposite side to be pressed upward to release the frame for folding. (Not easy to do if you're wearing flip-flops.) The Combi stroller has to be folded in on itself in a U-shaped configuration to stay locked in the folded position, and a small tab nearly hidden in the frame has to be located to lock it in the folded position or to release it for opening.

Highs & lows of light-weight portables

Highs. Turn on a dime, very manageable weight, and excellent performance for the most part. Lots of comfort features for baby, compact storage, carrying ease.

Lows. Prices often overinflated. Wheel and mechanical problems are common and small ones don't perform as well on rough or uneven terrain as larger-wheels. Low handlebars are less comfortable for tall parents; skimpy sunshields offer poorer protection. Could be harder to get complaints resolved with an overseas manufacturer.

Zooper's Waltz
($300)

This 17-pound stroller is for newborns and children weighing up to 45 pounds and has an extra-wide seat to accommodate big tots. The seat's 4-position seat back includes a full-recline option for use with infants onward and comes with a 5-point harness for both waist and shoulders. The frame takes two hands to fold, but folds flat for storage. There is suspension on both the front and rear wheels with front ones that swivel or lock straight forward. The ventilated canopy includes a viewing window, and there is a somewhat small, but serviceable, storage bin underneath. Extra accessories include a rain shield and a leg-warming boot. The frame accommodates Graco SnugRide, Peg Perego Primo Viaggio, Britax Companion, and Evenflo's On My Way infant-only car seats in the rear-facing position (sold separately).

Peg Pérego's Pliko P3 Classico
($339)

A favorite of parents, the 16-pound P3 is designed for use by children from 6 to 36 months and weighing up to 45 pounds. It uses a sturdy, lightweight aluminum frame with a carry handle on the side that folds compactly with one hand and can remain standing when folded. Plush seat padding is removable and hand-washable. The backrest offers 4 recline positions, and there are 2 footrest positions. A 5-point harness holds the baby at both waist and shoulders. The generous canopy adjusts to different shielding positions and has a vinyl peek-in window for viewing the baby below. The front play tray can be opened and shut like a gate or completely removed. The cushioned grip-style handles are curved for wrist comfort and extend up to 3 inches for taller parents. Front wheels swivel or lock into a forward-facing position with suspension on all 4 double wheels. A built-in rear footboard allows a standing tot to ride. Auxiliary straps are available from retailers to allow an infant-only Peg Pérego Primo Viaggio car seat or a Navetta bassinet to be fastened into the stroller frame (both sold separately).

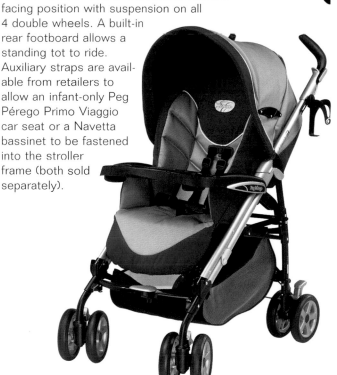

Maclaren's Techo XT
($310)

When it comes to weight, this nimble 14.2-pounder for use from birth to 33 pounds can't be beat! It offers 4 recline positions and a 5-point padded harness with 3 slots in the seatback for adjusting harness height. Its grip-style handles are cushioned and extend 1½ inches for taller parents, and there are several rear storage pockets. The deep, folding canopy has a UV-protected window for looking down on the baby. The padded leg rest can be adjusted to different angles for baby comfort. There are dual wheels on all sides with a swivel lock on those in the front. Minor drawbacks (other than its hefty price) are no front tray, a smallish underside bin that is difficult to access when the seat back is fully reclined, and its awkward folding maneuver that calls for pushing down on one lever with a foot and pressing up on another (which could be uncomfortable if you're wearing sandals or flip flops), and its not being able to stand when folded. Mind the X joints in the rear, too, that stabilize the frame but could conceivably capture small fingers during the folding process.

MULTI-COMPONENT SYSTEMS

These are the elite, trendy, head-turning Bentleys in the world of baby wheels. They are ingenious inventions that most likely represent the wave of the future when it comes to stroller design. A well-designed and sturdy folding frame with thick wheels is used to support a variety of seat components, including an infant bassinet and seats in several sizes. The seats are designed to recline to multiple positions and can be placed facing either toward the parent or outward.

Most offer a variety of optional accessory packages, such as diaper bags, foot muffs, weather and insect shields, zippered carry bags, and color-coordinated diaper bags. Plus, parents are given a wide choice of fabric colors, so that components can be mixed and matched.

Expect astronomical prices for these newfangled inventions (around $800 and up). Competitive pressures in the marketplace are likely to bring down prices, but they will also give rise to imitators that will offer similar designs and features, but at lower prices, in the years to come.

Bugaboo's Strollers
($530–$900)

The costly Dutch Bugaboo system has hit the U.S. by storm, and you can expect less-expensive knockoffs from other manufacturers to show up in years to come. The key words for strollers in the series are strong, maneuverable, and adaptable. The Bugaboo line uses sturdy but lightweight aluminum tubing and air-filled tires—large wheels on one end and smaller, swiveling ones on the other. Except for the Bugaboo Bee, a more traditional, folding stroller with a huge canopy and car seat adapters ($530), Bugaboo's other models—the Cameleon ($900), the Frog ($760), and the Gecko ($680)—offer a detachable 3-position, rigid-framed seat that locks into the stroller frame to face either rearward or forward. The Cameleon and Gecko also come with a detachable bassinet (carry cot) suitable for carrying reclined newborns and young babies. All have a huge removable canopy for shielding the baby from glare, weather, or curious onlookers. The units are available in a variety of color combinations from neutral tans to brilliant reds and oranges. Also included in the pricier versions are an under-seat bag, mosquito netting, a rain cover, a carry handle for toting the unit in a folded position, and a maintenance kit that includes an air pump and protective liquids and gels. A large series of optional accessories are available (also at top price), including a rather boxy diaper bag, a foot muff, a suspended cup holder, a gooseneck umbrella that serves as a sunshield, a wheeled board for tots to hitch a ride on the rear, a car seat adapter, and a transport bag. Definitely a lifestyle statement for the trendy and deeply pocketed parent.

Highs & lows of component systems

Highs. State-of-the-art flexibility allows you to change out components to suit the needs of your baby or child at any given stage in development. Seat components offer almost infinite positions, and they face forward or rearward, depending on how you lock them into their frames. Most of these strollers are very easy to steer. Multiple mix-and-match color options and numerous accessories allow you some leeway in choosing what you want to add to the mix.

Lows. Extremely costly. Assembling the unit and components can be a challenge until you get the hang of it. Components take up a lot of trunk space, and reassembling them in the parking lot or garage can be a hassle. The wide wheels that jut out from frames may make tight shopping situations awkward. Safety issues could arise when components fail to adequately lock into their frames or when hardware for components or frames fails. Pneumatic tires raise the issue of having a flat tire. You'll have to buy an adapter for an infant-only car seat separately.

UPPAbaby's Vista
($600)

Similar in its adaptability to the Bugaboo line, this welded aluminum stroller weighs in at nearly 25 pounds and is for use from birth through a weight of up to 40 pounds. It comes with both a flat-bed bassinet and a one-piece seat insert that adjusts to 3 different positions and uses a 5-point padded harness. Both bassinet and seat are covered in nylon fabric that is removable and machine-washable and line dried. The padded handlebar adjusts 4 inches for taller parents. The unit comes with a rain shield as well as a hand leash to keep the stroller from rolling away. There's a small fabric storage bin below. The frame folds readily with a single motion with the seat inside. Like Bugaboo strollers, the Vista has smaller wheels in the front and larger in the rear, but it uses rubberlike, cushiony tires with foam cores, rather than air-filled ones, so you never have to worry about having a flat. All wheels have shock absorbers. An optional car seat adapter and cupholder, a rear ride-along board for tots, and a zippered carry case are available options for separate purchase.

FULL-SIZE CARRIAGES/STROLLERS

At the top of this category are stately enameled carriages that can cost thousands of dollars—with giant spoke wheels, silver medallions, and leather straps to adjust the spring action—from prestigious old companies like Silver Cross. Far beneath this price point are multi-component carriage systems and carriage/stroller combinations that have adapted better to modern life. Nonetheless, there's no getting around their sheer bulk and awkwardness when it comes to dealing with their interchangeable bassinets and seats.

Granted, almost everyone has fantasies of pushing a baby carriage through the park with a tiny, exquisite baby inside. In truth, baby carriages are mostly a vestige of the past. They're heavy. They're bulky. They can't be stuffed into the trunk or hidden away in the hall closet, and they typify a kind of leisurely life reflected in turn-of-the-century paintings, rather than the high-speed in-and-out nature of our vehicle-dominated lifestyles.

> **❝ My baby was given an elegant, old-fashioned baby carriage by a doting aunt (who never had children). We only used it outside once or twice, but its springy rocking motion was a godsend indoors when our baby was fussy and needed to be soothed to sleep inside our apartment. ❞**

By federal regulation, only carriages and full-size carriage/strollers are allowed to fully recline into a flat bed position, and because of that, they answer the concerns of parents who want their newborns to have a protected cot on wheels. Along with the recline capability must come some means of covering the stroller portion of a carriage/stroller's leg openings to prevent the baby from wriggling out through one of the holes and strangling. Most manufacturers accomplish that with either a rigid footrest that folds upward and locks into a closed position or with mesh fabric that seals off the leg holes when a baby naps.

Highs & lows of full-size carriages/strollers

Highs. The bassinet or full-recline feature offers newborns a comfortable sleeping place during walks, and some models have carry cots that can be removed from the frame and used separately as a freestanding place for napping babies. The spring action of larger models can be very soothing to babies and can make for a smoother ride on rough surfaces. It may make a good resale item.

Lows. The fixed, nonswiveling wheels of the largest carriage styles require pushing down on the handlebar to lift the front wheels off the ground for pivoting in a new direction. (Let your nanny do the pushing!) Carriages/strollers are bulky and most are too heavy to lift comfortably in and out of car trunks. Definitely not suitable for shopping in stores, navigating narrow aisles, or for public transportation and airline travel.

Bumbleride's Queen B
($430)

The Queen B has the traditional look of a high-chassis carriage. A child seat comes standard with the stroller, but the bassinet accessory for smaller babies must be purchased separately. The seat offers 4 recline positions and has a 5-point adjustable safety harness with shoulder pads and an infant headrest. The footrest is adjustable and comes with a removable boot cover. All four 12-inch wheels have springy suspension, air-filled rubber tires with swivel front wheels. The handlebar adjusts from 30 to 42 inches. The chassis has a wire-mesh basket beneath the seat. The universal seat-belt adapter fits most infant-only car seats. An optional rain cover, plush seat liner, bassinet insert, and toddler seat are also available, as well as an accessory toddler seat that enables the stroller's frame to convert to a 2-seater for twins.

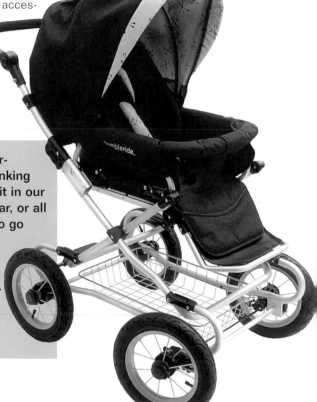

We bought a huge carriage/stroller without thinking about where we'd store it in our house, take it with our car, or all of the steps we'd have to go down just to take a walk with our baby. Big mistake. We ended up buying a second, lighter-weight stroller half the size that worked much better.

Stokke's Xplory
($800–$1,000)

The costly but adaptable Xplory has a frame constructed of aluminum and high-grade plastic. One model, the Xplory Basic, is simply the folding frame with a movable seat for children 6 months to 45 pounds, while the Xplory Complete adds a plush removable bassinet (0 to 6 months) that fastens onto the single, stalk-like arm of the stroller. The baby faces the parent in the bassinet, while the child seat can face either the parent or outward toward the world. The seat and bassinet units adjust to a series of heights, with the seat offering 3 rear-facing and 2 forward-facing positions. The circular handle for pushing the stroller adjusts for both height and angle. The unit comes with a canopy, a 5-point harness with padded shoulder straps, a rain cover, mosquito netting, and a matching shopping bag that fastens at the base of the frame for storage. (Note: Adjusting seat or bassinet heights takes practice.)

TRAVEL SYSTEMS

Travel systems are combination products. For $100 to $300, you get a color-coordinated, rear-facing infant car seat and its base, along with a fully functioning folding stroller. Adapters allow the stroller's frame to lock in the car seat (usually so the car seat faces you). Once a baby is strong enough to sit upright on her own and the car seat is no longer needed, the car seat holder is removed and the baby graduates to the regular stroller seat.

Highs & lows of travel systems

Highs. You may be able to save money by buying the package deal and get the two products for less than the individual price of each component when purchased separately. Being able to lift your baby from the car in his seat and click it onto the stroller's frame could be a plus. Having a matching car seat and stroller is an appealing concept.

Lows. You're locked into the infant-only car seat concept, when a convertible car seat may work better for your needs (see our discussion on pages 88 and 102.) And you're also committing yourself to the particular model of stroller that the manufacturer pairs with the seat, when strollers from other companies may perform the same function but be lighter, more maneuverable, easier to fold, or offer more useful features than the travel system's. (Since many strollers now have universal attachment systems for car seats, it may make more sense to shop for your baby's car seat and stroller as separate items based on their own merits.)

Graco's Metrolite Travel System
($200–$230)

This travel system includes an 18-pound aluminum-framed stroller and a Graco SnugRide Infant Car Seat, along with its stay-in-car base. The stroller part of the system offers a 3-position reclining seat and a 5-point harness with 2 slots for adjusting strap height. There's a height-adjustable handlebar with a parent console below that has 2 cup holders. The frame folds using a simple 2-step process and stands independently in the folded position. The large storage bin underneath has a rear spring-action fold-down lip for easy access. The system comes with a Graco SnugRide Car Seat, a rear-facing infant-only seat for babies weighing between 4 and 22 pounds and less than 29 inches tall. Both stroller and car seat have removable canopies.

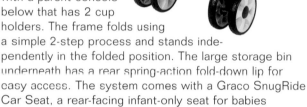
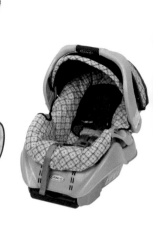

Baby Trend's Travel System
($160)

The 20-pound Baby Trend stroller portion of the travel system has an aluminum frame and is designed for use alone with babies from 6 months to 40 pounds. The removable and washable padded seat offers 2 recline positions. In front, there is a swing-away and removable child tray with cupholder and a fold-down canopy; in the rear, a parent console has a cupholder and covered storage compartment. The stroller uses a one-hand folding system and is self-standing when folded. The deep storage bin underneath has a spring-down lip for easy access. The stroller is adapted to carry the highly rated Flex-Loc rear-facing infant-only car seat, which is included in the system along with its base for the car. (You can review the car seat's features on page 101.)

JOGGING STROLLERS

Strollers for jogging or racing are descended from the bicycle and have the spoke wheels and large air-filled tires (12 to 21 inches in diameter) that are typical of bicycles. The larger the wheels are, the less drive is needed to move them along, the easier it is for the stroller to mount obstacles such as curbs or uneven terrain, and the more suited the stroller is to bringing a baby along for athletic jogging.

These large-wheelers enable parents to run while pushing the stroller in front of them. Their long, sleek frames protect parents' shins from striking the frame's rear axle while they're kicking forward. Not only do the strollers perform well on tracks and other level surfaces, but they can also manage trails and snow more smoothly than low-wheeled standard strollers do.

Typically, wheels are mounted on a welded triangle-shape frame that's constructed of aluminum, steel, alloy, or light and strong but costly titanium. The single wheel in the center front is sometimes smaller than the two wheels bringing up the rear. A hammock-style fabric seat is suspended in the center of the frame. **(Note:** The tricycle configuration of these strollers shouldn't be confused with smaller-wheeled imitators that simply mimic racers but aren't for running.**)**

Even though the inflated tires on these models offer some cushioning to protect small passengers from being jarred, newer designs now incorporate added shock-absorbing features, such as springs over either rear or all wheels, or springs buried inside a two-section frame in the front to allow it to bend slightly to cushion bumps.

The seat of the stroller may (or may not) recline to accommodate napping babies. The deeply angled fabric seat is designed to keep small fingers and hands from becoming captured in the wheel spokes turning nearby.

Most models in this class come with a 5-point harness system to strap the baby in—around the waist, between the legs, and over the top of each shoulder. On the whole, jogging strollers fall short when it comes to offering the basic seat comforts found with other types of strollers. You won't find much (if any) cushioning, padded headrests, rigid back supports, or ergonomically correct hip-to-knee seat lengths that would allow the baby's legs to relax comfortably on a footrest.

WARNING
Jogging strollers aren't for young babies!

Babies under 6 months of age shouldn't ride in jogging strollers. Babies this age have insufficient neck and spinal formation and strength to sit in the semi- to full-upright positions demanded by big-wheeled exercise strollers, or to withstand the jarring that occurs when the stroller hits rough spots at a high speed. Wait until your baby can sit well by himself before giving him rides.

The unit may have a single locking hand brake resembling a bicycle's, and some models add locking foot-operated brakes for added security when parking the stroller on an incline. Most also offer a wrist or waistband leash that attaches the stroller to the parent, as a protection to keep the stroller from getting away if the parent stumbles.

Sun canopies range in size and protective capacity depending upon model and brand. A deep or moveable canopy will help protect your baby from the sun and ultraviolet rays. Some canopies come with a vinyl window sewn into the roof to allow a parent to peer in on the baby.

Reflective tape may be sewn onto the front and back of the stroller and across the rim of the canopy so the stroller is

> **"Postpone buying a jogging stroller until your baby is mature enough and you've had plenty of time to recover from your C-section. I bought a deluxe model when I was pregnant, thinking how wonderful it would be to run with my baby. Then the thing just sat there and stared at me— a constant reminder of how tired and depressed I felt. It took months to feel up to trying it out. "**

more visible in low-light conditions. Mesh side wings on some models allow for better cross ventilation in hot weather, and they usually have small flaps that roll down like window shades to close the vents when it's windy or cold.

Many models offer mesh bins underneath for toting sweaters, diapers, and other paraphernalia. They differ in size from tiny to generous, depending, again, upon the manufacturer and model. Like strollers in other categories, you may find consoles between the handlebars for holding keys or a beverage and various pockets for baby toys or diapers. But as with other models, extra accessories add extra weight.

Most jogging strollers offer some type of front-wheel fender that acts as a shield to protect the baby from being splattered with mud and sand as the wheels rotate. Rarely, a model will offer a swivel-wheel option that allows the wheel to be unlocked from the straightforward position, to make steering easier in tight places; otherwise, the entire rear of the frame has to be lifted for a change of direction.

Although a swiveling front wheel may appear to be an impressive sales feature in the store, it's not as impressive on the track. If you fail to lock the wheel in the forward-facing position for running, you could risk an abrupt halt—as with shopping carts—when the front wheel shifts sideways.

Finding the best models

The best jogging strollers are relatively lightweight, have easy-to-remove wheels, and offer additional shock absorption beyond just air-filled tires. Handlebars should be the right height for the runner—high enough to prevent stooping but low enough that the pusher's arms are held in a comfortable, natural position.

Remember that these strollers are heavy and cumbersome and don't work well in tight spaces, such as store aisles. Trunk space makes a difference too, since you will probably be driving the stroller to where you plan to run. If you're only planning to take vigorous walks with your baby, a lighter weight, more maneuverable model will adapt better and be easier to manage.

Extra-wide (and extra-heavy) double-seat jogging strollers are available to accommodate two children, but attempting to push two children of different sizes could cause the stroller to veer, making it hard to keep on a straightforward line.

BOB's Ironman Running Stroller
($350)

The Ironman is designed for use by serious runners. Its 20.8-pound aircraft-quality frame features a cushioned multiposition handlebar, one-handed folding, a deep adjustable canopy. The seat has a 5-point harness and the seatback has 4 recline positions from upright to semi-upright; however, the stroller is not recommended for use until the baby reaches 3 to 4 months for strolling, and 6 months or older for jogging. Its 16-inch wheels have spokes and air-filled tires. The front wheel offers a fine-tune adjustment as well as an adjustable suspension system to help control veering. All wheels remove easily using a quick-release tab, for more compact storage. In addition to the locking rear-wheel brake, there is a bicycle-style slowing brake on the handlebar and a wrist strap to help keep the stroller under control. Note: The frame is adapted to hold most major infant seats, but we recommend that the stroller be used only for walking with a young baby inside. Other models in the series include SUS and SUS D'Lux models with thicker treads for off-road jaunts, and a double-seater named the Duallie. Accessories available for purchase include a diaper bag, a console unit for the handlebar, a weather shield, a sunshield, and a travel bag for toting the stroller.

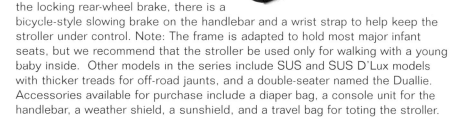

Dreamer Design's Rebound Jogger DLX (Deluxe)
($325)

This 24-pound stroller is for babies from 6 months to 100 pounds (or about 10 years). The stroller's welded aluminum frame folds readily with a 1-step trigger action. Its 16-inch bicycle-style alloy wheels with spokes and air-filled tires remove easily with a push-button action. There's also a suspension system on the frame above the front wheel to help reduce jarring. The cockpit-style seat and leg area are covered in removable, washable ripstop fabric with reflective stripes. The seat has a 5-point harness and a 30-degree recline using an adjustable back strap. There is a deep fold-down bubble-style canopy. The parent's padded handlebar adjusts from 43- inches to 52- inches. The unit offers rear foot brakes as well as a bicycle-style squeeze brake on the handlebar. It has a rear pocket, two bottle holders, and a small mesh-sided storage bin underneath.

Highs & lows of jogging strollers

Highs. Easy to push and a breeze for rolling over curbs, through snow or across puddles. A great way to get your exercise while giving baby a breath of fresh air, and most babies appear to enjoy riding up high and either snoozing or looking around.

Lows. More expensive than standard strollers. Dismantling the wheels from the hefty stroller frame in order to fit the whole thing into the trunk can be a challenge. The sharp seat angle of most models—even in the recline position—and the rough ride make these strollers unsuitable for babies under 6 months of age. The frame is too large and awkward for use in narrow spaces, such as in stores, in crowds, in cabs, or when using public transportation. As with a bicycle, rubber tires and inner tubes can go flat, so be prepared to use a pump and to make trips to gas stations or bicycle shops to fix tire or wheel problems.

Baby Jogger's Performance Single
($360)

The grandfather of all jogging strollers, this 24-pounder with a one-piece aluminum-and-steel frame is designed to accommodate children from 6 months of age up to 100 pounds in weight (or about 10 years of age). It's specifically designed for dedicated joggers and racers who plan to chalk up hours of running weekly with their babies in tow; and thus the huge bicycle-style 20-inch wheels with pneumatic tires that move swiftly and elegantly in true racing style. Adjustable fork tips enable fine-tuning of the front wheel's tracking. The tires have rear shocks to soften jarring.

Inside is a padded, easy-to-operate reclining seat with a 5-point harness, and a small underseat storage shelf. There is a handlebar brake as well as rear-wheel parking brake. The deep canopy can be adjusted for weather protection. The seat and canopy have removable fabric for hand-washing. Numerous accessories can be purchased separately, including a rain/wind shield or bug screen, inserts made of fleece, a tire pump, cushioned shoulder straps, a detachable umbrella, a zippered travel bag, a cupholder, and even an infant car seat adapter. Wheels remove with a push-button release for storing the stroller. The manufacturer offers a 1-year warranty on parts and a lifetime warranty on the frame.

MULTISEAT STROLLERS

If you're expecting twins or you have a small child and will be adding a baby, then a multiple seater is for you. Strollers that carry more than one child either place seats side by side or put one seat behind the other (tandem). Some tandems are available with more than two seats.

By necessity, side-by-sides usually have slenderer seats than those of standard strollers, so they can squeeze through 29- to 32-inch doorways. Their configuration is best suited for two children weighing roughly the same, since having a heavier child on one side may cause the stroller to veer.

Most tandems have the rear seat higher than the front one, in what is called stadium seating, to give the small rear passenger more foot room and a better forward view. Many tandems and some side-by-sides come with adapters that allow the frames to support infant car seats. Tandems are also available in long three-seat configurations. Some tandems offer seats that can be arranged to face rearward, forward, or toward one another.

Side-by-sides are often simply two stroller frames joined together by a center support post and a shared set of wheels in the middle. Each seat back usually reclines separately, and most seats have their own canopies, although some models stretch a huge canopy across both seats.

There are also two-seat jogging strollers with wide frames that suspend two seats in the middle. Some can even accommodate 3 children. (Check www.joggingstroller.com to see what's out there.)

Double-seaters, just like single-seaters, vary in quality and the amenities they offer. How well balanced or awkward a double is depends a lot upon the design and engineering skill of the manufacturer. Models can be exasperating and sometimes dangerous, especially when manufacturers treat them simply as very large regular strollers without dealing with the requirements of this type of stroller. When they are well executed, they operate smoothly and function well. When they're poorly made, they can be a nightmare to maneuver, fold, and store.

Stability and cornering are serious issues with double-seaters. A single, swiveling front wheel for the stroller can make maneuvering easier, but the tricycle-style configuration could be a dangerous trade-off, since a single front wheel may not be strong or stable enough to support the stroller in an upright position, especially when going over steep curbs.

> ❝ Our twins are expected in three months. We still haven't settled on a stroller for them. We've spent lots of weekends browsing in stores, and trying just about every stroller we can get our hands on. Nearly every stroller we've tried is poorly designed, unsafe, awful to use, or just plain ugly. ❞

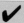 Checklist

Double stroller shopping

Here's what to look for when you shop for a double stroller. (Also see general information on the shopping list for single strollers, page 266).

✔ **Manageable weight and size.** Double-seater frames can be very heavy. Keep in mind that you're going to have to lift the stroller in and out of vehicles and manage it over curbs.

✔ **Infant car seat adaptability.** If you plan to use the stroller like a travel system, make sure the stroller's frame is designed to support one or two infant car seats of the brand you plan to use.

✔ **Seat comfort.** The stroller's seat backs should recline easily; and the more positions offered, the better. In tandems, the rear seat needs to be far enough away from the back of the front seat so that the front seat can recline without squeezing the baby in the back.

✔ **Maneuverability.** The stroller should roll straight ahead without veering. Can front swivel wheels be locked in the straightforward position? How easily does the stroller turn corners?

✔ **Canopy or sunshade.** Deep independent canopies for each seat are preferable to shallow canopies or a single canopy to cover both seats. Check whether the canopy must be removed before the stroller can be folded.

✔ **Storage.** The storage bin underneath should be large and easily accessible.

✔ **Safety restraints.** Both seats should have adjustable 5-point harnesses.

✔ **Secure fasteners.** If the seats can be removed for repositioning, make sure they lock securely in all positions, with no danger of accidentally detaching.

Highs & lows of multiple seaters

Highs. Let you push two or more children together. Sometimes could cost less than two comparable strollers. Many have comfortable reclining seats similar to single strollers. Some model frames can support infant car seats, until your babies outgrow them.

Lows. Large and bulky. Lifting, folding, and reopening can be major hassles. Some models are poorly designed and could even be unsafe. Vulnerable to bent frames and wheel malfunction.

Avoid:

✗ **Excess frame weight.** If the stroller weighs more than one-third of your body weight, seek a lighter model.

✗ **Hazards.** Beware sharp edges on the stroller's frame or seats. And a poor footrest for the rear seat could allow the child's leg to slip into the storage bin below.

✗ **Cramped quarters.** Make sure that both seats have adequate legroom, especially when the front seat is reclined.

✗ **Insufficient sun protection.** Small canopies won't protect babies from glare and sunburn.

Graco's DuoGlider LXI

(S210)

The 32-pound DuoGlider LXI is for babies from birth (when riding in infant seats) through 80 pounds total weight including both riders. It has a tandem configuration—one seat behind the other—arranged in stadium style with the rear seat placed higher than the front seat to provide adequate legroom and views for the rear passenger. The front seat partially reclines, while the rear seat can lie completely flat for an infant. The stroller is designed to carry 2 children of different weights with the heaviest child in the front seat, or 2 children about the same weight in either position. And both front and rear seat positions can support Graco's SnugRide infant car seat. Both stroller seats have padded 5-point harnesses and have their own folding canopies. Both seats have front trays that swivel to the side. The adult's handlebar is padded and comes with a console and cupholder. Double wheels in the front swivel or lock into the forward-facing position. The frame has a one-hand fold mechanism and is self-standing in the folded position. Its extra-large storage basket offers easy access from the rear.

Maclaren's Twin Triumph

(S325)

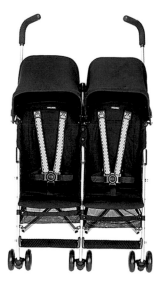

Weighing in at 21.6 pounds, this side-by-side works best with 2 children from 3 months of age up to 55 pounds each, for a total of 110 pounds. It offers two independent seats with their own canopies, multiple recline positions, and 5-point harnesses with three height-adjusting slots in the seat backs. The aluminum frame is one of the narrowest in its category (30 inches), making it slender enough to roll through most standard doorways. It has padded grip-style handles, but no parent cupholder or front trays for riders. There are 6 wheels with dual tires—all with spring suspension. In the rear are 2 small carry pouches and a small mesh storage bin. The frame has a convenient carry handle on one side. As with Maclaren's single strollers, this one folds with relative ease using push-down and push-up foot tabs, but watch out for the X joints on the rear frame that could capture small fingers during the folding process.

WHEELED CAR SEAT FRAMES

Rather than being a full stroller complete with a seat, these bare-bones stroller carriers are designed for only one purpose: to support most standard infant-only car seats. They use a variety of hardware configurations and/or straps to hold in the car seat, and once your baby outgrows the infant seat (usually between 8 and 12 months), the carrier will no longer be usable.

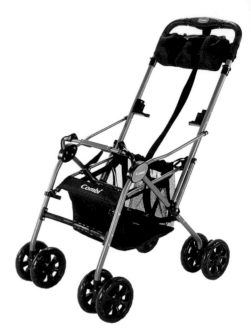

Combi's Flash EX Infant Car Seat Stroller Frame
($60)

Weighing in at only 10 pounds, the Combi Flash light-weight stroller frame is designed to hold most mainstream rear-facing infant-only car seats. It has dual front and rear wheels, with locking swivel wheels in the front. One-hand release makes folding and opening the frame a simple maneuver, and it locks in the folded position to self-stand and can be toted using an attached carry strap. The frame comes with a small elasticized storage bin underneath, and there's an attachable stroller pack with insulated bottle pockets.

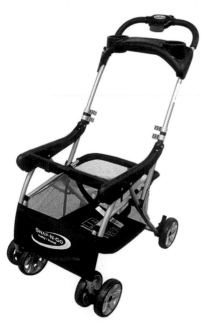

Baby Trend's Snap 'N Go Lite
($90)

Weighing 16 pounds, this easy-to-maneuver infant car seat frame comes with a generous and easy-to-reach storage bin. It has dual swiveling front wheels and folds compactly and easily using a single squeeze button on the stroller's handlebar. A longer (and heavier) Snap 'N Go Double model is available to carry 2 rear-facing infant-only seats.

Highs & lows of wheeled car seat frames

Highs. Lighter weight and less expensive than a stroller. Folds compactly, and some folded models are small enough to be carried onboard and stuffed in an over-head bin of an aircraft. Ample and easily accessed storage underneath most models. (Some larger double-seat frames are available.)

Lows. Requires an infant-only car seat and can't be used without it, which means it will be obsolete sometime late in the first year. May not offer the suspension of a full-size stroller or support all car seat models. The seat must be well latched into the frame or it could fall.

BICYCLE TRAILERS AND BICYCLE SEATS

If you enjoy bicycling, you probably wish you could bring your baby along. There are two inventions designed to do just that: bicycle trailers and bicycle seats.

Trailers are small two-wheeled zippered cabins covered in tent material, with vinyl or mesh windows on the side and single or double seats inside for babies and children. The units fasten to the rear axle of a bicycle with a long, rotating tubular arm. The cabin frame folds down for storage.

Bicycle seats allow babies to ride on the back of an adult's bicycle by providing a snap-on shell to support the child. The seat has straps to hold the child in.

Both inventions have their share of serious safety problems. There are reports of bicycle trailers turning over because of uneven pavement or of being struck in traffic. The cabins can get hot in warm weather and subject children to street-level carbon monoxide.

Bicycle seats have caused bicycles to fall over with the baby trapped in the seat, an accident that is most likely to happen when the bicycle is parked. Children have also sustained injuries when the seats have become dislodged from their bases or when a child's heels have been caught in the wire spokes of the bicycle's rotating rear wheel.

The hazards are severe and frequent enough that we feel we cannot recommend trailers and bicycle seats for use with babies and young children.

WARNING!
Bicycles and babies don't mix!

Think twice before purchasing or using a bicycle trailer or a bicycle-mounted seat. You may be putting your baby at serious risk of injury if the trailer or seat components fail or you crash or bump a vehicle with your children in tow. If you decide to purchase or use either of these products, make sure your child wears a properly-fitted helmet, and confine your rides only to off-road, even surfaces.

SAFETY CONSIDERATIONS

The U.S. Consumer Product Safety Commission estimates that over 12,000 babies and young children are hurt seriously enough each year to be rushed to emergency rooms as the result of stroller-related accidents.

Over 87 percent of the injuries happen when children fall from the stroller. Head injuries account for 22 percent of the injuries. Approximately 61 percent of the accidents happened in or near children's homes. Other injuries occur when strollers tip over, or when children outside the stroller fall into the stroller's hard, sharp parts.

In rare instances, children have had their fingers badly crushed by stroller components that have accidentally collapsed. Rarer still are cases where babies' strollers have been struck by vehicles when their parents pushed their strollers out in front of them into traffic.

Stroller recalls and certification

Strollers and other wheeled devices such as carriages, wheeled car seat frames, and bicycle seats and trailers are regulated by the U.S. Consumer Product Safety Commission (CPSC, www.cpsc.gov). Typically, one or two strollers are recalled every year when their components fail and cause children to be injured, although the injuries are seldom life threatening.

Manufacturers will usually issue a repair kit to correct the problem with a recalled stroller, although sometimes the entire stroller will be replaced with a new, safer model, or the manufacturer will offer to reimburse consumers for the value of the recalled unit.

For a comprehensive and up-to-date stroller recall list, go to www.recall.gov and search the CPSC link with either the product category "stroller" or by using specific search information based on the stroller's model name or other identifying information.

If it appears a stroller or other product has been recalled, it's important to note whether it falls into the specific model numbers or dates of manufacture for the recalled versions, since there may be stroller models with the same name that are perfectly safe and were not affected by the recall because they were manufactured at a different time or did not have the flaw. Note: Very dated recalled models may not be included in this list, even though used recalled strollers may still be in circulation.

Carriages and strollers are one of the product categories that are a part of the voluntary certification program overseen by the Juvenile Products Manufacturers Association (JPMA) and the American Society of Testing and Materials (ASTM). To have their products certified, manufacturers must submit them to a testing process to check for a variety of potential flaws and safety problems, and the strollers must also carry important safety warnings for parents.

Since the standard is voluntary, not all manufacturers participate in the certification process. Manufacturers whose products pass the testing process can place "JPMA Certified" seals on their products showing that they have passed rigorous safety and durability tests. Not all manufacturers choose to have their strollers certified, and even if a stroller is certified, there's no guarantee that it won't be recalled if a potential hazard turns up.

Stroller safety checklist

Here are some suggestions for mini-mizing stroller hazards.

✔ **Only use a stroller with a 5-point harness system.** A 5-point harness system, holding your child in not only by the waist and crotch but also by the shoulders, is safer than a 3-point system without the shoulder restraints. Keep straps adjusted snugly to prevent your child from standing up, slipping out from the seat, or leaning over and falling out.

✔ **Don't weigh down the handlebars.** Don't hook your purse or shopping bags over the stroller's handlebars. The stroller could tip backward, and injure your child.

✔ **Report near misses.** Report both potential accidents and real injuries, not only to the manufacturer but also to the Consumer Product Safety Commission's toll-free product-safety hotline, 800-638-CPSC(2772), or online (www.cpsc.gov).

✔ **Return malfunctioning strollers.** If your stroller folds accidentally, has sharp parts that could hurt your baby's fingers, has wheels that malfunction, or came with a broken safety harness, stop using the stroller immediately and return it to the store where you got it, for a replace-ment or refund.

✔ **Follow directions.** The directions that come with the stroller are important. They instruct you on the weight, age, and height limitations of the stroller and how to assemble it and adjust the harnesses.

They also tell you how to open, fold, and use it safely. And they should list every potential safety hazard and let you know how to contact the manufacturer if there's a problem. Store the instructions along with your sales receipt for the stroller in an easy-to-locate place.

✔ **Don't overload the stroller.** Use single-seat strollers with only one child and don't overload the storage bin or the stroller's seat by trying to carry heavy objects inside.

✔ **Use the brakes.** Engage the brakes whenever you park the stroller, to keep it from rolling away from you. (And never leave your child alone in a stroller.)

✔ **Exercise caution when moving into traffic.** Don't push a stroller out in front of you into traffic, especially from between parked cars. Always stand alongside your stroller at intersections and make sure turning and oncoming traffic can see you before you move into the street.

✔ **Mail in the registration card (or register online).** Strollers have faced numerous recalls. The manufacturer needs a way to contact you in case a dan-gerous flaw turns up.

✔ **Be careful in buying a used stroller.** If you purchase a used stroller, all com-ponents should be in good working order. Roll the stroller with a child inside to make sure it doesn't have veering prob-lems, and be sure to check that the stroller hasn't undergone a recall.

21

SWINGS & JUMPERS

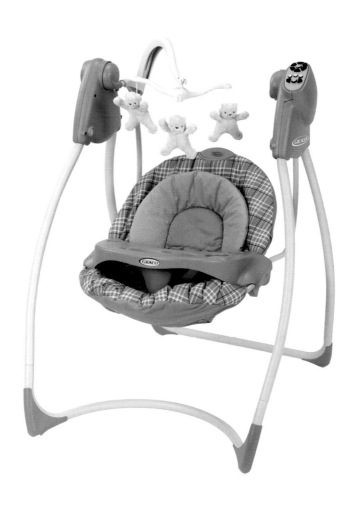

This chapter is all about suspended baby seats that offer your baby soothing rocking motions. You'll find our suggestions for buying an automatic indoor swing, an outdoor swing, or a jumper that suspends from a doorjamb. It has suggestions for making the best choice for your baby, along with detailed shopping hints and a discussion of important safety issues.

WINDUP AND ELECTRIC SWINGS

Getting into the swing of things

Ever since your baby was a small passenger inside you, he's been soothed by the to-and-fro motions of walking. In Grand-ma's day, a rocking chair supplied that sensation, but now there are automatic baby swings that with just the push of a button give your baby the back-and-forth motion that soothes him, but perhaps not the warmth and security of being held and cuddled.

Lots of parents call their automatic baby swings "supper savers." Babies tend to be their fussiest at adult dinnertime, and swings can be the saving grace that lets parents eat.

Swings come with a variety of frames. Older versions have tubular legs in an A shape on each side, joined by a crossbar across the top from which the baby's seat is suspended. A small motor on one side of the crossbar drives the back-and-forth rocking motion of the swing.

Newer "open top" models dispense with the A- frame and use a single arm underneath or behind the baby's seat to propel it. The absence of the top crossbar makes the seat easier to access for putting the baby in or taking him out of the swing's seat. Some open-top models allow the baby's seat to rotate so that the baby can move either back-and-forth or side-to-side, depending on which works best.

Choosing the right model

Mechanically, swings get their rocking motion using one of two drivers. Nearly obsolete windup swing motors have a handle on one side of the frame to tighten an internal spring with a ratchet that slowly loosens with each back-and-forth motion of the swing's seat. The swinging action continues for 10 to 15 minutes (or more) until the spring loses its tension and requires another winding.

Windup swings are the least expensive option, and some babies appear to respond to the hypnotic tick-tock sound the ratchet makes. Unfortunately, when it stops, babies usually wake up (sending parents racing to wind up the swing again).

Most swings today are battery- operated. A box on the side of the swing contains a small motor with nylon gears that drives the swinging action. Electric swings usually run on 4 to 6 C or D batteries that are good for several hundred hours of rocking before the swing starts to slow down. Motors vary in strength, and most simply lose power over time. It usually takes a minute or so for the swings' small motors to build up speed when getting started, but a few good pushes can rev up the motion.

Almost all swings offer several choices for rocking speed. However, most swings don't adapt to different baby weights very well. How fast or slow a swing moves depends on the weight of the baby, the length of the swing's supporting poles, and whether the windup is losing tension or the batteries or motor are wearing out.

Small, lightweight babies will be rocked faster and in a wider arc, while heavier babies will churn back and forth more slowly and with less oomph.

Electric models are quieter than windup versions, but all electric versions make a constant whirring sound. Separate light and music actions may require an additional set of smaller batteries that are fed into an overhead or tray compartment. A few electric models also come with power cords with adapters for plugging the swing into a nearby outlet, a major plus.

Seats usually have several reclining options. The instruction manual that comes with the swing will show you how to adjust the seat to accommodate your baby. Most seats use a 3-point harness that has belts for the waist and between the legs, although some upscale models now offer 5-point harnesses that fasten waist, crotch, and shoulder belts into a single buckle.

Seats usually have a bar or tray across the front of the seat and a post between the leg holes to help hold the baby in. Most seats come with a padded fabric seat cover that can be removed for washing. In some instances, the swings are unsafe without the pads. Thicker seat padding, trendy fabric, and added options often increase the price.

Some models are heavily cushioned and are more like semi-reclined well-padded baby bassinets designed for young babies before they're able to sit up on their own.

When to Buy

From 1 1/2 to 4 months of age to soothe a fussy baby or save dinnertime.

Others come with both a regular seat and a rectangular bassinet/baby bed that are interchangeable on the frame.

Keep it simple

Year by year, swing manufacturers add extra features to try to lure parents into buying them; and every year, prices rise on the heavily outfitted models. Some come with toys or light shows embedded in the tray in front of the baby or novelty mobiles with lights and toys that rotate above the baby's head. A virtual jukebox of sounds, offering up to 12 tunes, is built into some top-of-the-line models.

The extra embellishments not only cost more money (and eat up more batteries); but they also stimulate the baby, rather than soothing and lulling him to sleep. Some highly sensitive babies may be unnerved by all the action. And mastering the push buttons on the side of the swing to control the volume, swing time, tune choices, and swinging speeds can take some doing.

Our suggestion: Go with a simple battery-operated model that has adequate seat padding, a deep recline, and well-fitting seat belts—and forgo the rest. A little motion stimulation in a swing is probably good for your baby; but walking with him, talking to him, and rocking him in your arms are superior, more baby-sensitive ways to provide soothing.

Six shopping strategies for buying an automatic baby swing

For most parents, buying a swing is an act of desperation. With one out of five babies labeled "excessively fussy" these days, you may be at your wits' end and willing to pay *anything* to stop the fussing.

Before you shell out a lot of money for one of these automated soothing devices,

remember that your baby will probably be content to be in one for only about 3 months— 5 months max—and some babies can't stand them at all. Once your baby starts to sit up, he's likely to try grabbing the side poles, which could end in disaster.

Remember, too, that most standard-size swing frames eat up a huge amount of living-room real estate. If your family lives in a tiny apartment, you may want to explore alternative options for meeting your baby's motion needs, such as using a grown-up rocker or glider that lets you sit down, too, or an infant seat with a much smaller footprint that offers similar rocking and vibration motions for less space (and money). (Infant seats are discussed starting on page 78).

1. Shop around. Most large discount chains, such as Toys "Я" Us and Babies "Я" Us, offer a variety of swing models from which to choose. If you bring your baby with you, try out different seat configurations, belts, recline features, etc., and divide the swing's price by three to get a sense of how much it's going to cost per month for the luxury of owning one. Used swings are okay if they're in perfect working order, with no broken components.

2. Compare prices. Once you've settled on the brand and model you want, search around on eBay and other online e-tailers as well as at the big discount chains for the best bargains. **Note:** A price on the Internet may look really great until you factor in shipping and handling costs for such a large item. They usually don't show up until you've taken out your charge card and are seriously committed to placing the order.

3. Read the fine print. Know in advance

what the return policy is for the swing in case your baby hates the contraption. You don't want to get stuck with it 15 days later when you had to return it in 14 to get a refund.

4. Ask for help. A baby swing is more of a luxury than a dire necessity. If you've shot your baby budget, consider hinting broadly to your folks. Tell them how your neighbor's baby loves his, and you're sure your Bumpkins would really enjoy one, too, if you could only afford one.

5. Keep your receipt, and register. Most stores will refuse to accept a returned product without a receipt. And as with all baby products, the manufacturer needs to know how to contact you in case a dangerous flaw turns up and there's a recall, so mail the registration card (or register online, if that's an option).

6. Read the directions! They'll tell you how to use the product safely and how to contact the manufacturer if you have any questions.

Avoid:

✗ **Space hog.** A large footprint that will eat up too much space in your living room.

✗ **Sharp edges.** Especially around the leg holes, these could scrape or cut your baby.

✗ **Poor-quality parts.** Flimsy seat belt or buckle.

✗ **Improper leg holes.** Leg holes higher than the seating area that could cut off circulation.

✗ **Irritating noise.** A model that recycles tinny birthday-card tunes over and over will irritate you more than baby's crying. (Most swings offer volume controls and on-off switches for sounds.)

✗ **Frame hazards.** Frame legs or feet that could cause you or others to trip.

✗ **Instability.** A rattly, unstable frame that could tip over easily.

✗ **Electronic overkill.** Too many lights, motions, toys, and other unnecessary add-ons that increase the price but not the soothing.

✔ **Checklist**

Automatic swing shopping:

Here are suggestions for buying an automatic swing
A "JPMA Certified" sticker on the frame or carton means the design complies with rigorous safety and durability standards maintained by the Juvenile Products Manufacturers Association.

✔ **Seat belt.** Sturdy, easy-to-adjust seat belt for waist and crotch.

✔ **Comfort features.** A well-padded head and seat area.

✔ **Recline.** A seat back that reclines deeply.

✔ **Removable bar.** A removable front bar or tray makes it easier to seat and remove your baby. (Affixed toys are unnecessary.)

✔ **Crotch post.** To keep the baby from sliding under the bar or tray ("submarining") and deadly entrapment.

✔ **Stability.** The swing's frame is hard to tilt or pull over.

✔ **Folding.** Folds easily and compactly for storing.

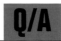

Q Since our baby was 3 weeks old, he seems to want to be held all the time to keep from crying. I'm wondering if a swing would cure his colic?

It might or might not, depending upon what's causing your baby's discomfort and how sensitive he is to outside stimulation. While some babies love the back-and-forth motion a swing provides, some highly sensitive babies are unnerved by it. We suggest trying out a friend's swing with your baby before making the plunge. If your baby is in pain for some reason, no amount of motion will work for very long.

Q A friend wants to give us a baby swing for a shower present, but I feel we need other things more — like a good car seat or a high chair. Should we accept her gift, or is there a graceful way to bow out and have her give us what I think our baby will need?

Here are three options: (1) Accept the swing, try it out with your baby, and if it works to free your hands and soothe your baby, be grateful. (2) Hopefully the gift giver will be thoughtful enough to put a receipt for the gift in the package so you're free to return it for a refund or an exchange. **(Note:** Some stores put a 14- to 30-day limit on returns, so you may be forced to return it before your baby gets a chance to try it out.) (3) Tactfully tell your friend that what you *really* need is a car seat (or other product) by name and model number, and hope she isn't offended by having her generous offer declined. Most likely, she'll understand.

"There's not that much difference between our jungle-themed swing in turquoise and green with flashing lights and monkey sounds (the "Rolls-Royce" of the baby swing world) and one we could have picked up at a yard sale. We just didn't figure that out until our baby was 6 months old and didn't need it anymore. **"**

Highs & lows of automatic baby swings

Highs. Most work like a charm when it comes to soothing babies in the early months.

Lows. Eat up a lot of space. Make whirring, tick-tocking, or tinny music sounds. Your baby may wake if you rewind the swing or it runs out of battery juice. Siblings often want to mess with the swing, and pets sometimes become aroused by them and attack them, injuring baby in the process. Motors are sometimes flimsy and weak, especially with used models, and gears wear out over time.

Quick tips

Slow down, baby! If you find the lowest swing speed is still too fast or too high for your baby, tuck a blanket behind him and let one corner hang out the back of the seat so the drag will slow it down.

Shop used swings, but with caution. You may be able to find a great deal on a used swing from friends whose baby has outgrown one, or by shopping garage sales or thrift stores. Inspect the swing carefully to make sure that the seat recline works well and that the tray, the seat belt, and other parts of the swing are intact and in working order. Be sure, too, to find out if there's been a recall for the model, and even if there hasn't, the U.S. Consumer Product Safety Commission will let you register your used swing online for notification if there's one later (www.cpsc.gov).

Plan to recoup your investment. Decide in advance that you're going to resell your baby's swing to another set of parents as soon as he tires of it. Try posting a notice at the grocery store or running an ad in your local paper. Then pack it up and move it out rather than carting it to the basement or attic to gather dust for years.

❝I suggest borrowing an automatic swing first to see if your baby takes to it. For us, it was just a big space waster.**❞**

❝Our low-end swing only had two speeds—fast and slow. We really used only one speed—fast.**❞**

❝My friends gave me their old baby swing, and it helped me keep my sanity during those first months! My son would nap in it and it would lull him to sleep on difficult nights (e.g., after I'd been rocking him for endless hours).**❞**

AUTOMATIC SWINGS

Graco's Luvin' Hug Swing
($80)

This trendy-looking swing has a curved open-top frame with removable, washable seat cover, and infant head support. The seat has a 5-point safety harness and the seat back offers 2 heights for the shoulder harnesses. It has a one-handed 4-position recline. There are 6 swinging speeds, and you have a choice of 15 classical music tunes or nature sounds. The front tray opens like a gate for putting baby inside and has a rigid post to prevent sliding out. The mobile has 3 soft toys on an arm that swings out of the way. The 10 minute timer has automatic shutoff. The smaller-than-usual frame folds compactly for storage. Requires 3 D batteries to run over 100 hours.

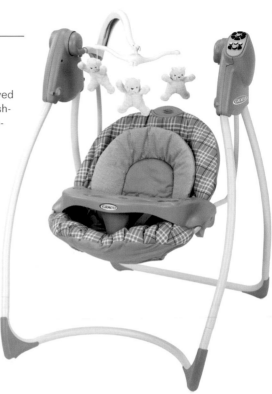

Fisher-Price's Baby Papasan Cradle-Swing
($100)

Parents have lots of praise for this swing, but it does constitute a rather hefty investment. It's loaded with comfortable padding, including an infant headrest, and the direction of the seat can be changed with the push of a button to provide either side-to-side or front-to-back rocking motion. The seat has a removable front toy bar/tray, and it reclines or sits up by repositioning the arm that holds the seat. An overhead mobile rotates and plays music, a feature that turns off after 7 minutes. Besides the fat price tag, the other major drawback is the 2 protruding feet that could present a tripping hazard for parents and other children.

Swing high! Swing low!

Outdoor baby swings are suspended plastic swinging seats for babies and tots who are still too young to hold onto the sides of regular swings. If you have a backyard tree with a sturdy horizontal limb or a deck with cross beams, you may want to consider installing one for your baby. Swinging is usually fun for babies and evokes a lot of great parent–baby interactions.

Most outdoor swings are quite simple and consist of a rigid molded seat shell with leg holes and a between-the-legs post in the front. A safety belt helps hold the baby inside. Weather-resistant ropes (usually plastic) or a combination of ropes and chains with S-hooks come with the swing to suspend it from a tree limb or crossbar.

It's up to you to decide how high or low you want the swing to be. Usually, putting the swing at your waist level is the most convenient option for lifting the baby in and out of the seat. Adult supervision is always required.

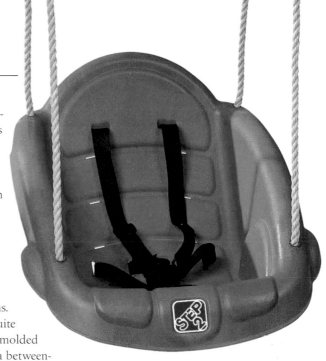

Step 2's Toddler Swing
($20)

For children aged 9 to 36 months, this swing uses weather-resistant rope and has molded handles in the front for easy pushing. The swing's 5-point harness, though a little difficult to latch and unlatch, securely holds the baby in place. Ventilation holes in the swing allow airflow around the child and drainage. Some assembly required. Available in several colors.

When to Buy

9 months and up to 40 pounds, depending upon the model. (Always follow the manufacturer's age and weight guidelines for your swing.)

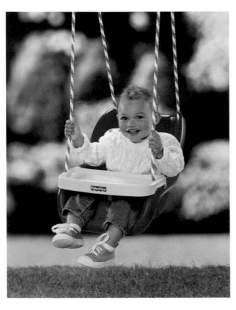

Fisher-Price
Infant to Toddler Swing
($20)

A high-backed molded swing for babies
6 to 36 months. It comes with a 3-point
restraint system (shoulders and crotch)
and a front tray that can be pulled up
the ropes for putting the baby inside.
The newest model can recline to give
better neck and head support to babies
as young as six months. The rimmed
tray acts as an armrest and can hold
toys or snacks when the seat is not in
motion.

Highs & lows of outdoor swings

Highs. Fresh air and sunshine (in moder-
ation) are good for babies, and they are
usually calmed by being outdoors. They
especially enjoy the rhythmic motion of
the swing and the playful interactions
with parents that swings evoke.

Lows. Swing surfaces get dirty, damp, and
may rot in the outdoor air. A tree limb
must be strong enough, even enough, and
low enough to support the swing. Some
swings may have sharp holes or edges that
could cut a baby's finger or limbs. The
baby is in danger of falling out if there's
no seat belt to hold him in place, or of
sliding under the tray if there is no
between-the-legs post. Other children
playing around the swing could be struck
by the swing while it's in motion.

Avoid:

✗ **Poor finishing.** Sharp edges and
unfinished seams or gaps that could capture a limb or head.

✗ **Flimsy ropes and fasteners.** Could
allow the swing to fall.

✗ **Flimsy belt.** Could allow your baby to
get captured in leg holes or tumble out.

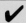 # Checklist

Outdoor swing shopping

If you have the outdoor space and a sturdy tree limb or structure with a wooden crossbar over soft ground or a cushiony surface, a baby swing may be a fun add-on, since babies are thrilled at the rhythmical motion and parent-baby play that swings evoke. Here's what to look for when shopping for a swing.

✔ **Comfortable seat.** The right dimensions for your baby.

✔ **Seat belts.** A necessity for holding your baby safely in place.

✔ **Rear head support.** To help prevent whiplash.

✔ **Between-the-legs post.** To keep the baby from sliding out.

✔ **Cleanable, weather-resistant materials.** To withstand rain and grime and be easily hosed down.

✔ **Smooth, sturdy ropes.** Durable, but smooth enough not to chafe the baby's hands or arms.

✔ **Strong fasteners.** Fastening hardware should be sturdy and all seams double-stitched to prevent fraying.

JUMPERS

Jumping into action!

Jumpers are designed for pre-walking babies who are strong enough to sit up unassisted. They're useful for only a small window of time: between when your baby confidently sits up on his own and before he takes his first steps. Once a baby can walk, a jumper will feel more like a trap than a plaything. But . . . during that golden moment of development, some babies seem quite delighted to be in a seat that lets them jiggle up and down on their own.

Jumpers fasten onto the top ledge of wooden doorframes using spring-action tong-shaped clamps. (If your doorways aren't framed in wood, you can't use one.) Springs or thick bands of rubber attach from the top clamp to straps attached to a baby-size seat.

The seat is positioned so that the baby's feet touch the floor, enabling him to bounce the seat each time he bends and straightens his legs. Not all babies enjoy being in bouncers, and some get dizzy from all the swinging and swaying. And almost all babies hit the side of the doorway with their heads or get their hands hurt between the seat and the doorjamb at least once.

When to Buy

8 months to 24 pounds (or walking, whichever comes first). (Always follow the manufacturer's age and weight guidelines for the jumper.)

Five shopping strategies for jumpers

Because they are not used for very long, jumpers are rarely available in baby shops or big discount stores; but you may be able to find one online, and some manufacturers sell them directly to the public from their Internet sites. (See the *Resource Guide* starting on page 338 for a long list of Internet e-tailers.) Before you buy, here are some precautions you need to take.

1. Check your baby's skills. Your baby shouldn't use a jumper unless he's a strong sitter and can do so without using props or his hands to hold himself upright. We suggest 8 months or older.

2. Shop around. Once you decide on the jumper model you want, conduct an Internet search to find the e-tailer with the best price, the lowest shipping costs, and the most reasonable return policies, to make sure you can return the jumper if it doesn't fit your door jamb or your baby doesn't like using it.

3. Put everything in print. Print a copy of the Internet page advertising the product, as well as your order form, in case the product doesn't arrive or you decide to return it. Write down when the product arrives, too.

4. Read the instructions carefully. Manufacturers offer parents critical safety information in their instruction brochure, so make sure to read it completely before your baby uses the jumper.

5. Don't keep it if it doesn't fit. It's unsafe to use a jumper that doesn't fit your baby or that allows him to fall to the side. It's also dangerous to try to rig up a jumper on something other than a preinstalled doorjamb. Just return the product instead.

E & I's Bungee Baby Bouncer
($30)

The unique bellyband on this jumper adjusts to baby's size and closes with both strong Velcro and a buckle, and since there's no wiggle room, as with traditional bouncer seats, baby is protected from veering sideways or falling forward. The crotch fastens onto the belt with double snaps. Babies' arms fit between double straps on each side that connect to a wooden crossbar. A sturdy rubber cord fastens to the doorframe clamp.

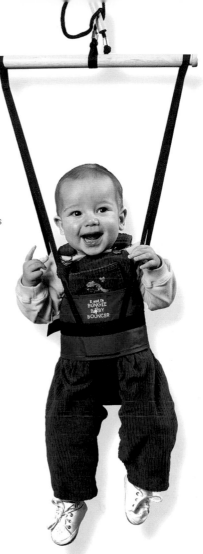

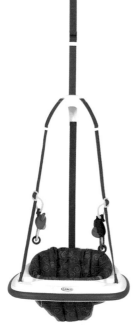

Graco Doorway Bumper Jumper
($35)

For babies weighing less than 25 pounds and able to sit upright unassisted, this jumper's seat frame has cushioned bumpers on all sides to protect the doorway (and baby's fingers). The three-strap configuration helps keep the seat stable. The spring-action, no-mar clamp adjusts to various doorframe sizes and can be tightened and locked once it is in place. The unit comes with 2 soft removable toys that attach using rings. **Note:** It has no seat belt, although the depth of the seat should help to keep baby inside.

Checklist

Jumper shopping

If you've decided to give a jumper a try with your springy child, here are our suggestions about what to look for when you shop for one.

✔ **Sturdy clamp.** The clamp should be metal rather than plastic and have a strong spring that won't allow the clamp's tongs to release accidentally or to slip off the wooden door frame. The tongs should have nonslip tips to keep them in place.

✔ **Strong spring or rubber band.** The spring or rubber band for bouncing should be sturdy and fastened well to the clamp and the seat's straps.

✔ **Thick, sturdy straps.** Straps should be made of tightly woven, heavy material with double or triple stitching where they fasten to other components.

✔ **Nonslip strap adjusters.** Buckles that allow the straps to be adjusted should hold without slipping.

✔ **Comfort features.** A seat that's well padded, especially around the leg holes, to protect the baby's legs from pressure or chafing.

Highs & lows of jumpers

Highs. Some babies are excited about being able to make their seats jiggle.
Lows. Useful for only a limited amount of time. Won't work on all doorways. Components sometimes break or fail. Serious safety problems, including knocking into the doorway, require constant supervision.

Avoid:

✗ **Poor construction.** Flimsy clamp, springs, or rubber bands.

✗ **Wrong size seat.** Seat too large, giving baby's body leeway to fall sideways or forward.

✗ **Poor finishing.** Poorly sewn attachments for springs and straps.

SAFETY CONSIDERATIONS

Every year, automatic baby swings and jumpers are involved in about 1,600 injuries serious enough for emergency-room treatment. The injuries usually happen when babies fall out of the swing or jumper and crack their heads on the floor.

Babies may fall out of automatic baby swings when they aren't belted in properly, especially when the swinging front tray is left open or when a component, such as a frame leg, support, or seat breaks.

Jumper injuries happen when components fail and babies crash into the sides of the door jamb or fall to the floor, or when parents place the wrong age or weight baby in the device. When used with babies whose bodies aren't sufficiently mature, a serious and even deadly form of whiplash is possible from being jarred too vigorously in the jumper. Sometimes jumpers' clamps or springs work loose or break, or the seat may be so shallow or have such large leg holes that a baby can fall out. (Never try to jerry-rig a jumper on a door jamb without a frame.)

Automatic swings and jumpers are especially dangerous when other children attempt to put the baby inside or take him out. Or they push the swing or jumper, stressing components to the breaking point or causing automatic swing frames to tilt and fall over.

In some cases, older babies have been too active or large for swings and jumpers, causing them to break. An older baby can grab a swing's sidebars and manage to pull himself out. More rarely, babies' legs have turned blue when seat rims for swings and jumpers have cut off circulation, or their arms have been bruised when they've struck swing components going in or out.

Outdoor-swing accidents happen when the swing tips over in front or the seat belts break, causing the baby to fall and sometimes resulting in serious head injuries. The most serious accidents happen when the baby falls onto hard surfaces such as hardened soil, wood, brick, or asphalt.

Sometimes babies suffer from serious and potentially fatal whiplash because they are too young to be using an outdoor swing, or children play roughly with them. The product is designed only for babies who can sit unassisted—6 to 8 months of age—and who don't exceed the manufacturer's recommended maximum weight. And sometimes other children are injured when they roam into the pathway of the swing and are struck by it. Outdoor swing components sometimes break, and swing ropes deteriorate with weather and age, causing them to fray or to become splintery, which can hurt a baby's hands.

All swings for babies should have waist belts to help hold the baby in. Swings have sometimes been recalled by the Consumer Product Safety Commission (CPSC) when components fail, posing the risk of injury to babies.

Product recalls and certification

Recalls have happened for automatic swings, outdoor swings, and jumpers. So before you purchase any used products in these categories, be sure to look up the product's recall history, and contact the company to make sure that the product has been changed following the recall to ensure that hazards have been repaired and newer versions are safe. Recalls can be searched by going to www.recalls.gov and entering the product category or specific model name in the site for the Consumer Product Safety Commission (www.cpsc.gov).

Automatic swings come under the Juvenile Products Manufacturers Association (JPMA) voluntary certification program that has been developed in cooperation with the American Society of Testing and Materials (ASTM). Jumpers and outdoor baby swings, however, are not part of the certification program at the time of this writing.

A "JPMA Certified" sticker displayed on the product or the box indicates that the swing's manufacturer has had representative models in the line tested and that they comply with certification requirements. It does *not* mean that the specific product your baby is using has been individually tested for flaws or that the product is fail-safe. A variety of certified products have undergone recalls when they were shown to have major baby-harming flaws or components that failed.

Safe use tips

Here are some tips to make sure your baby is safe when using an automatic baby swing, a jumper, or an outdoor swing.

✔ **Follow instructions.** Be sure to follow the manufacturer's instructions to the letter, especially in assembling and installing the product correctly and closely following guidelines for your baby's age and weight. Discontinue use as your baby nears the upper weight limits for the device.

✔ **Don't start too early.** Jumpers and outdoor swings shouldn't be used unless your baby is able to sit unassisted and without using his hands for at least 5 minutes or more.

✔ **Take protective measures.** Place a soft rug or cushioning under these products to protect against the potential for falls, and always use safety belts if they are supplied with the product, rather than relying on the product's front tray or shield to hold your baby inside.

✔ **Never leave your baby's side.** Keep within arm's reach of your baby at all times, and keep children and pets at a safe distance. Always stand directly in front of or behind the jumper when your baby is seated inside, to ensure that his movements don't cause him to strike his head or smash his fingers on the edge of the doorway. Don't attempt to use a jumper like a swing or let children play with the baby while he's seated in it, since either of these things could detach the jumper from the doorway, causing the baby to fall.

✔ **Don't attempt to repair a broken product.** Frequently inspect the components of these products to be sure they are in working order. Immediately discontinue using any product that is broken and contact the manufacturer, rather than trying to repair it yourself. If there's the potential for baby injury, report the product failure to the Consumer Product Safety Commission as well as to the manufacturer (and consider holding on to the malfunctioning product—or photos of the problem—as evidence).

✔ **Don't overdo.** Your baby's neck and back can stand only so much upright sitting before tiring. And some babies get a form of motion sickness from springing around too much in jumpers. Except for automatic swings with reclining seats, limit the use of upright seats to under 15 minutes at a time (or less if he loses interest or complains).

✔ **Be careful with batteries.** If you use a battery-operated automatic swing, frequently check the batteries. Sometimes they can leak fluid that can cause chemical injuries. Battery leaks inside the battery compartment can also cause damage. Remove the batteries if you plan to store the swing for any length of time. Don't mix old and new batteries or different types of batteries (alkaline, standard, or rechargeable). Don't try to recharge regular batteries that aren't designed for that purpose, and don't dispose of used batteries in a fire—they could explode or leak acid.

22

TOYS

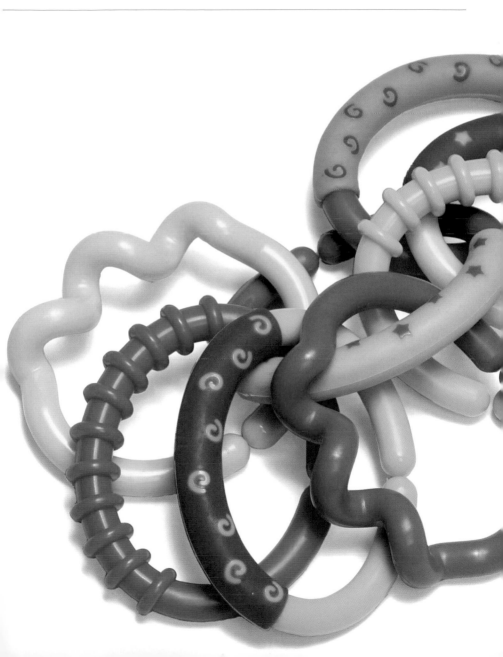

Parents are the best playthings for babies! But toys can introduce your baby to colors, textures, and special experiences. The best toys for your baby are safe, sturdy, and fit your baby's size and stage of development. This chapter will help you shop wisely for baby's playthings. You'll find a variety of toy examples and important toy safety tips.

EVERY DAY IS PLAY DAY!

Do babies really need piles of toys?

Probably not, but most parents are convinced even before their babies arrive that toys are indispensable. The truth is your baby will develop into a perfectly healthy and smart child even if you never bring a single store-bought toy into your home.

It's the play part that's important for a baby, and toys are simply tools to encourage that. They can't make your baby any happier or smarter, and, as you're likely to discover, a baby's favorite pastime doesn't involve a toy at all. Young babies who are just starting to pull up their heads would rather look at their mom's face than a doll or mobile. Babies working on their grasping and banging skills are as happy, if not happier, with a spoon and a kitchen pot than a solid-gold rattle.

People are babies' favorite playthings. Playing with your baby means talking to her, snuggling her, walking her around the house, or strolling her around the neighborhood. That's the kind of entertainment babies really love and thrive on.

If nothing else, showering your baby with piles of oddly shaped, cute—or sometimes useless and annoying—plastic and wood objects, some of which repeat the same tinny sounds over and over, can certainly be educational for you. It teaches you organizational skills, how to remove batteries, and how to keep focus in the face of annoying distractions.

The giant toy industry

Grown-ups love giving babies toys. The Toy Industry Association estimates that infant toys are a $3.2 billion market. Fewer than five retail chains account for 60 percent of toy sales. Small mom-and-pop toy stores, and a few mini–retail chains that typically charge more for toys, account for the remaining 40 percent of sales. Big-box stores like Wal-Mart are the largest sellers of toys, while Toys "Я" Us, is the toy industry's largest dedicated retail toy outlet.

Mozart or Mom?

Beware of toys, CDs, or television programming that promise to boost your baby's IQ, to enrich your baby's brain, make her smarter or "educate" her. A 1993 study sparked a sensation by claiming to document the so-called Mozart effect that suggested that children exposed to music at young ages developed higher IQs than those who were not; and soon after, toys playing classical music were bought in droves by success-driven parents.

A series of more recent and well-documented research studies have debunked the Mozart-effect myth. In fact, so-called "baby stim" toys may have exactly the opposite effect on baby's intellectual growth than that hoped for by eager parents. That's because sitting a baby in front

of a product deprives babies of much-needed parent–baby experiences.

Parents' sensitive responses to baby signals—holding, carrying, and talking with their babies—are the bedrock of baby learning. It's stimulation through these multiple sensory channels that provides a wide array of sights, sounds, textures, tastes, sensations, and aromas all at once that are ideal for fostering baby learning.

Local parent–baby play opportunities

Taking a parent baby class is a great way to get out and get moving with your baby. You both gain stimulation, socialization, and stretches. Just as fitness clubs for grownups have spread across North America, special classes and clubs for parents and babies are springing up everywhere.

Parents in large metropolitan areas may be able to choose from a broad range of mom-and-me activity programs and classes, including Gymboree, stroller exercise groups, playgroups, swimming classes, parent-and-baby postnatal yoga groups, gymnastics, and even disco groups for tots and moms. Libraries and large bookstore chains such as Barnes & Noble often offer story hours for different age groups. Some forward-thinking hospitals, YMCAs, YWCAs, and university child-development centers also offer ongoing mother–baby support and activity groups.

Note: The tuition for commercial classes may be expensive, especially if special gear is required. Class quality depends greatly on the teacher's skill and experience. And you may find that the class you want may not be scheduled at a time that's good for you and your baby. (Or it may work with your baby one

---

Quick tip

Don't let your baby play with used toys unless you know they're in perfect condition, the right age range for your baby's safe use (look the toy up on the Internet), and they haven't been in a recall (www.recalls.gov).

week but not the next.) Ask about having a free visit or two before you commit to a long-term contract.

Most major cities have free parenting newspapers listing local activities for babies and children, and local Internet sites are accessible for most major cities. Look for the newspapers at the entrance to your local library, and search parents' resources online using the keywords "directory," "parents," and the name of your city. (A reference librarian can help you.)

Protecting your child from lead

Lead ingestion is associated with children's behavioral problems, learning disabilities, hearing problems, and growth retardation. It is estimated that in the U.S. approximately 930,000 children between the ages of 1 and 5 have seriously elevated blood lead levels.

Babies are exposed to lead when they gnaw on lead-containing metal products, such as brass keys and key rings; when they chew on toys containing lead; or when they're exposed to lead dust in soil, and dust or paint chips laced with lead that are found in old houses and antique furniture.

If you are concerned that your baby has been exposed to lead, then a simple blood test from your doctor may help to determine if there are elevated lead levels in her blood. Should lead show up in your baby's body, it will be important to find and eliminate the source of your baby's exposure.

In addition, your physician may also suggest increasing the iron and calcium in your child's diet (which can be depleted by lead), frequent mopping of your house with a damp mop to minimize lead dust, frequent hand washing, and discouraging your baby from chewing on and ingesting nonfood substances such as toys and objects that

 # Checklist

Toy shopping

Here's what to look for when you're buying toys for your baby.

✔ **Age appropriate.** Follow the manufacturer's age guidelines to the letter. They're veiled safety warnings, not developmental guidelines.

✔ **Intriguing to the baby.** Babies love a variety of textures and colors, and they're intrigued by faces in a mirror, including their own.

✔ **Baby activated.** The best toys require the baby to do something. Look for toys for banging, touching, tasting, stacking, and rolling.

✔ **The baby dimension.** Hand toys should be small enough to be grasped by tiny hands, but not so small that they can be swallowed and choked on. (See baby choking discussion on page 241.)

✔ **A part of life.** Sometimes everyday objects hold more appeal for babies than fancy, costly toys. Consider enriching your baby's play life with metal pots and lids, thick-handled wooden spoons, puppets and stuffed dolls made from socks, and picture albums with plastic pages that display photos of relatives and cutouts of animals.

could contain lead. Ongoing monitoring and medication may also be required if seriously high lead levels are found.

Plastics, chemicals, and baby toys

There is continuing concern, especially among consumer and environmental groups, that some chemicals used in manufacturing plastic baby toys and baby bottles could potentially be toxic to babies. Particularly in the spotlight are soft plastic toys that babies like to chew on, such as teethers, molded squeeze toys, and waterproof baby books that could release chemicals when they interact with babies' saliva.

The concern is that phthalates (pronounced "thall-eights") could potentially interfere with body hormones that regulate maleness and femaleness in fetuses and infants, and it is possible that they might affect the liver, kidneys, lungs, and developing testes if they are ingested in high enough levels.

In the vast majority of cases, human exposure to phthalates falls very far short of the experimental doses shown to cause harm to animals. The chemical industry and toy manufacturers strongly dispute that there is scientific basis for concern; but in the meantime, the city of San Francisco and the European Union have banned phthalates in children's toys, and half a dozen state legislatures are considering similar measures.

Our suggestion is to avoid off-brand imports and stick with baby toys from mainstream manufacturers who are likely to frequently test their products for safety.

Avoid:

✗ **Baby too young.** A "too-old" toy may go unused and get underfoot; but more important, it may pose a safety hazard. Buy and use toys only in the manufac-turer's recommended age range.

✗ **Don't open packages in the car.** It's not a good idea to let your tot tear into a toy package as soon as you get in the car. Today's toys are packed securely enough to sustain a drop from a skyscraper. Wait until you get home, where you can open the package properly. Then carefully inspect the toy to ensure it's safe, with no small parts or ones that could come loose, before handing it over to your baby.

✗ **Steer clear of DVDs or video games, even if they claim to be educational for babies.** In 1999, the American Academy of Pediatrics recommended no "screen time" at all for babies under the age of two, because the more time a baby watches a screen, the less time he or she is engaged in the human interaction that is so crucially important to brain growth and development. Your money would be better spent hiring a neighborhood 8-year-old to come over and make goofy faces.

TYPES OF BABY TOYS

So you want to buy your baby some toys. What to get?

As you shop for your baby, always remember that you are your baby's favorite toy. While toys may not prepare your baby for Harvard, they do teach a baby about the object world—about shape, color, texture, cause and effect (open a door and see what's inside; push something and it will roll). They can also help your baby practice focusing her eyes on moving objects and enhance her reaching and grasping skills.

So what kinds of toys do babies like? It actually depends on the baby's personality, and gender. Female babies tend to prefer toys that have a lot of color and texture, while males' brains are hardwired to prefer things that move. But every baby's different—one baby's favorite toy can be another baby's big yawn.

Following is a roundup of some popular toys that have been recommended by parents.

Mobiles

The point of a mobile, in theory, is to give baby something to look at and listen to as she wakes up or as she tries to fall asleep. Mobiles usually fasten onto the crib's side bar with a clamp and have a long arm that reaches out into the center of the crib, where small stuffed toys or painted images slowly rotate to the sound of music above the baby's head.

Simple mobiles use windup music boxes with a small rotator bar to provide both the sounds and the motions. The most sophisticated versions are battery operated or electric and present a huge array of noises, motions, and graphics, and may even offer a remote control option so you can start it going without baby even knowing you're there. Some are compatible with MP3 players, letting parents program the soundtrack. But that's overkill, especially since babies usually want to be picked up and held by their parents, not left alone, even with the most intriguing light and sound show. Mobiles even frighten some babies!

Mobiles should be used only during the first five months of a baby's life and removed as soon as she begins to roll over or tries to get on all fours. Then they should be removed from the crib and put away, since the toys and strings that are attached to mobiles can entangle the baby. (See safety considerations, starting on page 336.)

Rattles and noisemakers

These days, rattles come inside plush toys, in the form of plastic or wooden rings, or as components that snap onto activity centers, floor gyms, and car seats. You can shake and move a rattle about 6

Inexpensive baby playthings

Playthings don't have to be expensive or come from toy stores to be fun for your baby. Here are some readily available playthings for parent–baby fun.

INSTEAD OF	TRY
Crawl-through tunnels	Cardboard boxes with both sides open.
Rattles and drums sealed	Wooden spoons and pots and pans, or plastic containers with dried beans inside (make sure the seal is tight).
Hand puppets	Cotton socks with faces drawn on the toes.
Baby DVDs and TV shows	Bribing neighborhood children to play brief baby games.
Shape sorters	A shoebox with a hole in the lid.
Activity centers	Nursery rhymes, finger games, and Itsy Bitsy Spider.
Water play	A turkey baster, plastic cups, and containers in a baby bathtub.
Telephone talk	An old telephone with the wires removed.

to 8 inches from your baby's face to let her eyes follow it, and a rattle can also be used during tummy time to encourage your baby to reach for it. Later on, rattles and noisemakers may be fun on stationary activity centers or for stroller bars.

Teethers

Teethers, the human version of puppy chew toys, are designed to be held and gnawed on as baby begins to cut teeth, usually between 3 and 8 months. They generally look like small gel-filled necklaces or cushioned bracelets or beads, and some can be chilled to help soothe swollen gums. Shop for mainstream brands from known and trusted toy manufacturers that don't use phthalates in plastic toys, and avoid inexpensive imports or teethers that appear flimsy. Some gel-containing teethers have been recalled when they broke, exposing babies to toxic liquid. Don't freeze the teether—the cold can burn a baby's gums. (A cold washcloth—used with your constant supervision—works just as well.)

Soft and fabric toys

Every animal on the planet from aardvarks to zebras has been sculpted, stuffed, and covered with fluff. Most stuffed animals in the world are manufactured in China on behalf of American companies. Because "plushies" seem to get cuter all the time, you can expect to buy, inherit, and receive piles of them as gifts before your baby enters kindergarten.

Stuffed or puffy animals (and quilts) should be kept out of your baby's crib because they pose a suffocation hazard, and toddlers will use them as props for climbing out. Instead, use your baby's animal menagerie as part of your nursery decor. Sit them on a colorful shelf far away from baby's reach, or suspend them in a mesh hammock, also well out of reach.

As your child grows, she'll probably pick a few choice critters to favor as "lovies," ignoring the rest. It's a good idea to limit the number of stuffed animals you keep out for general use, storing the others out of sight (or donating them to charity).

Soft fabric toys are another genre of soft toys that are excellent for baby play. They're the worms, flower faces, and baby-sized fabric balls that offer a variety of textures, colors, and crinkling sounds to intrigue small explorers. The best versions, such as those made by Kids ii, offer bright colors, whimsical patterns, and a variety of unexpected sounds or textures.

Electronic toys

Battery-operated toys talk, roll, light up, giggle, dance, make music, sing the alphabet, do the hokey-pokey, or mimic computers or telephones or cell phones. While a baby may be momentarily intrigued by one or even giggle at it, some babies may find them startling or overstimulating. Older toddlers may like playing the same sounds and lights over and over, to the consternation of their parents. (See our battery warnings on page 337.)

Play gyms

For babies lying on their backs, arches hold suspended toys, mirrors, and other playthings that babies can bat with their hands and feet. Most gyms fold compactly and some offer foot-activated noises.

WARNING

Magnets can be fatal

Magnets found by young children stuck on refrigerators or buried in the back of alphabet letters or inside toys can be swallowed or aspirated by babies and young children. If more than one magnet is swallowed, the magnets can attract each other and cause intestinal perforation or blockage, both of which can be fatal. Keep all magnet-containing products away from your baby!

Our favorite tot-toy choices

Here's a list of perfect toys for little "movers and shakers."

Push toys. Miniature shopping carts, popcorn poppers, toy vacuum cleaners and lawnmowers, and stable ride-on trucks for walkers.

Hand toys. Toys with bumps, textures, and animal sounds just the right size for toddler hands.

Soft balls. Soft, fat balls that fit perfectly between a tot's arms for rolling or tossing.

Big Shape sorters. Soft stackers with fat doughnut shapes to put on and off. Simple shape-sorter boxes to drop blocks into. Wooden pounding toys for tots.

Nontoxic crayons. Chunky toddler-size sticks for drawing on paper, but watch out for scribbling on tables, walls, and books.

Soft puppets. Bright puppets with exaggerated features to "talk" to baby. (Be sure eyes are well fastened on and fur won't come off when mouthed.)

Bathtub toys. Toys that float or pour, and a suctioned net to store them in.

BABY TOY IDEAS BY AGE

✱ Birth to 8 weeks

Babies exploring sight and sound
Toys for this age provide visual and auditory stimulation through colors, shapes, lights, voices, and music.

Fisher-Price's Miracles & Milestones Track & Play Center
($32, birth and up)

A crib toy with a bold, smiling face that slides across the top, lights that blink, music, and a gentle female voice that says, "Hello, Baby," that's activated when the baby spins a black and white checkered roller. Can be used later as a lap toy with shapes of different textures to touch, a ladybug clacker, a purple squeaker, and a mirrored spinner. On/off, volume control, and three modes of play. Requires 3 C batteries (included).

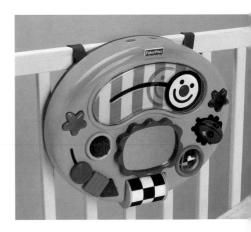

Manhattan Toy's Baby Whoozit
($10, birth and up)

A 6-inch circle-shaped 2-sided soft toy with simple black and white graphic designs on one side and a friendly face that squeaks, rattles, and crinkles on the other. Made of satin, velour, terry, felt, and fuzzy fake fur, so there are plenty of textures for a baby to touch. Attaches with a Velcro loop to crib, stroller, diaper bag, or other toys.

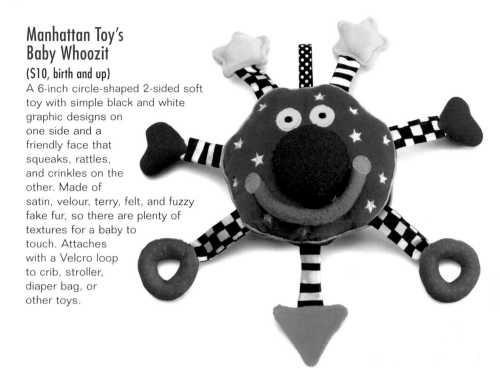

Taggies' Little Taggie
($25, birth and up)

An interactive "lovie" (that's mom slang for a carry-around cuddle toy) based on the observation by two moms that babies and kids love to rub satin edges, clothing labels, and tags. The 12-inch x 12-inch fleece blanket has 20 tags of unique patterns and textures along its edges for babies to examine, mouth, and touch. Tags can be used to attach the blanket to a stroller, car seat, diaper bag, or other toys.

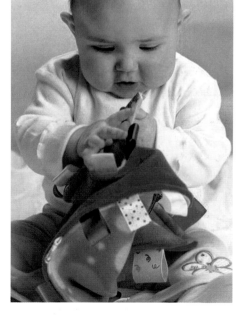

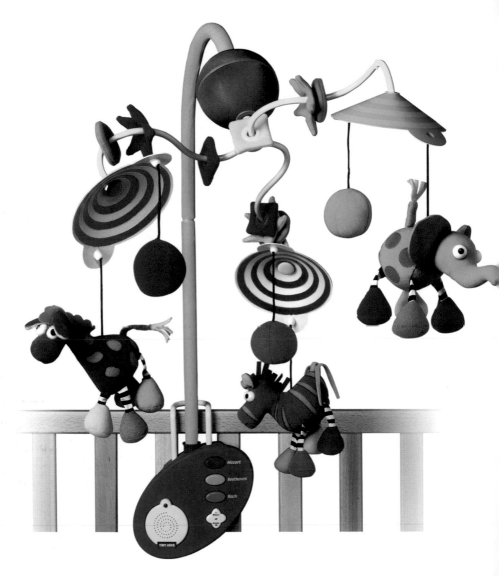

Tiny Love's Symphony-In-Motion Deluxe Mobile with Remote

($40, birth to 5 months)

Bright high-contrast circles and stars, and a horse, an elephant, and a giraffe dangle from three wobbly, curving arms that spin and rotate in a constantly changing pattern. Mobile plays classical music of varying tempos, including Mozart, Beethoven, and Bach, and can be activated from across the room by a remote control. Runs on 3 AA and 3 AAA batteries (not included). Assembly required.

Learning Curve's Lamaze My First Mirror

($20, birth and up)

Child-safe baby mirror in a red soft frame attaches with Velcro loops to a foam wedge that is covered with different textured and colored cloth for baby to explore, including lime green, purple, orange, and black-and-white zebra-striped fabrics. Mirror slips out of frame for cleaning; wedge and frame are also washable.

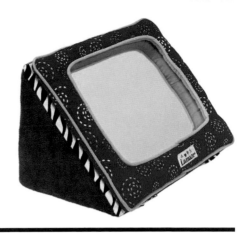

✱ 8 weeks to 6 months

Babies learning about their arms, legs, and mouths

Toys for this category include dangling objects for baby to bat at, toys that encourage eye–hand coordination, and ones that encourage head-raising, controlled movements, and rolling.

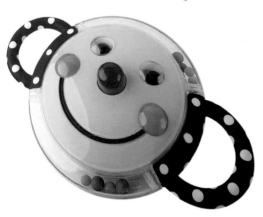

Tiny Love's Gymini

($60, 0–10 months)

The Gymini is a 3-dimensional activity gym for baby to use while lying on her back. The borders of the play mat can be closed to provide a baby more security, or opened to allow more space. The adjustable Kick & Touch response pad makes music with baby's contact. The padded, hanging arches hold 5 removable, hanging toys and a large mirror to encourage baby to lift up her head and see their reflection. Can be folded for storage. Requires 3 AA batteries (not included).

Sassy's Smiley Face Rattle

($7, birth and up)

Two handles for ears, a red nose that beeps, eyes, and beads that rattle—a great invitation for exploration! The mirror on the back also invites the "where's baby?" game.

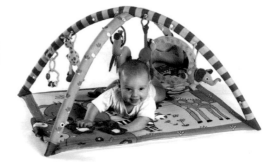

Small World Toys' IQ Baby Knock Knock Blocks
($26, birth to 36 months)
Eight soft-sided building blocks and eight foam triangle wedges for baby to stack and build. Blocks are made of multiple fabrics and come with peekaboo windows and doors that jingle, crinkle, and rattle. Wedges are covered in bold black-and-white graphics.

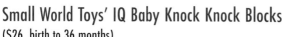

Manhattan Toy's Skwish Classic
($15, birth to 12 months)
Colored wooden beads move and slide on bright rods, making pleasant sounds. Easy for babies to grab and squish, black nylon cords return the rattle-type toy to its original shape time after time.

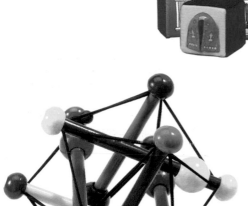

Infantino's Ring-a-Links
($4, birth and up)
Teethable textured links that attach to a car seat, diaper bag, stroller, baby's other favorite toys, or to each other. Set of eight includes two yellow and orange links with spiral tops, two green and blue ribbed links, two purple and blue links with raised stars, and two with orange and yellow gummable swirls.

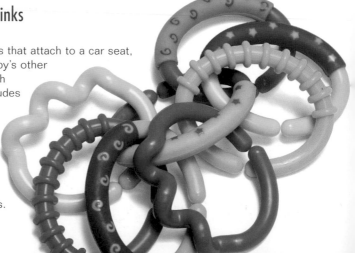

Learning Curve's The First Years Massaging Action Teether

($8, 6 months and up)
A big blue ring handle with a green and purple textured spinner connects to a yellow star with lines, bumps, and ridges that gently vibrate when baby bites down on them. PVC-free and includes a lifelong, nonreplaceable battery.

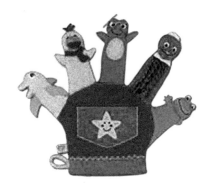

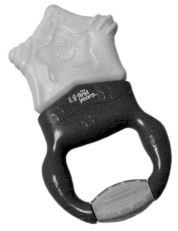

Baby Einstein's Discover & Play Washglove

($9, birth and up)
A finger puppet bath glove in a foam-filled cotton-and-polyester-blend fabric, with a different Baby Einstein character on each finger—a dolphin, a duck, a turtle, an octopus, and a frog. There is a star pocket on one side, a baby-safe mirror on the other, and a loop for hanging it up to dry.

✳ 5 to 9 months

Babies developing core body strength and coordination

This category includes cause-and-effect toys, toys that encourage using both hands together, toys that promote the emergence of language, and toys that reinforce object permanence.

Little Touch's LeapPad

($30, 6 to 36 months)
A read-aloud learning system with three skill levels for exploring shapes, animals, colors, and first words. Level one exposes the baby to music and sounds, level two introduces word play and early language, and level three adds rhyming and other preschool readiness skills. Includes *One Bear in the Bedroom* and a parent guide. Additional books and cartridges can be purchased separately.

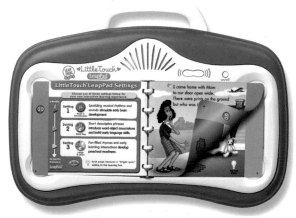

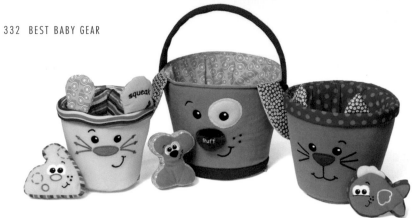

Infantino's Bucket Buddies

($16, 6 months and up)

Three soft-sided character buckets that crinkle, squish, and rattle, with three corresponding toys for put-and-take play, peekaboo play, nesting, and stacking. Includes a blue doggie bucket with a blue bone, an orange cat bucket with an orange fish, and a yellow mouse bucket with a yellow piece of cheese.

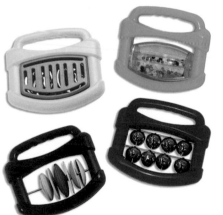

Edushape's Mini Orchestra

($22, 6 months and up)

Four sturdy baby-size hand instruments that introduce a variety of sounds, including rainbow-colored beads that spin in a clear plastic drum, eight jingle bells, yellow and green plastic dishes that clip-clap, and a tambourine-like rattle that produces a ringing sound.

Sassy's Who Loves Baby? Photo Book

($7, 6 months and up)

A washable plastic book that holds up to six interchangeable photographs, such as baby month by month, photographs of a baby's family, the baby in different moods, or pictures of colors or first words.

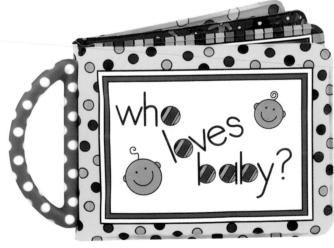

✱ 6 to 10 months

For crawling babies
Toys that encourage babies to practice grasping skills, crawling, pulling to stand, and cruising.

Sassy's Fascination Station
($8, 6 months and up)

This 6-inch Ferris wheel spins, rattles, and has a small mirror. It also attaches to a high chair or stroller tray when it's placed in its suction-cup base. Multiple patterns include stripes, polka dots, and a grinning smiley face.

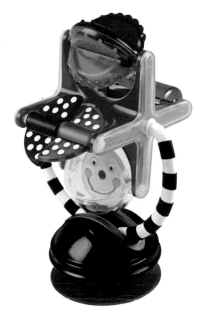

Little Tikes' Wide Tracker Activity Walker
($20, 6 to 36 months)

An activity center with a circular red-and-yellow spinner, a caterpillar clacker, and a clicking bee, this later converts into a push toy with an easy-to-grasp handle, a wide, stable base, and parent-controlled speed adjustment. Doors on the front hold stackable blue, yellow, and red plastic letters, which the baby can deliver. Assembly required.

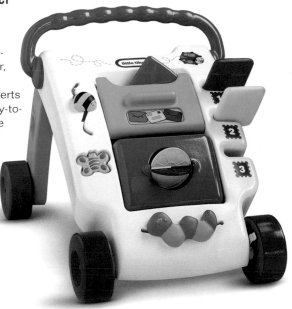

Edushape's Sensory Ball
($10, 6 months and up)

A bright knobby-textured ball that is easy to push, grab, and hold. It rolls in an unpredictable wobbly pattern that is fun to chase.

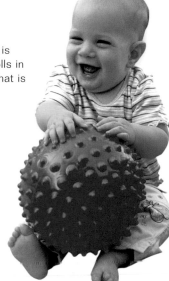

Chicco's Shape Sorter Drum
($25, 6 to 24 months)

Made of colorful, durable plastic, this shape sorter has openings for a green square, a red rectangle, and a blue circle. Turn the toy on its side and it becomes a roll toy for a baby to toddle after. Turn it again and the baby can play with the smiling drum by banging on it, or by pressing one of three buttons that produce musical melodies, drumbeats, or quirky sound effects. On/off and volume-control switch. Requires 2 AA batteries (included).

✱ 9 to 15 months

For babies beginning to walk

Toys in this age range help babies develop coordinated movement for walking. They also encourage them to practice the pincer grasp and continue to develop and master previous skills.

Sassy's Stacking Cups
($5, 9 months and up)

Four durable see-through plastic cups in bright colors and patterns stack into a tower, or nest inside of each other. They can be banged together or used in the bathtub for water play. Each cup is rimmed with a chewable thick plastic ridge.

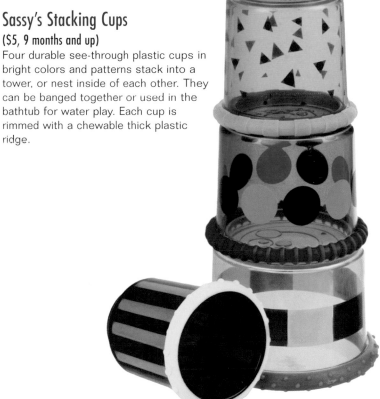

SAFETY CONSIDERATIONS

The number of babies and children injured by toys continues to rise. According to the estimates of the U.S. Consumer Product Safety Commission (www.cpsc.gov), over 77,000 babies and children younger than five years old are injured seriously enough every year in toy-related accidents to be rushed to emergency rooms.

Airway obstruction—choking and suffocation—is the leading cause of unintentional death from injuries for babies under one year of age. Small toys, those with small removable parts, and those that break into pieces pose the greatest choking hazard to babies and young children. This hazard is related to a baby's tendency to put everything in her mouth, and since a baby's airway is smaller than an older child's or adult's, it can be easily plugged up by a swallowed object, leading to rapid suffocation.

Strangulation happens when toys with strings, straps, or cords longer than 7 inches wrap around a child's neck, cutting off her air supply. Of special danger are toys that are suspended across a baby's crib, such as a mobile or play gym, that can wrap around a child's neck, cutting off her air supply. Loops of blind cords also pose a danger when they're left within reach of the crib or a standing baby. Wheeled toys are another source of baby injuries and deaths when babies topple down staircases or are outdoors and roll themselves into bodies of water or into the path of vehicles. Constant supervision is required!

Toys for children of all ages are regulated by the U.S. Consumer Product Safety Commission. To protect from choking on, inhaling, or swallowing small objects, a regulation bans toys and other products for babies and small children if the items have small parts or could produce small pieces if they broke. Other regulations address sharp points on toys; the dangers of lead, usually found in paints; and the hazards of other toxins. The regulations also address how toys are labeled and the warnings they carry to ensure that parents know to avoid toys that could be unsafe for babies, such as small figures, latex balloons, and small balls.

Toys are frequently the subject of recalls. If you're unsure of a toy's safety, perhaps because you bought it used, you can visit www.recalls.gov on the Internet to access CPSC's recall site. You can then perform a search of general toy recalls by category or home in on a specific toy by model name.

Safe use tips

Here's a list of hazardous toys to avoid to help keep your baby safe.

Small balls. Small balls, including marbles, that are less than 1¾ inches wide pose a particular hazard to young children when they become lodged in a child's airway, blocking off her air supply. The balls are commonly found in vending machines and in toy packages designed for older children. Federal law requires that small balls be labeled with a warning, but that has not prevented the death of about seven children a year in the U.S.

Balloons. Uninflated or broken latex balloons are the leading cause of suffocation deaths in children—more than 100 babies and children have been killed by them in the U.S. An accident typically happens when a child chews on a piece of a broken balloon as if it were a piece of gum or tries to blow up the balloon but sucks it into her windpipe instead. When the balloon is inhaled, it can form a perfect seal over a baby's airway and lungs. Don't let your child play with inflated or deflated latex balloons.

Suspended toys and wall hangings. When baby gyms, mobiles, exercisers, kickers, and other toys are suspended from one side of a crib or play yard to the other, they can hang babies because of their vulnerable soft throats and airways. A baby's head is so heavy in comparison with the rest of her body that it may be impossible for a baby to right herself once her neck gets entrapped in the suspended toy. Most at risk are babies who are just starting to get up on their hands and knees. Take down suspended toys as soon as your baby shows signs of pulling up or crawling. Keep nursery wall hangings well out of your baby's reach, too, especially if there are small parts or strings that could cause choking or get entangled around your baby's neck.

Quilts and puffy toys. Even though they may appear to be made for babies, pillows, quilts, comforters, sheepskins, crib bumpers, pillowlike stuffed toys, and other soft products can suffocate your baby and don't belong in her crib. Be especially cautious about inexpensive stuffed toys such as the types you win at fairs or that come from vending machines. They may have loose eyes or hair that could choke a baby.

Hard toys in the crib. When your baby begins to pull up using the crib's bars, remove any hard toys or those fastened on the crib's side that could be used like steps for climbing out of the crib, which could lead to a fall and serious head injuries.

Battery-operated toys. Battery compartments sometimes leak caustic acid, especially when a baby gnaws on the toy. Make sure battery compartments are babyproof and moisture resistant. Batteries can sometimes cause a toy to be heavy, and if dropped could injure the baby. Shop carefully, watch for excess weight, and inspect the toy frequently for leaks or a loose battery compartment cover.

23

WEB RESOURCES

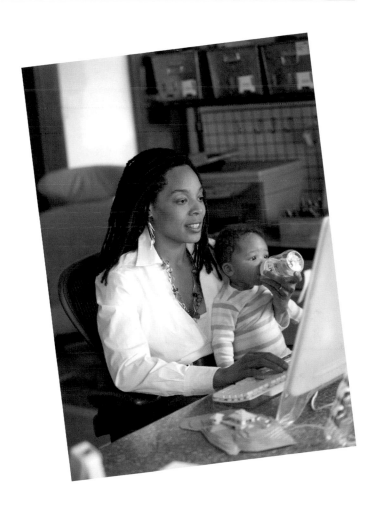

Here's a collection of some of the most popular Internet sites for searching out information on baby products. There are loads of places to visit, whether you're looking for product reviews, places to order stuff, or federal and not-for-profit organizations, where you can research baby-product safety and report product failures.

SHOPPING IN CYPERSPACE

Shopping online for baby products, toys, and clothes can be fun. It's certainly convenient and exciting to have boxes delivered to your door like birthday presents, but you may want to compare product prices with local stores, and especially the mega-store chains.

There are thousands of Internet sites selling baby products. Unfortunately, it's sometimes hard to tell the difference between sites that offer objective consumer and parenting reviews and those that offer pseudo-information or post bogus parent reviews with a hidden agenda to sell their products.

Even though ordering products from e-tailers and the sites of big-store chains with Web sites could be a great way to capture a bargain on baby clothes and gear, you'll need to factor in the shipping and handling costs. You may discover that you'll come out even or perhaps a little ahead by buying things locally, especially if they're marked down or on sale. We suggest that you not agree to back-order goods from the Internet. You could get stung if a car seat or crib takes months to arrive or your baby has outgrown the clothes you ordered.

Be cautious about buying from overseas vendors. Shipping prices may be exorbitant, there may be long delays, and currency exchanges may make the product a lot more costly than it appears at a glance. Sites like www.oanda.com convert currencies so you'll know what you'll really be paying in U.S. dollars. One clue for the country of origin for a Web site can be found in its Web address. Sites ending in .uk are British, those with .au are Australian, .fr are French, for example.

Protecting your personal info

As we mentioned at the beginning of the book, if you don't want to be inundated with junk mail offering everything from baby formula to infant life insurance, exercise caution when giving away your e-mail address when you "join" by signing in.

Keep a small address book next to your computer to hold all of your user names and passwords, and make each of your passwords a long string that combines both alphabet letters and numbers to make it more of a challenge for hackers to steal your identity.

When you sign up to join online parenting "clubs," or to get a username for ordering goods, don't ever give away your phone number unless it's mandatory—otherwise be prepared for lots of dinnertime solicitation calls. And be sure to sign up for your state's "do not call" registry, which is usually administered by the office of the attorney general of the state. Being on the registry is not fail-safe, and companies still routinely dial the prohibited numbers or deliver automatic prerecorded messages in an attempt to induce you to return the call.

Still, if putting down some personal information is the only way to access bulletin boards and chat rooms, you may feel that the extra hassle of being a target for junk calls and junk mail may be worth it. A good strategy is to maintain two (or more) separate e-mail addresses—one for your "real" e-mail and the other, which you don't need to check often, as a destination for solicitations and unwanted "sale" notices.

Internet shopping checklist

Here are our suggestions for having a successful online shopping experience.

■ **Know the return policies.** If you don't want to get stuck with a product you hate or one that's flawed, make sure you know what the seller's conditions are for returning the product, including the time limits for doing so. This information may appear in an FAQ (Frequently Asked Questions) section.

■ **Read the privacy notice.** Make sure that your identifying information will stay private and not be used by any other site or distributed to "cooperating partners" or makers of products that "may be of similar interest."

■ **Say "no" to future special offers.** Unless you want your e-mail address junked up with unwanted ads and solicitations every week, always uncheck the "Yes, I'd like e-mails of special offers" or other statements that leave you open to solicitation.

■ **Use secure sites.** When you get to the place where you are to enter your credit card information, look for these indications of a secure Web site: There should be a closed gold padlock at the bottom right of the screen, and the address of the site (in the white box at the top of the screen) should begin https:// (with an "s" at the end) instead of just http://.

■ **Write down the Web address and customer service number.** That way you'll be able to track purchases and complain if purchases are late in arriving.

■ **Calculate the shipping costs, then back out.** Before you jump to the "complete-the-order" button, weigh how much it will cost to get the product delivered to your door. Then seriously consider cancelling your order if the seller's shipping and handling charges aren't aligned with actual UPS or FedEx delivery charges, or if shipping makes the product cost nearly as much as you would pay locally.

(Getting the product from a local store also means you can return it without the hassle of having to pack it and possibly footing the shipping bill.)

■ **Use the same credit card for all purchases.** That way you can quickly spot fraudulent or unauthorized charges.

■ **Print your order from the Web sites and the e-mail confirmation of the order.** You may discover you need these documents to prove that the e-tailer received and is shipping your order, verify the e-mail address of the customer service contact, record the date of the order, and track your package with an order confirmation number. You may need to refer to them later if the package fails to show up, is the wrong product, or is missing parts. Store your printouts in a folder or use a 1-gallon plastic zippered bag to keep all of your purchase documentation in one place.

■ **Watch out for imposters.** Never give your credit card information or other identifying numbers, such as your Social Security number or passwords, in response to an e-mail query, even though it may sound like your bank, your service provider or one of the companies you've done business with in the past. Legitimate businesses will never ask you to do that, but impostors will emulate the exact business or bank and try to convince you that something is wrong with your account in order to harvest your identity and credit card. Submit this sensitive data only by using secure, encrypted Web sites.

■ **Report fraud immediately.** If something doesn't look right and you believe your credit card is being used fraudulently for purchases or to open new accounts (identity theft), immediately notify your credit card company to close any accounts that you believe have been tampered with or opened fraudulently. Contact any one of three of the major consumer reporting companies (their Web sites include www.equifax.com, www.experian.com, and www.transunion.com) to place a fraud alert on your credit report to prevent new illegal accounts from being opened in your name. Contact the FTC using their toll-free hotline for help: 877-382-4357. An ID Theft Affidavit, available online from the Federal Trade Commission (www.consumer.gov/idtheft), will help you in disputing new, unauthorized accounts. Use the ID Theft Affidavit also to file a police report in your district.

■ **Report bad businesses.** Report sour interactions with e-tailers to the Better Business Bureau at www.bbb.org and register complaints on the "contact us" forms with the bad companies.

Internet sources about baby products

The entries in this section are designed to serve as an at-a-glance guide to Internet resources that are all about baby products. These are good places to start when you're looking for reliable consumer information on baby products.

These listings and reviews were current at the time of publication. If you encounter a dead link, try using key words to conduct a search using your favorite search engine (Google, Yahoo, MSN, Mamma, etc.). Remember that Web sites can sometimes change addresses or close down, and new sites spring up almost daily. If we've missed any of your favorite sites or you're with an organization that would like to have its address listed here, please write us in care of our publisher, and we will try to include your address in the next edition.

Major Baby-Product Manufacturers

This is a list of the most well-known manufacturers of baby products. For more information on manufacturers, go to the Juvenile Products Manufacturers Association's Web site: **www.jpma.org.**

4moms
Baby bathtubs and bathing accessories.
888-434-MOMS (888-434-6667)
www.4momsonline.com

Ameda (See Hollister, Inc.)

Amy Michelle
Diaper bags.
303-279-0690
www.amymichelle.com

Angelcare
Baby monitors.
800-430-0222
www.angelcare-monitors.com

Angelguard, Inc.
Infant car bed.
330-723-5928
www.angel-guard.com

Angel Line
Baby furniture.
856-678-6300
www.angelline.com

Aprica U.S.A., Inc.
Strollers, high chairs, baby carriers.
877-8-APRICA (877-827-7422)
www.apricausa.com

Arms Reach Concepts
Bedside bassinets.
800-822-4690
www.armsreach.com

Avent America (see Philips Avent)
Baby bottles and feeding accessories.
630-350-2600
www.aventamerica.com

BABYBJÖRN (Baby Swede)
Soft carriers, potties, diaper bags.
866-424-0200
www.babybjorn.com

Baby Einstein
Educational DVDs and infant products.
818-549-7456
www.babyeinstein.com

Baby Jogger Company
Large-wheeled jogging strollers.
800-241-1848
www.babyjogger.com

Baby Trend
Strollers, car seats, travel systems, play yards, high chairs.
800-328-7363
www.babytrend.com

Badger Basket Company
Bassinets and changing tables.
847-381-6200
www.badgerbasket.com

BOB Strollers
Running strollers and accessories.
800-315-3039
www.bobgear.com

Bravado! Designs
Nursing and non-nursing bras and breast pads. Available in extra-large sizes.
416-466-8652
ww.bravadodesigns.com

Britax Child Safety, Inc.
Car seats and strollers.
888-893-2447
www.britaxusa.com

Bugaboo
Imported multi-component strollers.
212-645-2340
www.bugaboo.com

bumGenius
Reusable diapers and covers.
888-332-2243
www.bumgenius.com

Bumbleride
Strollers.
619-523-5422
www.bumbleride.com

Bummis Inc.
Reusable diaper covers, Kokkoon
car seat bag.
888-828-6647
www.bummis.com

Bungee Baby Bouncer
(See E and I Inc.)

Cardinal Gates
Metal gates and safety items.
770-252-4200
www.cardinalgates.com

C&T International/Sorelle Furniture
Baby furniture importers.
201-531-1919
www.sorellefurniture.com

Chicco U.S.A., Inc.
Strollers, high chairs, soft carriers, play
pens, toys.
877-4-CHICCO (877-424-4226)
www.chiccousa.com

*Child Craft Industries (includes
Legacy brand)*
Cribs and furniture.
812-206-2200
www.childcraftindustries.com

Colgate Mattress Atlanta Corp.
Crib mattresses and special-size pads and
mattresses.
404-681-2121
www.colgatekids.com

Combi USA
Strollers, car seats, play yards, high chairs,
diaper bags.
803-802-8416
www.combi-intl.com

*COSCO
(See Dorel Juvenile Group)*

Crown Crafts Infant Products, Inc.
Baby bedding and soft carriers.
800-421-0526
www.ccipinc.com

Delta Enterprise Corp.
Cribs and baby furniture, strollers.
800-377-3777
www.deltaenterprise.com

Dex Products, Inc.
Baby safety and comfort products.
800-546-1996
www.dexproducts.com

Diaper Dude
Diaper bags for dads.
310-487-4705
www.diaperdude.com

Discovery Toys
Developmental baby toys.
800-341-8697
www.discoverytoysinc.com

Dorel Juvenile Group
(Cosco, Safety 1st, Eddie Bauer)
Large variety of baby products from car seats to strollers, high chairs, and play yards.
800-457-5276
www.djgusa.com

Dreamer Design
Jogging strollers, accessories.
800-278-9626
www.dreamerdesign.net

E and I Inc.
Bungee Baby bouncer
800-853-6001
www.bungeebabybouncer.com

Eddie Bauer
(See also Dorel Juvenile Group)
Baby clothes, diaper bags; car seats manufactured by Dorel Juvenile Group under the "Eddie Bauer" name.
800-625-7800
www.eddiebauer.com

Enfamil
Baby formula.
800-BABY123 (800-222-9123)
www.enfamil.com

ERGObaby
Baby/child fabric carriers.
888-416-4888
www.ergobaby.com

Evenflo Co. Inc.
Wide variety of baby products, including strollers, car seats, baby carriers, and the famous "Exersaucer."
770-455-6879
www.evenflo.com

Fancee Free Manufacturing, Inc.
Women's bras and lingerie, including nursing bras.
800-325-5088
www.fanceefreemfg.com

First Years, The (See Learning Curve)

Fisher-Price
Baby toys, baby seats, high chairs, strollers.
800-828-4000
www.fisher-price.com

Fuzzi Bunz Diapers
Reusable pocket style diapers.
866-DRY-BABY (866-379-2229)
ww.fuzzibunz.com

Gerber
Baby clothing and feeding supplies.
800-4-GERBER (800-443-7237)
www.gerber.com

Go-Go Babyz
Strollers, car seat attachments.
408-219-7810
www.gogobabyz.com

Graco Children's Products
Wide variety of baby products, including moderately priced strollers, car seats, and play yards.
800-345-4109
www.gracobaby.com

Guardian Angel
Metal window guards.
800-445-2370
www.angelguards.com

Handi-Craft Co. (Dr. Brown's)
Baby bottle with a straw inside and breast pumps.
800-778-9001
www.handi-craft.com

H. J. Heinz
Baby food.
800-872-2229
www.hjheinz.com
www.heinzbaby.com

Hollister, Inc. (Ameda)
Hospital-grade, electric breast pumps.
877-99-AMEDA (877-992-6332)
www.myhollister.com

Hoohobbers
Moses baskets, diaper bags, crib bedding.
773-889-1466
www.hoohobbers.com

HUGGIES
(See Kimberly-Clark Corp.)

Infantino, LLC
Baby toys and soft carriers.
800-365-8182
www.infantino.com

Inglesina U.S.A., Inc.
Imported strollers, high chairs, changing
bags, and accessories.
877-486-5112
www.inglesina.com

InStep-Schwinn
Running strollers and bicycle trailers.
608-268-8931
www.pacific-cycle.com

International Playthings, Inc.
Developmental toys.
800-631-1272
www.intplay.com

Jane USA
Imported strollers and car seats.
415-824-1237
www.janeusa.com

Jeep
(See: Kolcraft Enterprises, Inc.)
800-453-7673
www.kolcraft.com/jeep/

JJ Cole Collections
Car seat and stroller accessories,
diaper bags.
435-787-1657
www.jjcoleusa.com

J. Mason Products
Wide range of baby products, including
inexpensive and moderately priced
strollers, high chairs, and play yards.
800-242-1922
www.jmason.com

Johnson & Johnson
Baby bathing supplies (including creams,
soaps, and shampoos) and baby formula.
800-526-3967
www.jnj.com

Joovy
Strollers and running strollers.
877-456-5049
www.joovy.com

Kel-Gar Inc.
Safety products, car seat and stroller
accessories, bath accessories.
972-250-3638
www.kelgar.com

Kelty Kids
Backpacks for carrying baby, strollers,
diaper bags.
800-535-3589
www.kelty.com

KidCo, Inc.
Safety gates, home safety items, running strollers.
800-553-5529
www.kidco.com

KidKusion Inc.
Child safety and bath products.
800-845-9236
www.kidkusion.com

Kids II
Baby seats and toys.
770-751-0442
www.kidsii.com

Kimberly-Clark Corp (HUGGIES)
Disposable diapers and pull-up pants. Baby skin care products.
800-544-1847
www.huggiesbabynetwork.com

Kolcraft Enterprises, Inc.
Wide variety of baby products, including strollers, high chairs, mattresses, and play yards. Maker of "Jeep" baby products.
800-628-6875
www.kolcraft.com

Kool-Stop International Inc.
Running strollers and bicycle trailers.
800-586-3332
www.koolstop.com

Kushies Baby
Baby accessories, layettes, and apparel.
905-643-9118
www.kushies.com

L.A. Baby
Cribs, bassinets, mattresses, gliders, small cribs, crib bedding.
800-584-3094
www.lababyco.com

Lambs & Ivy
Baby bedding and gifts.
310-839-5155
www.lambsandivy.com

LeapFrog Enterprises Inc.
Educational toys for babies and children.
800-LEAP (800-5327)
www.leapfrog.com

Learning Curve International/ The First Years
Makers of toys for babies and children.
800-704-8697
www.learningcurve.com

Lego Baby/Lego Systems, Inc.
Toys for toddlers and children.
800-453-4652
www.lego.com

Little Tikes
Children's climbing and ride-on toys.
888-832-3203
www.littletikes.com

Maclaren U.S.A., Inc.
Upscale imported strollers and carriages.
877-442-4622
www.maclarenbaby.com

Manhattan Toy
Innovative toys for babies and children.
612-337-9610
www.manhattantoy.com

Maya Wrap, Inc.
Baby and child fabric wrap carriers.
888-MAYAWRAP (888-629-2972)
www.mayawrap.com

McKenzie Kids (See *Mommy's Helper*)

Medela, Inc.
Breast pumps, breastfeeding accessories, bras.
800-435-8316
www.medela.com

Metromamma
Baby carrier and baby wrap.
702-353-2053
www.metromamma.com

Million Dollar Baby
Baby cribs and furniture.
323-728-9988
www.milliondollarbaby.com

Mobi Technologies, Inc.
Mobicam infant monitor.
818-771-1620
www.getmobi.com

Mommy's Helper–McKenzie Kids
Diaper bags and diaper-bag kits, potty training aids, safety products.
316-684-2229
www.mommyshelperinc.com

Morigeau-Lepine
Cribs, beds, gliders.
970-845-7795
www.morigeau.com

Munchkin, Inc.
Feeding, bathing, teethers, travel, safety items.
818-221-4246
www.munchkin.com

Mustela
Baby and mom skin-care products.
800-422-2967
www.mustelausa.com

My Brest Friend–Zenoff Products
Nursing support pillows.
415-421-5300
www.mybrestfriend.com

Nestlé (Good Start)
Baby formula.
800-547-9400
www.verybestbaby.com/goodstart/

North American Bear Co., Inc.
Baby soft toys and mobiles.
800-682-3427
www.nabear.com

North States Industries
Safety gates.
763-486-1754
www.northstatesind.com

Oi Oi Baby Bags
Diaper bags and stroller accessories.
877-905-3800
www.oioi.com.au

Over The Shoulder Baby Holder
Adjustable, fabric baby slings.
800-637-9426
www.overtheshoulder.com

Pali
Wooden cribs and furniture.
919-781-4285
www.paliitaly.com

Patchkraft, Inc.
Infant bedding and nursery accessories.
201-833-2201
www.patchkraft.com

Pediped, Inc.
Soft leather baby booties and shoes.
800-880-1245
www.pedipedbabyshoes.com

Peg-Pérego
Imported strollers, carriages, high chairs, car seats.
260-482-8191
www.perego.com

Peter Potty
(See Visionaire Products)

Philips Avent
Baby bottles, feeding accessories.
630-350-2600
www.aventamerica.com

Playtex Products, Inc.
Baby bottles, diaper disposal system, skin-care products.
203-341-4181
www.playtex.com

Prince Lionheart, Inc.
Soft carriers, feeding devices, safety products.
800-544-1132
www.princelionheart.com

Procter & Gamble (Pampers)
Disposable diapers.
800-285-6064
www.pampers.com

Protect A Bub
Stroller sunshades, inserts, rain covers, swaddling wraps.
212-570-1670
www.protect-a-bubusa.com

Pu Digital
Potty seats and accessories.
850-567-9585
www.flipnflush.com

Regal Lager, Inc.
3-wheeled strollers, feeding products, changing-table pads, back packs, other infant products.
800-593-5522

R.E.I.
Sporty backpacks for carrying tots.
800-426-4840
www.rei.com
www.regallager.com

Robeez Footwear
Soft-soled leather footwear from birth to 4 years.
800-929-2623
www.robeez.com

Ross Products division of Abbott Laboratories
Baby formula.
800-986-8510
www.ross.com
www.welcomeaddition.com

SafeGuard
Child seat.
317-867-8166
www.safeguardseat.com

Safety 1st
(See Dorel Juvenile Group)

Safe-Lok
(See Mommy's Helper)

Sassy, Inc.
Innovative baby toys, safety devices, monitors.
616-243-1042
www.sassybaby.com

Sherpani
Backpack baby carriers.
720-214-2194
www.sherpani.us

Simmons Kids
Crib mattresses and vinyl products.
770-512-7700
www.simmonskids.com

Simplicity For Children
Bassinets, baby furniture, play yards,
portable cribs, swings.
610-685-6900
www.simplicityforchildren.com

Sorelle Furniture (See C&T
International)

Stokke, LLC
Imported strollers, other baby
products.
678-627-0246
www.stokkeusa.com

Stork Craft Manufacturing, Inc.
Cribs, dressing tables, gliders, other children's furniture.
877-274-0277
www.storkcraft.com

Storksak Diaper Bags
Diaper bags.
866-354-9944
www.storksak.net

Summer Infant, Inc.
Baby bouncers, bedrails, bath products,
gates, monitors.
401-671-8550
www.summerinfant.com

Sunshine Kids Juvenile Products
Car seat and car and stroller accessories.
888-336-7909
www.skjp.com

SwaddleDesigns, LLC
Swaddling and receiving blankets, security blankets, baby burpers.
206-525-0400
www.swaddledesigns.com

Sweetpea of California
Nursery and juvenile furniture
and bedding.
628-578-0866
www.sweetpeacal.com

Tiny Love–The Maya Group
Innovative baby toys.
888-TINY-LOVE (888-846-9568)
www.tinylove.com

Tough Traveler
Framed carriers for transporting baby.
800-GO-TOUGH (800-468-6844)
www.toughtraveler.com

TrendyKid
High chairs, infant seats, toilet adapters,
toilet-training accessories.
888-TRENDY-K (888-873-6395)
www.trendykid.com

UPPAbaby
Strollers, video monitors, safety items,
sunshades.
800-760-8060
www.uppababy.com

Vermont Precision Woodworks
Baby and child furniture.
802-888-7974
www.vermontprecisionwoodworks.com

Visionaire Products/Peter Potty
Makers of Peter Potty, a flushable training urinal for boys.
312-997-2310
www.peterpotty.com

Zooper
Imported strollers, high chairs, safety gates, rockers, hook-on chairs.
888-742-9899
www.zooper.com

Baby Product Consumer Information

About.com – Baby Products
Information about various categories of baby products and links to important sites.
www.babyproducts.about.com

Baby Bargains
The home site for Alan and Denise Fields' Baby Bargains. Up-to-date information on baby-product manufacturers, baby product glitches, plus candid baby-product reviews from the authors and lots of parents.
www.babybargains.com

Better Business Bureau
Gathers complaints on bad and untrustworthy businesses to help alert consumers.
www.bbb.org

Car-Safety.org
Excellent resource for parents about car seats; has a buying guide for safe cars and car seats, LATCH car seat information, and an FAQ (frequently asked questions) on safe seat installation.
www.car-safety.org

Car Seat Data
Detailed information on car seats for infants and toddlers, including important car seat links and a compatibility database to help decide what seat to buy.
www.carseatdata.org

Consumer Federation of America
A not-for-profit consumer's organization concerned with product safety.
www.consumerfed.org

Consumer Reports
Site for Consumers Union, the premiere product-information source. Provides free articles on baby products and subscription-only access to baby product ratings.
www.consumerreports.org

Consumer Search
Compiles objective reviews on a wide variety of baby products using various consumer sites. (Search by product model.)
www.consumersearch.com

Dr. Toy
Site for Dr. Stevanne Auerbach, a noted child-development expert. Offers annual reviews of toys for babies and children. A great source for ideas about innovative, stimulating toys.
www.drtoy.com

Don's Car Seat Page
A noncommercial, outline-style guide to child passenger safety on the Web.
www.milenko.com/carseats

Epinions
The place to visit before you buy! Candid reviews of baby products from other parents. (But watch out for the "halo" effect—parents bragging about great $800 strollers, for example.)
www.epinions.com

Oppenheim Toy Portfolio
A great source for solid, objective reviews of toys for babies and children.
www.toyportfolio.com

Parents' Choice Foundation
Selects, approves, and gives awards for outstanding toys, media, and materials for babies and children.
www.parents-choice.org

SafetyBeltSafe U.S.A.
The best Internet source for information on car seat safety. Take a look at the technical section.
www.carseat.org

Seat Check
A free locator for children's car seat inspection services.
www.seatcheck.org

Toy Industry Association (TIA)
The professional organization of toy manufacturers, with a tab for toy safety tips.
www.toy-tia.org

General Baby Products

Amazon Baby
A large collection of baby products in this newly emerging e-tail area for Amazon. Some products offer ratings from purchasers.
www.amazon.com/baby

Babies "Я" Us
Wide selection of baby products from this mega baby-gear retailer. Occasional specials or free shipping offers.
www.babiesrus.com

Baby Age
A somewhat limited collection of baby furniture and strollers.
www.babyage.com

Baby & Me Boutique
A well-chosen collection of quality baby products.
www.babyandmeboutique.com

Baby Ant
Nice collection of cribs, clothing, changing tables, etc.
www.babyant.com

Baby Because
Careful selection of eco-friendly and organic products for babies.
www.babybecause.com

Baby Box
Luxurious products— fun to look, even if you can't afford to buy.
www.babybox.com

Baby Mine
Baby clothes and bedding, including organic cotton goods.
www.babyminestore.com

Baby Outlet
A baby-gear department store online.
www.thebabyoutlet.com

Baby Style
A huge selection of baby clothes and upscale pricey baby products.
www.babystyle.com

Baby Universe
An online department store for a wide variety of baby products.
www.babyuniverse.com

Baby Zone
An online resource for new parents. Information on local events near you. Check out the "free stuff" tab.
www.babyzone.com

Bobux
A source for soft leather shoes for crawlers, creepers, and new walkers.
www.bobuxusa.com

Buy Buy BABY
A big online baby-product source.
www.buybuybaby.com

Carousel Designs, Ltd.
Pricey bedding ensembles (don't use the quilt!) in bright patterns; also sheets in special sizes for bassinets, and other off-size mattresses and pads.
www.babybedding.com

The Children's Place
A specialty children's retailer with quality merchandise and accessories at a great value from newborn to preteen.
www.childrensplace.com

Diaper Bags
A dot com for surveying lots of diaper bags in different materials, colors, and styles.
www.diaperbags.com

Eddie Bauer
Offers diaper bags and some car seats, with links to sites that sell other Eddie Bauer licensed products.
www.eddiebauer.com

Fisher-Price
Has an age-appropriate guide to toys; plus information on developmental stages and play tips.
www.fisher-price.com

GAP
This well-known brand of mall shops offers baby and kids clothing online. Great sales.
www.gap.com

Gymboree
Baby and child specialty clothing retailer. They also offer mom-and-baby classes for fitness, arts, music, and more.
www.gymboree.com

In Fashion Kids
A wide selection of colorful, cute baby outfits, especially for holidays and special occasions, at affordable prices.
www.infashionkids.com

JCPenney
Baby clothes and furniture. Occasional sales.
www.jcpenney.com

Kid Stock Inc.
Baby and children's clothes and equipment.
www.kidstockmontana.com

The Kids Window
Chic European baby clothes worth drooling over.
www.thekidswindow.com

Lakeshore Learning Materials
An educational supplier—toys for developmental learning for babies and young children.
www.lakeshorelearning.com

Lands' End
Excellent diaper bags, plus quality baby clothes and carriers.
www.landsend.com

Lil Diaper Depot
Organic cotton and eco-friendly products especially for mom and baby.
www.lildiaperdepot.com

Little Shoes
Shoes and clothing for tots and children.
www.littleshoes.com

Magic Moments Christening Collection
The place to go for an exquisite christening gown for your son or daughter.
www.magicmomentschristening.com

Maukilo European Toy Collection
Colorful, clever European toys for "the baby who has everything."
www.maukilo.com

Modern Seed
Limited selection of modern-style furnishings for kids, including cribs.
www.modernseed.com

My Little Ducks
An all-boy clothing site, from newborns onward.
www.mylittleducks.com

Natural Baby
A good source for reusable diapers and diapering aids.
www.naturalbaby-catalog.com

Net Kids Wear
A wide range of baby products, including clothing, cribs, strollers, car seats, and more.
www.netkidswear.com

Nordstrom
Mall store online—carries clothes and diaper bags, and upscale baby duds.
www.store.nordstrom.com

Old Navy
Mall store online—has great deals on infant and toddler gear.
www.oldnavy.com

Oliebollen
Euro-style baby duds and toys.
www.oliebollen.com

One of a Kind Kid
European and American designer clothing for babies and children, including smocked dresses and rompers.
www.oneofakindkid.com

One Step Ahead
Both a catalog and an online store of carefully chosen baby products with an emphasis on uniqueness and quality.
www.onestepahead.com

Oompa Toys
A wide assortment of imported toys, many in wood and fabric.
www.oompatoys.com

Organic Bebe
Organic cotton baby clothing.
www.organicbebe.com

Potty Training Tips
Sells a wide array of potty-training products with accompanying how-to tips.
pottytrainingtips.com

Rattle & Roll
A boutique of upscale baby products.
www.rattleroll.com

Red Envelope
A boutique-like site for unique baby gift items.
www.redenvelope.com

Right Start
A discriminating choice of car seats, strollers, safety items, and nursery aids.
www.rightstart.com

Robeez
Clever, stylish leather baby booties and shoes.
www.robeez.com

Safe Beginnings
Sells safety products as well as parenting books and videos.
www.safebeginnings.com

Sears
A selection of baby products, sometimes with good items on sale.
www.sears.com

Sensational Beginnings
Both a catalog and a Web site for well-chosen baby toys at each stage.
www.sensationalbeginnings.com

Shower Your Baby
Big collection of baby hard goods, including strollers, cribs, and other nursery items.
www.showeryourbaby.com

Smarter Kids
A great source for age-specific baby toys.
www.smarterkids.com

Stroller Depot
Strollers of all kinds, stroller accessories, car seats, and a variety of other well-chosen baby-gear items.
www.strollerdepot.com

Target
Online site for the huge retail chain; offers trendy baby clothes, products, furniture, and accessories.
www.target.com

Toys to Grow On
A great site for developmental toys that also offers birthday gift ideas.
toystogrowon.com

Tutti Bella
Pricey designer baby and kids duds with definitive boy and girl looks from birth onward.
www.tuttibella.com

Wal-Mart
Great prices on cribs, strollers, diapers, baby clothes, and more.
www.walmart.com

Baby Shower Resources

Baby Center
A huge baby information source with lots of ideas on baby gifts, baby showers, and fun baby-shower games.
www.babycenter.com

Baby-Shower.com
Shower themes, shower planners, gift ideas . . . everything baby.
www.baby-shower.com

Baby Shower Central
Printable games, themes, supplies
and recipes.
www.babyshowercentral.com

Baby Shower Games, etc.
Games, etiquette, supplies, and even suggestions for coed showers.
www.baby-shower-games-etc.com

The Baby Shower Site
Commercial site selling baby-shower
products.
www.thebabyshowersite.com

Product Information
For Special-Needs Babies

4MyChild
Provides resources and information for
parents caring for children with special
needs.
www.4mychild.com

American Foundation for the Blind
Help for parents with visually handi-
capped babies, including a great review of
stimulating baby toys. (Enter the search
word "baby.")
www.afb.org

Association for Retarded Citizens
Offers a state-by-state resource guide on
benefits, support, and services for families raising children with intellectual and
developmental disabilities.
www.thearc.org

Columbia Medical Manufacturing
Offers adaptive equipment, such as special car seats, seat extenders, and buckle
guards.
www.columbiamedical.com

Dragonfly Toys
Toys for children with disabilities.
www.dragonflytoys.com

KidSource Online
"Newborns: Disabilities" contains a huge
list of links and articles for parents.
www.kidsource.com

LD Online
Provides parents of children with learning
disabilities with tools, products, articles,
and online support.
www.ldonline.org

*Marion Downs National Center
for Infant Hearing*
This site from a national organization to
support parents of babies and young children who are deaf or hard of hearing
contains informative articles, links, and a
parent support group locator.
www.colorado.edu/slhs/mdnc/

National Down Syndrome Society
The organization's mission is to enhance
the quality of life and to provide support
for individuals with Down syndrome and
their families.
www.ndss.org

*National Early Childhood Technical
Assistance Center*
Help and information on how to connect
with the early intervention services and
adaptive equipment provided for babies
and toddlers through the federal
Individuals with Disabilities Education
Act (IDEA).
www.nectac.org

National Fathers Network
Sources and support for fathers of babies and children with disabilities.
www.fathersnetwork.org

Through the Looking Glass
A California clearinghouse for parents with disabilities.
www.lookingglass.org

United Cerebral Palsy
A leading source of information on cerebral palsy, with a collection of informative articles about CP in infancy.
www.ucp.org

Parent-Advice Sites

Baby Center
A huge baby information source with lots of ideas on baby gifts, baby showers, and fun baby-shower games.
www.babycenter.com

Baby Place
A starting point for information on pregnancy, birth, and babies.
www.baby-place.com

Center for Early Education and Development
Contains a series of excellent articles on baby development.
education.umn.edu/CEED

Huggies Baby Network
Sponsored by Huggies, this commercial site contains lots of information on parenting babies as well as chat boards.
www.HuggiesBabyNetwork.com

iParenting
Recalls, parenting news, chat boards, experts, and "iParenting University" with subscription courses in pregnancy, breast-feeding, and baby care. Sponsored by *Pregnancy* and *Baby Years* magazines. Also available in Spanish.
www.iParenting.com

Mocha Moms
A support group for stay-at-home mothers of color. Members participate in weekly meetings, potluck dinners, and community service projects.
www.mochamoms.org

National Child Care Information Center
Provides useful technical information for parents about early care and education. NCCIC partners with the Child Care Bureau.
www.nccic.org

National Network for Childcare
Sponsored by the U.S. Department of Agriculture's Cooperative Extension system, this site offers informative articles about babies, including discussions of childcare issues and options.
www.nncc.org

National Resource Center for Health and Safety in Child Care
Licensing requirements for childcare centers, state-by-state.
nrc.uchc.edu

Parenthood.com
A comprehensive source: directory of pregnancy, parenting, and childcare articles and Web sites. Categories include childcare, education, health, fatherhood, finance, nutrition, organizations, safety issues, product recalls, infertility, and online shopping. Accesses chat rooms, discussion boards, support groups, and family home pages.
www.parenthood.com

Parents Place
This branch of iVillage includes a pregnancy section that features articles, charts, message boards, and a newsletter option.
www.parentsplace.com

Pump Station
Educational breastfeeding information from lactation consultants; plus, a variety of pumps, nursing bras, and breastfeeding supplies for sale.
www.pumpstation.com

Stroller Strides
Fitness support group to help moms get back into shape after baby. Perfect for the mom who doesn't have time for the gym.
www.strollerstrides.com

The Compleat Mother
Information on breastfeeding, childbirth, parenting.
www.compleatmother.com

The Happiest Baby
Dr. Harvey Karp's site offers information and products to soothe crying, fussy, and/or colicky babies.
www.thehappiestbaby.com

Urban Baby
Offers local Web sites for major cities that include bulletin boards, calendars of events, local resources, and shopping information.
www.urbanbaby.com

Children's Health & Safety

American Academy of Pediatrics
Valuable information on immunizations, important health issues, and an annual "Family Safety Guide to Car Seats."
www.aap.org

Child Welfare League of America
Offers parents useful information concerning the health and welfare of infants and toddlers.
www.cwla.org

KinderStart
A giant source for parenting information with lots of links to info on common childhood concerns.
www.kinderstart.com

National Safe Kids Campaign
A national not-for-profit organization for preventing unintentional childhood injuries with more than 300 state and local coalitions, many of which offer safety-seat inspections.
www.usa.safekids.org

Mother Risk
Sponsored by the Canadian Health Network, this site offers information on how to protect yourself and your baby from health risks, and includes research updates and discussions of occupational hazards, smoking, and substance abuse.
www.motherisk.org

Zero To Three
A not-for-profit organization to promote the healthy development of babies and toddlers. Great infant development information.
www.zerotothree.org

Family Vacation Help

About.com – Travel with Kids
Features articles, links, deals, and a newsletter on traveling with children.
www.travelwithkids.about.com

Baby's Away
Rents baby equipment, including cribs, strollers, toys, rocking chairs, gates, potty seats, and even DVDs and players for 30 "destination resort" locations.
www.babysaway.com

Carousel Press
A travel publisher's Web site that provides family-oriented travel information.
www.carousel-press.com

Family Travel Times
An online subscription newsletter that gives the scoop on resorts, motels, and attractions for kids and families.
www.familytraveltimes.com

GoCityKids
This site offers great things to do for baby and you when visiting major cities.
www.gocitykids.com

Rascals in Paradise
A travel agency dealing with resorts and tours for families traveling with babies and children. They'll arrange for flight, hotel, car rental, and other needs.
www.rascalsinparadise.com

Federal Agencies

The U.S. government has lots of sources to help parents with baby-related issues, including baby products and baby-product safety. Here's a list of the major agencies offering valuable information for parents.

Centers For Disease Control and Prevention (CDC)
1600 Clifton Rd., NE, Atlanta GA 30333.
800-311-3435
www.cdc.gov
Offers information on children's illnesses, and also infant and child growth charts to help you predict your child's height and weight growth for any given month.

Federal Trade Commission (FTC)
FTC Consumer Response Center, Room 130, 600 Pennsylvania Avenue, N.W., Washington, DC 20580.
877-FTC-HELP (877-382-4357)
www.ftc.gov
www.consumer.gov/idtheft (for identity theft information)
A federal consumer-protection agency that helps to protect individuals and businesses from illegal or fraudulent exchanges. It also maintains a database of identity theft reports and offers a formal complaint form for use in clearing your name.

Food and Drug Administration (FDA)
5600 Fishers Lane, Rockville, MD 20857
888-INFO-FDA (888-463-6332)
www.fda.gov
Branch of the U.S. Department of Agriculture that regulates baby food and baby skin-care products. Site offers brochures on baby feeding and health.

National Center On Birth Defects and Developmental Disabilities
NCBDDD, 1600 Clifton Rd., MS E-87
Atlanta, GA 30333
770-488-7160
www.cdc.gov/ncbdd
Offers information on developmental disabilities, jaundice, birth defects, and other childcare and parenting topics.

National Highway Traffic Safety Administration
NHTSA
400 Seventh Street SW
Washington, DC 20590
888-327-4236
www.nhtsa.dot.gov
Oversees the safety of car seats for babies and children. Lists recalls of car seats and offers buying guides, installation tips, and other pertinent car seat safety information. Some offerings in Spanish.

U.S. Consumer Product Safety Commission (CPSC)
U.S. Consumer Product Safety Commission
Washington, DC 20207
800-638-2772
www.cpsc.gov
The federal agency in charge of monitoring and regulating products, including those for babies and young children. It issues product recalls and accepts parents' reports of unsafe products.

Parenting and Consumer Information Magazines

Most of these sites offer searchable archives of past articles, including baby development and baby product, clothing and toy features.

American Baby
www.americanbaby.com

Baby Talk
www.babytalk.com

Child
www.child.com

Compleat Mother
www.compleatmother.com

Consumer Reports
www.consumerreports.org

Consumers Digest
www.consumersdigest.com

ePregnancy
www.epregnancy.com

Family Fun
www.familyfun.com

FitPregnancy
www.fitpregnancy.com

Mothering
www.mothering.com

Parenting
www.parenting.com

Parents
www.parents.com

Pregnancy
www.pregnancymagazine.com

Vegetarian Baby & Child
www.vegetarianbaby.com

INDEX